DENTAL ETHICS
AT CHAIRSIDE

DENTAL ETHICS AT CHAIRSIDE

THIRD EDITION

PROFESSIONAL OBLIGATIONS AND PRACTICAL APPLICATIONS

David T. Ozar
David J. Sokol
Donald E. Patthoff

Georgetown University Press
Washington, DC

The publisher is not responsible for third-party websites or their content. URL links were active at time of publication.

Printed in the United States of America

Library of Congress Cataloging-in-Publication Data

Names: Ozar, David T., author. | Sokol, David J., author. | Patthoff, Donald E., author.
Title: Dental Ethics at Chairside : Professional Obligations and Practical Applications / David T. Ozar, David J. Sokol, Donald E. Patthoff.
Description: Third edition. | Washington, D.C. : Georgetown University Press, [2018] | Includes bibliographical references and index.
Identifiers: LCCN 2017029349| ISBN 9781626165526 (hardcover : alk. paper) | ISBN 9781626165533 (pbk. : alk. paper) | ISBN 9781626165540 (ebook)
Subjects: LCSH: Dental ethics.
Classification: LCC RK52.7 .O96 2018 | DDC 174.2976—dc23
LC record available at https://lccn.loc.gov/2017029349

♾ This book is printed on acid-free paper meeting the requirements of the American National Standard for Permanence in Paper for Printed Library Materials.

19 18   9 8 7 6 5 4 3 2   First printing

Printed in the United States of America

Cover design by Trudi Gershenov.

In the memory of our parents,
Clarence and Anita Ozar,
Benjamin and Rae Sokol, and
Don and Joann Patthoff,
and for our wives,
Lorraine,
Carol, and
Deborah,
and our children,
Kate and Anne,
Susan and Scott, and
Erica, Alex, Adria, and Chelsea.

Contents

Preface

Most people, surveys show, still trust the health professionals who serve them, even in this cynical age, and dentists are still among the most trusted of health professionals. It is important for a dentist to keep this fact in mind and to reflect often on its implications, especially when dental practice seems to be changing so much. For the dental profession and many other professions face strong pressures from many sources to mirror the patterns of thinking, valuing, and acting that characterize the competitive marketplace. It is hoped that, in the minds of the large majority of dentistry's patients, the principal realities of dental practice are still what they have long been: that dentists have the knowledge and skills needed to serve their patients' oral health needs and that dentists are professionally committed to using this expertise according to the profession's ethical norms and for the well-being of their patients. But each dentist, each dental professional organization, and our society's oral health community as a whole needs to carefully study and reinforce these commitments if the larger community's trust in the dental profession is to remain strong.

There is encouragement for ethical conduct within the dental profession. But there is still relatively little assistance available to dentists for judging what conduct is ethically best in a complex situation. Few dentists have had extensive training in professional ethics, in dental school or elsewhere, and effective continuing education programs on ethical concerns in dental practice are few and far between. Many dentists' personal resources for professional-ethical reflection are considerable, and many have thoughtful peers, spouses, and friends to whom they can turn when particularly pressed. Few, however, would deny that they have often chosen a course of professional action while sensing that they had not given the matter all the ethical reflection it deserved and that they frequently did so because they ran out of ideas about how to consider it. Most dentists, we believe, would appreciate the chance to examine some additional ideas and well-developed intellectual tools to use in reflecting on the professional judgments and choices they must make.

Today, more faculty members assigned to teach or mentor dental students in dentistry's ethics and the skills they need to grow in professionalism are seeking relevant training than in the past. But they continue to struggle to find adequate time in the schools' curricula to enable their students to complete the first steps to learning dentistry's ethical norms and carrying them out in practice in the clinic.

This book is written for the sake of these students and their teachers and for practicing dentists who want to enrich their understanding of dentistry's ethical norms and reflect more deeply on how to live and practice them. It is also written in the hope that people outside the dental community would consider it important to understand what professional-ethical reflection in dental practice is about. But in one respect it is written first of all for the sake of dentistry's patients, who—for the most part—still trust their dentists to be not only competent but ethically adept in their professional practice as well. If this book can contribute to the continued fulfillment of their trust by contributing to dentists' fulfillment of their professional-ethical commitments, it will have accomplished its principal goal.

The reader will note that a number of words and phrases that have well known meanings in standard speech are capitalized throughout this book. Whenever such words or phrases are capitalized, it is because they are being used in a context that points to a particular aspect of dentistry's professional ethics. The phrase "Ideal Relationship," for example, points to a specific component of ethical dental practice and in fact, as chapter four explains, to a specific kind of relationship that the ethical dentist strives to bring about with every patient. The same is true of the phrase "Normative Picture" introduced in Chapter Two, "Central Practice Values" introduced in chapter three and developed in detail for dentistry in chapter five, and so on.

This third edition has been completely revised and updated from the previous editions. It would have far less to offer without the contributions to its first and second editions from their coauthor, the late David J. Sokol. Many of his contributions to the previous editions remain in this one. This third edition, like its predecessors, could not have been written without the encouragement, support, and valuable insights of our three families and of many colleagues. We are also particularly grateful to the students and patients who have taught us so much. We are grateful to the members of the American Society for Dental Ethics, especially the late Tom Hasegawa, as well as Larry Garreto, Anne Koerber, Larry Jenson, Bruce Peltier, Phyllis Beemsterboer, Jerry Winslow, and Pam Zarkowski. We are grateful to Steve Ralls, David Chambers, and the officers and members of the American College of Dentists and to Roger Winland and the editorial staff of the Academy of General Dentistry. We are grateful to Richard Brown and the staff of Georgetown University Press; to Frank Catalanotto and the American Dental Education Association; to Laura Bishop and Martina Darragh of the Bioethics Research Library at Georgetown University's Kennedy Institute of Ethics; to colleagues in the Academy for Professionalism in Health Care; the West Virginia Dental Association; the American Dental Association's Council on Ethics, Bylaws and Judicial Affairs; the West Virginia Eastern Panhandle Dental Society; to the Loyola University Chicago Philosophy Department; and to the faculty and administrators of the former Loyola University of Chicago School of Dentistry for their continuing support over the years.

1

⁕⁕⁕⁕⁕

The Dental Profession
and Professional Ethics

INTRODUCTION

Dentistry is a profession. Its members and students take this description of dentistry very seriously. Many practitioners of other occupations also call themselves "professionals." The adjective "professional" is also frequently used by advertisers and marketers to describe services and products that have nothing to do with someone's being a member of a profession. When used in these ways, the term "professional" doesn't mean much more than "well made" or "well performed."

For dentists and those studying to become dentists, however, dentistry as a profession has far more meaning than this. They would view themselves very differently if dentistry were not a profession. Calling dentistry a profession does not just say something about well-made products and exceptional services. Dentistry's being a profession says something about dentists. It says they have made important commitments, not just to themselves and to one another but to the society at large as well. It says there are norms of conduct that they are going to live by in their relations with their patients, with one another, and with the larger community, norms that have been developed and shaped by generations of ongoing collaborations between the profession and the larger community. It says there are standards of competence that dentists will adhere to in their practice, standards based on an established body of expertise that dentistry as a profession has developed over time for the benefit of the community and that it continues to improve on.

This is a book about dentistry as a profession. It is about the commitments that a person makes when becoming a member of this profession and that a dental student should therefore be incorporating into his or her life in order to become a dentist. There is much literature and ongoing research on the knowledge base and technical skills needed for dentists to practice competently as their experience, knowledge, and technology advance and they continue to improve the technical aspects of their practices. But learning more

1

about the ethical commitments at the heart of being a professional and improving one's living of them also takes time, attention, and practice. The knowledge base of this aspect of professional dentistry, though, is much larger than the list of dos and don'ts of an ethics code. There are also practical relational skills and important skills of effective ethical thinking to be learned, internalized, and improved on. For this knowledge and these skills need not only to be freely committed to but to become matters of habit, which means a person needs to develop the skills of self-formation to continue to grow as a person and as a professional. The aim of this book, then, is to add to the reader's knowledge base about dental ethics and dental professionalism and to describe some of the most important skills needed to grow in it.

The decisions a dentist or a dental student or any of us make involve not only questions about *oughts* and *shoulds* but also questions such as, What kind of person am I? and, What kind of person do I want to become? Addressing these questions carefully will often make our best responses to the *oughts* and *shoulds* much easier to identify. In this book, as in most professions, the concept of *professionalism* will be used to remind the reader of the importance of regularly asking questions such as, What kind of dentist am I? What kind of dentist do I want to become? What kind of person am I? What kind of person do I want to become?

What is professionalism? The concept *professionalism* is sometimes used in the negative—that is, with emphasis on what is missing when someone's behavior falls short of the most minimal ethical standards of a profession, when the person's conduct is such that it is hard to think of the person as acting like a member of that profession at all. It is obviously unprofessional in this narrow sense for a dentist to ignore an overhang in order to keep patients moving more quickly through the office or to inform patients only of treatments the dentist finds most profitable. The specific aim of this book, though, is to take seriously the idea that dentistry is a profession and that this says something about *who a dentist is* rather than merely implying that their services are *well performed*.

The focus of this book, then, will be on professionalism as something positive, something to be aspired to in everything a dentist does. Professionalism in this sense refers to the internalized and habitual ways of thinking and acting that characterize the life and practice of the most admirable members of the dental profession. Among these ways of thinking and acting are the distinctive skills of dental practice: First are those skills that are often called "technical" by which a dentist employs his or her professional expertise to actually benefit a patient, but equally important are *ethical* skills—skills in the realm of values and conduct, especially in the context of the dentist's relationships to patients and others.

This book will focus primarily on this second aspect of dental professionalism. It will offer descriptions of the ways of thinking and acting that the ethical dentist aspires to, those that constitute admirable professional-ethical conduct. It will examine cases from dental practice that, though they are fictionalized, describe typical ethical challenges that dentists encounter in their practices and that focus on the most important ethical skills (that is, the relational skills, the skills of ethical thinking, and the skills of self-formation) that a dentist needs to develop into habits in order to grow in professionalism.

A SAMPLING OF ETHICAL ISSUES IN DENTAL PRACTICE

Practicing dentists are already aware of the kinds of ethical issues that arise in day-to-day practice. Most dentists already have established habits of ethical conduct that they have built up over years of practice and careful self-assessment. These enable them to focus on relating effectively to their patients and doing technically competent work without having to stop and carefully think through each ethical issue that arises—even though a new dental student observing these situations might well have to look at them very carefully. Even the wisest and most ethically experienced dentists, however, encounter new situations that require careful ethical thinking. The concepts and skills explained and demonstrated in the following pages, then, can be very helpful in these situations.

Many readers of this book, however, will be dental students, including dental students early in their programs who are not yet working directly with patients. A representative sampling of ethical decisions that almost every practicing dentist faces regularly, then, seems useful here:

1. When examining a new patient, a dentist finds evidence of poor dental work. What should the dentist say to the patient? Should the dentist contact the previous dentist to discuss the matter? Should the dentist contact the local dental society?

2. Should a dentist ethically advertise that his or her practice will produce "happy smiles" as well as quality dental care? Are legal branding names that imply healthy smiles ethically acceptable?

3. Should a dentist tell a patient that his or her teeth are unattractive, with a view to recommending aesthetic treatment, when the patient has not asked for this opinion and has indicated no displeasure with his or her appearance?

4. Is it ethical for a dentist to decline to offer treatment to a patient for financial reasons? How ought dentists deal with those whose oral health needs are not covered by their insurance or government programs?

5. What is the proper relationship between a dentist and other dentists in the same community?

6. How ought a dentist deal with an adult patient who cannot fully participate in decision-making about care? Does this depend on the reason for the patient's inability to participate? What ought a dentist do when the guardian of a minor patient or of an adult who cannot fully participate in decision-making refuses to approve the ideal therapy for the patient?

7. What obligations does a dentist have, and to whom, when the dentist learns that another dentist is substance dependent in a manner that likely affects the care he or she is providing?

8. What is the proper relationship between a dentist and other health care professionals who care for the same patient? What should dentists require of the dental hygienists and dental assistants whom they employ? What are the obligations of dentist-employers toward employed dentists and these other groups?

9. Is it ethically important for a dentist to be an active participant in organized dentistry?

10. Does the dental profession as a whole have ethical obligations, and, if so, what are they? Are there ethical characteristics and skills that a profession should aspire to, especially in its relationships with the larger society? Do dentistry's professional organizations have ethical obligations as representatives of the dental profession, and, if so, what are they?

This is only a representative list of ethical questions that dentists regularly ask; there are many more. This book offers dentists a systematic account of professional ethics in dental practice that can help them understand issues like these and judge wisely about them.

ETHICAL QUESTIONS AND LEGAL QUESTIONS

Many of the issues that dentists encounter, like the examples above, have legal as well as ethical ramifications. In addition to dental school and continuing education courses there are numerous books and journal articles available to help dentists act within the law and protect themselves from lawsuits and other legal risks. Questions of professional ethics, though, are different from questions of law. They have a different basis and approach matters in a different way. In addition, many questions about a professional's ethical commitments concern matters where law has no opinion.

The most important ethical standards, in fact, are more fundamental than law. That is, laws can be either ethical or unethical, but the converse is not true. A clear-thinking person will thus try to ask the ethical question first and the legal question only later, and one of the first questions about any law that a thoughtful person will ask is whether or not it is an ethical law, both in what it requires in general and in how it applies to a particular case. If it is not ethical, then being ethical may require a person to work to change that law or, possibly, if the matter is important enough, to even conscientiously violate that law or engage in civil disobedience to change it. These facts about law and ethics do not mean that law is unimportant. It means that ethical questions are different from and more important than legal questions. An occasional comment about the law will be made in this book when it illuminates the ethical issue being examined. The focus of this book, though, is on professional-ethical questions in dental practice, not on law. Regarding genuine legal issues, other sources should be studied, and on specific questions, a good lawyer should be consulted to determine what the law (in each particular jurisdiction) requires and how best to protect oneself from legal risk.

CHOOSING TO BE AN ETHICAL PROFESSIONAL

This book will examine many of the ethical issues that arise in dental practice; it will also offer guidelines to assist dentists in determining *what is the ethical thing to do* as well as *what will support a dentist's growth in professionalism*. Its primary aim is not, then, to persuade anyone to be ethical or seek to grow in professionalism. This is not because no carefully reasoned arguments can be made to support being ethical, either in general or in one's professional practice. There are two other reasons. First, such arguments, when they are well constructed, are complex and abstract and therefore well beyond the scope of this book. Second, most people do not, ordinarily, choose to become ethical or decide to grow in the ethical practice of their profession simply because someone has offered them a carefully reasoned argument about it. Rather, they do so from complex reflections about the sort of person they want to be, the qualities of the people in their lives whom they admire and want to be like, the communities with which they want to be identified and to which they choose to owe allegiance, and the efficacy of different courses of action and patterns of life in relation to these goals. This book does not pretend, then, to replace reflections of this sort. The most a book like this can hope to do is contribute to such reflections by articulating the values to which individual dentists and the dental profession as a whole are committed, as well as the ideals to which they aspire as professionals, and by identifying the kinds of skills needed to achieve these goals.

PUBLISHED CODES OF CONDUCT AND ETHICS COMMITTEES

Most dental organizations, such as the American Dental Association, the Canadian Dental Association, regional and local associations, and the various specialty organizations, have published codes of ethical conduct to guide dentists in ethical practice. Many have ethics councils or committees that offer either formal opinions or informal advice to dentists on difficult ethical questions.

This book is not offered as a commentary on these codes or on the work of these committees; much less is it a competitor to them. It aims to accomplish a different and (in some ways) more basic function. Those who draft, approve, and interpret professional codes and opinions have ideas about the nature of the dental profession and the ideals, goals, and values on which these codes and opinions are based. Codes and opinions, however, do not—and, in practice, cannot—articulate these underlying and more complex ideas in a systematic way. A book like this—which does offer a systematic account of the nature of dental professionalism, dentistry's ideals, its goals, its values, and the implications of these for ethical practice—can, therefore, be very useful. It can facilitate and encourage discussion of these more basic aspects of dentists' ethical commitments. It can thus foster the development of a dental community that can become much more reflective and articulate on ethical issues, both internally and in its deliberations with the larger society. In addition, the dental community can then formulate codes and contribute to the work of ethics committees in ways that are more likely to be helpful in guiding ethical practice.

HABITS

Dental professionalism was described above as the internalized and habitual ways of thinking and acting—along with the relevant skills—that characterize the life and practice of the most admirable members of the dental profession. It is important, then, to ask why the ways of thinking and acting that constitute professionalism are specifically described as "internalized and habitual." One reason is the extremely important role that habits play in every part of our lives. Most of the actions we perform in life are not the product of careful and self-conscious deliberations about how to act. Most of our actions are done without careful reflection at the time; they are done from habit. Ordinarily, the vast majority of our actions are the product of various habits of acting, perceiving, valuing, and so on. Indeed, it seems clear that we could not function psychologically if most of our actions were not products of our habits; a dentist who needed to stop and evaluate every alternative way of acting every time he or she picked up an instrument or began to speak to a patient certainly could not practice effectively.

This does not mean that actions done from habit, however, are unconscious or irrational. Even if they are not carefully reflected on at the time, the habits these actions come from are themselves, for the most part, available for careful reflection and subject to thoughtful choice (hence the word "internalized" in the definition of professionalism). That is, if we choose, we can usually identify the habits that mostly shape a particular action and examine them. We can, then, compare them with alternative ways of acting, perceiving, and valuing; we can thus make a judgment about whether this is a habit we want to keep or one to try to change so that our future actions are based on habits more suited to what we judge best for that set of circumstances. One of the principal goals of technical training—and the hours and hours of practice that fill dental students' lives—is that the students will, in fact, eventually make all the necessary, basic skills of technically competent practice matters of habit.

This point about habits is particularly important in a book about ethics and growing in professionalism. Dentists who are admirable ethical professionals become so because of their conscientiously developed habits of acting ethically more than because of noteworthy individual actions. It is because of these conscientiously developed habits that they can be depended on—by their patients, by other dentists, and by the larger community—to do the right thing in almost every situation. The goal of a professional's striving to become a better professional is necessarily, then, a matter of establishing and maintaining the right ethical habits. That is, if we judge, on the one hand, that acting in a certain way under certain circumstances is the ethical thing to do, we should be working to support a habit of acting that way in that kind of situation. And, on the other hand, if we have acquired a habit that takes us in a different direction, we should start working to change that habit. The goal should be that we habitually do precisely that which we would judge is the ethical thing to do if we actually were to stop and deliberate carefully about it.

Throughout the book, however, to keep things from getting unnecessarily complicated, the cases and other examples offered will usually focus on the specific action that a dentist ought to undertake in a particular situation rather than on habits as such. In each instance, the reader should reflect, then, not just on the individual case described but also on the habits of perceiving, valuing, and acting, of which the case is an example. It is these habits, more than the particular actions in the case, that constitute the real subject matter of this book.

THE TERMS "MORAL" AND "ETHICAL," "OBLIGATION," "NORM," AND "STANDARD"

Some people use the word "moral" to mean one thing and the word "ethical" to mean something slightly, or even quite a bit, different; but people who use these words with different meanings often do not explain the difference and perhaps may not even notice it themselves. Unfortunately, there is no pattern of separating the meanings of these two words that is widely and consistently used or is commonly understood. As a result, serious misunderstandings can result from people's differing use of these words. So it is important to explain how the words "ethical" and "moral" will be used in these pages. In this book these two words will be treated as synonyms, and they will be used to mean only that the issue, question, reflection, or judgment to which they apply concerns what ought or ought not to be done or how a person/professional ought to live. More detailed or more complicated distinctions within this general arena of discussion—for example, the kinds of obligations there are and their relevance to some situation at hand—will be explicitly made when they are needed.

For the same reason, the words "obligation," "norm," and "standard" will be used only in a very general and interchangeable way in these pages. Saying someone has an obligation will simply mean there is something the person ought or ought not to do. Saying a particular norm or standard is relevant to a situation will simply mean that ethical thinking about the situation can identify certain ways of acting in the situation as ethically better or worse than others or that some other source of guidance about how one ought or ought not to act in the situation is available. The source of such guidance may be the dental profession's commitments to the larger society, the content of dentistry's ongoing dialogue with the larger society about dentistry's ethics, some other general source of dental ethics more specifically, or of ethics/morality more generally. More detailed or more complicated distinctions among the sources of such guidance or among the resources for professional-ethical reflection will be made explicit as needed.

DO ETHICAL QUESTIONS HAVE ANSWERS?

There is a widespread view within our society that questions about what ought to be done have no correct answers or, what amounts to the same thing, that one answer to a moral or ethical question is just as good as every other answer. There is no time to examine this fundamental issue carefully in this book. Instead, for our purposes, it will be most productive to simply say the matter is at least an open question. That is, on the one hand, no one has yet succeeded in demonstrating that there are no correct answers to moral questions, although people do have different views on many moral questions. On the other hand, there are some moral or ethical questions on which the level of agreement, even among people from very diverse backgrounds, is quite impressive. Yet, so far, no one has demonstrated to everyone else's satisfaction that one particular ethical system provides all the correct answers to ethical questions.

We do hope, of course, that pursuing this inquiry, looking for answers, and developing resources for answering ethical questions about dentistry will prove valuable. At the very minimum, and as a starting position, we can confidently assert that there is no good reason to believe this project represents a waste of effort. This is what is implied when we say, regarding the query about whether ethical questions have correct answers, that the matter is at least an open question.

Moreover, with regard to ethical questions about the conduct of members of a profession, the proposal being made here is that the content of a profession's ethics is the product of an ongoing dialogue between that professional group and the larger society. This dialogue is a social fact; it takes place, though, in many different venues and is an ongoing process, as will be explained in chapter 2. This means that many questions about the content of dentistry's ethics and what counts as dental professionalism do have answers because there is a significant consensus within this dialogue.

SOURCES OF PEOPLE'S GENERAL ETHICAL VIEWS

The contents of dentistry's ethics and what counts as dental professionalism have their source, then, in the ongoing dialogue of the dental community and the larger society. But people's general ethical views have many sources. People learn various parts of their ethical views from their family and other important figures in their upbringing, their formal education, their informal life contacts (both prior to maturity and afterward), and the culture of the society at large, as well as specific social and occupational groups, religious upbringing during their youth, their religious commitments as adults, and personal reflection throughout life.

Reasons will be offered, at various points in this book, for holding that a particular ethical standard is rightly included in dentistry's ethics. Such reasons will sometimes be based on what it means for dentistry to be a profession; at other times they will depend on more general ethical views. Because of the diverse backgrounds of those who read this book and the variety of general ethical views represented among them, the authors acknowledge that the reasons offered for saying that a particular ethical standard is rightly included in dentistry's ethics may be challenged. The authors hope that the general ethical positions taken in this book will at least resonate with people's experience—either experiences that the reader has actually had or others' experiences that the reader can, nevertheless, understand because of similarities to those of their own.

WHO WRITES A BOOK ON DENTAL ETHICS?

It might seem that to write a book on ethics the authors would have to think they have the answers to people's questions about how they ought and ought not to act. Most people, probably including most readers of this book, however, are quite suspicious of anyone who tells them how they ought and ought not to act. Even if correct answers to professional and other ethical questions are possible, most of us doubt that there are experts, in the usual sense, in these matters. So what kind of person writes a book on dental ethics?

As the authors of this book, we do not claim to be experts about what people ought and ought not to do. We believe that objectivity (the move away from subjectivity) in professional and other ethical judgments, as in all judgments, is increasingly achieved as one's judgments are grounded in a broader and broader base of human experience—both one's own experience and the experience of others. The experience that is relevant to the discussion of ethical issues, including professional ethics, is not exclusive to any particular group. All humans can learn from each other on these matters. In this sense, while there are no "experts" (in the usual sense) on professional or other ethical matters, every person who reflects carefully on his or her experience has expertise to share with others.

As the authors of this book, then, we view ourselves as fellow inquirers with all those who are concerned with understanding ethical issues in the dental profession specifically and in other areas of human life. We have had the benefit of a number of years of study in this field and of contact with many other thinkers who have studied these issues closely, and have worked with many of the practitioners who have served on professional ethics committees. We have also had the benefit of extensive feedback on the first and second editions of this book. This third edition distills, like the first two, what we have learned so far and what we want to share with others who are interested. It aims above all to assist its readers in doing their own careful reflection and broadening the range of experience on which their reflections are based. It also aims to widen the circle of inquirers who share a common base of experience and reflection on dental ethics and professionalism.

In other words, we have written this book because the issues of dental ethics and professionalism raise important questions, the answers of which require far more collective wisdom than is available without as broad a dialogue as possible. The goal of this book is to broaden and deepen this dialogue, within the dental community and in the community at large, on the important issues of ethics and professionalism that arise in dental practice.

Professional Ethics, Professionalism, and Patient Trust

CASE: GRIND IT OUT!

Jack Williamson, a fourth-year dental student, has just returned from a visit and interview at the main office of a prospective employer, Dr. Edward Prentice. Dr. Prentice runs three dental offices and plans to open a fourth in the summer. He has been interviewing senior students from dental schools in the state to help staff his new office.

Like many dental students today, Jack Williamson will graduate with very large debts. There is little chance a bank will loan him the money to start up his own practice, as his father was able to do. Jack's ailing father, unfortunately, had to sell his practice early, when Jack was in high school, and Jack's wife's job and the couple's desire to remain near his aging parents make a move away from the city unacceptable at present. So Jack is looking for a job in the area. As soon as Jack walks into the students' common room, everyone knows he had been out on an interview. "Nice suit, Jack! Are you trying to upgrade the clinic? Too much boring white?" says Len Billings, another fourth-year student. "How did it go?"

"A little weird," Jack answers. "Do you know where I was? Prentice's Smile Centers."

"I've seen the ads. 'Quick appointments when you need care; short waits when you get there.' What's it like?"

"Very cushy. The new place is going to look like the Taj Mahal. All the newest technology, too. That part was pretty interesting."

"What's the other part?" asks Becky Lissen, another classmate.

"The part about taking care of patients," says Jack. "I spent about an hour and a half at the Oakville Boulevard place—that was Prentice's second office. It's where he has his private executive office. The number of patients there was huge, and more were waiting for treatment. It looked like 'grind it out' was the motto."

"What do you mean?" asks Sandra Teng, another fourth-year student.

"I saw six dentists—three guys and three women, much like us, probably just out of school—working as fast as they could. They had the latest technology and lots of assistants, but all were set for speed and volume. They might as well have had 'grind it out' tattooed on their foreheads."

"Is Prentice pushing them that hard?" asks Len. "Anyway, what did you expect? If they didn't want to start their own practices, or couldn't afford to do it, then they probably had to take what they could get—just like some of us will have to. But you can handle that, Jack. Any of us in our group could. We all know how to work hard, and we're pretty fast, too. I mean, unless Prentice is some sort of jerk. So what's the problem?"

"He wasn't a jerk, Len, and hard work doesn't bother me either. I've worked for plenty of bosses who pushed me hard on the job, not to mention the kind of pressure on all of us here in this place. No, it's the quotas that got me, Len. They have target numbers, a certain amount of billable work per patient, per hour, per day, and so on, and they're judged by it. Prentice is very clear about that. It's simply what's expected. Once, while Prentice was on the phone, I saw one of the guys who was between patients. I went into his operatory and asked if there is a big push to get patients in and out or to pressure them into buying lots of care. He looked to see who could hear him first, then he leaned into my ear and said, 'Grind it out or get your butt out of here. That's the story.'

"I said that Prentice didn't seem like a bad guy, and he said, 'Oh, he's not nasty about it. In fact he's a very friendly sort of guy, but that doesn't change the expectations. He doesn't have to be nasty—he's in charge. He hires and he fires. If someone doesn't perform, they get the boot—and it doesn't take long for Prentice to figure it out. His data and contracts are iron tight.'"

"Do they do unnecessary care?" asks Becky. "Are the dentists there supposed to trick patients into thinking they need something they don't? Are they doing treatments without getting patients' consent? How do they handle all that?"

"I asked Prentice something about that after he got off the phone. I said I noticed the impressive volume of treatment and wondered how patients reacted to that or if it made for a lot of stress for his dentists."

"What did he say?"

"He said something about clear expectations making for good employee relationships. And if I came to work for him and wanted to know where I stood, I could easily figure it out myself by just comparing my work to the target numbers. He said that would make things very clear between us—as it does for all the people who work with him. As far as the patients, he said of course they had to give consent before they were treated. That's the law, and he certainly doesn't want his employees breaking any laws. He was very clear about that and added that he has a team of lawyers that keep up with all the legal changes and come in periodically to keep everyone up to date. He said a lot of practitioners don't bother to pay for that advice and put themselves at risk. He was really proud that he was protecting his employees that way."

"Maybe so, but what about pressuring patients?" asks Becky. "It doesn't seem like they're talking with people the way I'd want to talk with them, or even how I'd want any doctor to talk to me."

"He said patients know very little about dentistry. Some of them think they do from what they read online, but in the end they all depend on dentists to tell them what they need, and that's how his dentists create a high volume of work. He said he didn't want his dentists telling patients they needed things that would harm healthy teeth. That wouldn't be good dentistry, and the third-party payers he contracted with wouldn't pay for it anyway. But that still leaves a lot of leeway. So I asked him, 'Like what?' He gave the example of an amalgam showing signs of wear. They always recommend replacing it if it's within the patient's insurance contract limits. They don't recommend patching or repairing any tooth with a second or third amalgam, or even a large first amalgam, if a crown can be placed, and so on. He said some insurers don't always agree, but the goal in his offices is to offer patients the best that dental technology and expertise can provide—and that way we all go away happy. He also mentioned discolorations and other aesthetic things. He said lots of things can be proposed as needing work without lying to patients, and patients always have the right to accept or reject the recommendations.

"He has regular mandatory meetings with his dentists about how to become better salespeople. He said dental schools don't know how to teach good business. They try, but the market and technology keeps moving and they can't keep up with all of it. For one thing, it's expensive, and all dental schools have limited budgets. Lots of times they think they're getting a deal with a company who gives them something free, but then they get stuck with old equipment or something from a failing business trying to dump some old product or a long service agreement on them just so students might buy it when they graduate. He said if I came to work for him, I would really have a chance to work with the best and the newest equipment."

"I'm still struggling with how they do patient education," says Sandra. "If they were really educating patients, patients would be told that some of these things are not serious reasons for treatment, at least for most people. Some people can't afford a crown on their budgets. My brother needs one and can't even pay for the one I want to do on him to finish my competency requirement here at school. Anyway, there are often less expensive options than a crown, too."

"I asked about that," says Jack. "Prentice said patient education was important. Doing it was good dentistry, but doing it right takes time. But most patients won't sit still for it once they know the meter is running. Most just come in to get their teeth fixed, and his dentists fix them. That's what customers are interested in, he said, and that's what he's interested in. 'One of the reasons patients like it,' he said, 'is that they can come in, get the work done, and get out—just like our ad says: Quick appointments when you need care. Short waits when you get there.'"

"Then those patients don't really know what they're consenting to," says Becky.

"Maybe," says Jack, "Prentice said if a patient started asking for information that was going to take more than a minute or so to answer, then their practice was to politely tell those patients that they have to wait till another time or make other arrangements with one of their hygienists or patient managers, who are trained to do that kind of education. He said his dentists should, of course, gladly offer to answer their questions and, if a patient is interested, they offer the patient a separate contract for educational services that would start the meter running. If people aren't interested, then they're advised to go down the street. It's just the same as what they do with people who aren't captured in Prentice's third-party contracts but aren't willing or able to pay up front for exams and emergencies. They tell them to find a different dentist."

Imitating Prentice's confident and self-assured manner, Jack quotes him: "We have to be realistic here, Jack. The rule of the marketplace is caveat emptor: Let the buyer beware. We never lie to patients. We only plant seeds and make recommendations. So if the recommendations are well made, carefully made, they can work very effectively and help sell treatments that will keep our numbers high. That's what we expect of everyone in my offices, myself included. If we all follow through on that, we all make a good living out of it. Anyone who isn't interested should work someplace else. If you want to be idealistic, you can always participate in our yearly one-day free clinic. I can't tell you how good it makes me feel when I see those people really appreciating what we do for them that day. It's a voluntary day and we encourage all our dentists to do it. It's a win-win—one of our best community marketing events."

"I couldn't work in a place like that," says Becky, "even if they do seem to care about people and community needs."

"It bothers me, too," says Jack. "But a dentist has to make a living like anybody else, and my debt numbers are really starting to scare me—especially when the practicing dentists who come to teach in our clinic talk about what it's really like out there."

"Lots of dentists make a good living without doing it that way," says Sandra. "Did anyone there even mention doing what is best for the patient? That's what we've been taught, that the patient comes first. It doesn't sound like patients come first there—it's their wallets or their insurers' wallets that come first. It seems like those with no wallets are just left hung out to dry—except for the yearly free clinic thing."

"Did you ask Prentice about that?" asks Becky. "I mean, that it seems unethical to practice that way?"

"Not exactly, but he could tell I was having a problem. As I was getting ready to leave he looked at me and said he once had that student idealism about dentistry when he graduated but that it soon went away when he had to practice in the real world." Jack starts to imitate Prentice again: "Remember, if your patients in the school's clinic don't pay, it doesn't come out of your pocket. When it comes from your pocket, things won't look the way they did in school. No one is out there saying, 'Dentists are good people and do a lot of good, so let's make sure they can pay their debts, get their fair share, and earn a good living.' You'll learn very quickly that you have to make your own way. We all do. I've found a way to do that and to practice technically good dentistry at the same time. I don't hire bad dentists. I don't even interview bad dentists, Jack, only dentists in the top half of their class. That's because bad dentistry is bad business. But if you don't see that dentistry is first off a business, if you keep that idealism, Jack, then you're going to be living in La-La Land. You're welcome to try it if you want, but I think you'll find out very quickly that it won't hold up. You're free to look elsewhere, of course. There are plenty of corporate arrangements like mine, and we're all trying to tie into the whole health care picture, but mine's the best."

"That's sure a long way from what I've been taught," says Becky. "And he doesn't seem to be like any of the dentists I've really admired. I think it's unethical to practice like that."

"Maybe it isn't your ideal," says Len, "but maybe it's realistic. It's a different world out there from what it was thirty years ago, when the dentists we admired as kids were starting up. Most could graduate without huge debts, get a loan from a bank, and set up a lucrative practice. My uncle and maybe lots of others like him did that back then, and even if their borrowing, considering inflation, was close to ours now, they still did fine. But it's not that way anymore. I mean, not in today's climate. Insurance contracts and government policies are going to keep changing—and not in ways to help people like us. My debts are as big as Jack's, and the rest of you are probably in the same boat. Those guys back then could still be idealistic and still make a good living because they didn't have all these outside forces pushing on them. Maybe some of us will be lucky enough to end up in private practices that are still like the good old days. But you sure can't count on it."

"I'm not competing with Jack for a job," Len continues. "I'm going back to Minnesota. So I can hope Jack gets lots of offers so he can stay here in town. But suppose that Prentice likes Jack and makes him an offer, and suppose Jack doesn't get any other offers to choose from. Jack's dentistry is excellent, and he's a good guy and all that, but are you saying, Becky, that Jack shouldn't take Prentice's job? Maybe Prentice is a little extreme with the ads and the marketing and everything. But he doesn't practice bad dentistry. He doesn't harm people, and patients still have to consent to every treatment his dentists do for them. And he has some concern about the community, those in need, and the bigger health picture. Are you saying that it would be unethical for Jack, or any of us, to work for a guy like Prentice if the alternative is worse, like maybe not practicing dentistry at all?"

"It may mean some hard choices," says Sandra, "but if you stand for something, then you have to draw the line somewhere."

"Yes," says Jack, "the line has to be drawn. But where?"

TWO VIEWS OF DENTISTRY

Dentistry has long prided itself on being a profession, and dentists routinely describe themselves as professionals. Dentists, in fact, can clearly claim several of the most common characteristics of professions and professionals for themselves: (1) Dentists possess a distinctive expertise that consists of both theoretical knowledge and skills for applying it in practice. (2) Dentists' expertise is a source of important benefits for those who seek their assistance. (3) Because of their expertise, the larger society accords dentists, both individually and collectively, extensive decision-making authority in matters pertaining to it.

But there is a fourth widely accepted characteristic of a profession that requires careful examination here. There are two sides to this characteristic. One of these is professional ethics. Most people, both inside and outside of professions, hold that professional ethics is a central characteristic of a profession. Professions and professionals, therefore, have special obligations that other members of a society don't necessarily have. When a group becomes a profession, this view holds, it is precisely in doing so that it undertakes certain obligations to the rest of society. Similarly, when an individual becomes a professional—becomes a member of a profession—it is precisely in doing this that he or she undertakes the obligations that we summarize in the phrase "professional ethics." The other side of this fourth characteristic is trust—trust on the part of the people who are receiving professional services and trust by the society at large that the needs and well-being of the persons being served by the profession will be the primary goal of the profession as a whole and of each of its members. This commitment to give priority to the well-being of the persons the profession serves is often stated in the dental literature as "the patient *always* comes first." This way of stating this commitment does not serve any profession well, because the "always" asks more than any human can reasonably commit to. Thus, as chapter 6 will explain, it is sometimes a complicated matter to determine what this priority of the person or group receiving professional services requires. But such qualifications aside, most people—both inside and outside of our society's professions—hold that such trust is a central characteristic of society's relationship to each of its professions and that the basis of this trust is the profession's and its members' adherence to the profession's ethical standards.

Is dentistry a profession, then? Are these things true of dentistry and of dentists? Clearly dentistry has a distinctive expertise that enables it to respond dependably to people's oral health needs, and our society has been granting dentistry professional authority in matters of oral health for more than a century. But is this true about professional ethics and trust?

Many people would say, "Of course dentistry is a profession. Of course dentistry and its members are committed to and actually adhere, with only occasional exceptions, to an appropriate set of ethical standards. They are professionals who have earned the trust of those to whom they provide professional services." But others have challenged this view, claiming that it is an incorrect description of dentists and dentistry. Therefore, it is important to ask, before going any further, whether it is true that dentistry as a whole, as well as each individual dentist, has specifically *professional* obligations. If not, then a study of professional ethics at chairside can be very brief; for it need only be long enough to demonstrate that there is no such thing. If the dental community and individual dentists, however, do have specifically professional obligations—if Jack, Becky, Len, and Sandra in the case that began this chapter are right in thinking that they will have special obligations because they are dentists—then it is important to understand why this is so, even before asking more specifically what these obligations are.

To this end, it will be useful to contrast two fundamentally different pictures of dentistry. The Normative Picture holds that there are special norms that apply to dentistry in our society and that dentists therefore do have special obligations precisely because they are professionals. The other picture can be called the Commercial Picture. It claims that dentistry is no different in principle from any other activity in the commercial marketplace, with some people or organizations offering a product for sale in the marketplace and other people or organizations purchasing it from them. The following two sections will contrast these two ways of looking at dentistry in detail.

Dentistry: The Commercial Picture

The Commercial Picture, as indicated, takes dental practice to be no different in principle from the activity of anyone who produces and sells his or her wares or services in the commercial marketplace. The dentist has a product to sell and makes such arrangements with interested purchasers as the two parties are willing to make. Depending on one's view of the marketplace and society's control of the marketplace, there may be some fundamental obligations that all participants in the marketplace have toward all other participants. The usual list of these would include obligations not to coerce, cheat, or defraud other marketplace participants. Note that these are all obligations to *refrain* from acting in these various ways, in contrast with obligations to act positively in some way regarding others. In fact, obligations to *refrain*—for example, to refrain from coercing, cheating, or defrauding others—are the only kind of obligations that are ordinarily thought to be relevant in marketplace participants' dealings with one another. According to the Commercial Picture of dentistry, then, dentists do not have any obligations to *act positively* toward anyone else, including their patients, except insofar as a dentist voluntarily makes specific commitments to act in certain ways toward those individuals or groups. From this it follows that, according to the Commercial Picture of dentistry, the fact that a person is a dentist and a member of the dental profession has no moral/ethical import of its own. Dentists are like all capable humans in that they have an obligation to refrain from violating others' liberty by not coercing, cheating, or defrauding them. After that, any other obligations that a dentist might have will be the result of specific, voluntary arrangements between dentists and other participants in the marketplace, especially the dentists' patients.

According to the Commercial Picture, then, dentists have no special obligations to their patients and therefore no obligation to give priority to their patients' needs and well-being. From this it follows that the principal reason for patients to trust their dentists to ordinarily place the patient's needs and well-being ahead of the dentist's other interests is also missing from the Commercial Picture of dentistry.

According to the Commercial Picture, then, dentists' expertise and the application of it to the lives of patients is a commodity that dentists sell and patients buy, analogous to any other commodity bought and sold in the marketplace. The dentist is a producer; the patient is a consumer. Their entire relationship consists of communications about the commodity and its price, some agreement regarding an exchange (if an agreement is achieved), and then the actual exchange of the agreed-on commodity for the agreed-on price.

From the Commercial Picture point of view, the dentist and the patient are simply self-interested participants in the marketplace. That means that, in their principal relationship, they are first and foremost competitors, for each is trying to obtain from the other the greatest amount of what he or she needs or desires while giving up as little as possible of what he or she is offering in exchange. As a consequence, the proper criterion by which the dentist determines what sort of services to provide to the patient is not necessarily whatever will best meet the patient's need or best serve the patient's well-being. Instead, according to the Commercial Picture, the dentist determines what services to provide on the basis of whatever services the patient is willing to pay for and, among these, whichever ones will give the dentist the greatest return for the least cost in terms of the dentist's time, effort, money, satisfaction, and so on.

In fact, in the Commercial Picture the patient's needs and improved well-being play only a secondary role in the dentist's judgments about which services to offer a patient. The Commercial Picture, in short, focuses above all on determining, "What's in it for me?" or, as dental marketing consultants often put it, WIFM.

Of course, patients' needs and well-being do frequently function as motivators for patients to part with their money in return for a dentist's services. So dentists quite reasonably attend to patients' needs and well-being whenever doing so is useful in this way. But the patient's needs and well-being have no other significance for a dentist or for dentistry in the Commercial Picture. They certainly are not something about which a dentist or the dental profession has obligations, except insofar as these obligations are the products of explicit contractual arrangements with individual patients or other parties (e.g., insurance companies or other third-party administrators).

Of course, the dentist ordinarily communicates judgments to patients regarding their need for professional services; patients often know very little about good dentition and oral health themselves. But in the Commercial Picture the thoughtful patient would view the dentist's recommendations about treatment primarily as efforts of good salesmanship, efforts by the dentist to motivate patients to purchase services. The case might be made that the obligation to refrain from coercing, cheating, and defrauding others means that sellers are obligated to refrain from outright lies to potential buyers. But it is still the case that a dentist's recommendations for services are in principle identical, according to the Commercial Picture, to any other salesperson's efforts to get potential purchasers to buy. Thus, a dentist's recommendation that the upper-left first molar needs a two-surface amalgam restoration is no different in principle, according to the Commercial Picture, from a shoe salesperson's comment that the customer looks good in a particular pair of shoes. If the outcome of a particular dentist-patient encounter were to leave the patient no better off or even in a worse position than before but it maximized the dentist's interests, it will still be a successful relationship according to the Commercial Picture of dentistry, provided the dentist did not coerce, cheat, or defraud the patient. Similarly, according to the Commercial Picture, dentistry as a whole profession and dentistry's professional organizations have no particular obligations to the patients the profession serves, nor do they have any special obligations to the larger community as a whole simply because they are called "professional" groups and their members are called "professionals." (The leaders of these organizations will, of course, have certain contractual commitments to their members, depending on how the duties of the leaders' offices have been defined and agreed on, but these are not obligations to present or future patients of the profession nor to the community at large.)

Admittedly, it is possible to find examples of conduct conforming to the Commercial Picture on the part of some individual dentists and in the conduct of some patients, and certain other groups within our society explicitly espouse this view of each of the professions. Nevertheless, it is a premise of this book that the Commercial Picture does not provide an accurate account of the dental profession in our society today. The vast majority of dental professionals and the vast majority of members of the community at large do not accept the Commercial Picture of the dental profession any more than they accept it for any of the health professions. Instead, they accept an alternative picture of the dental profession, which will here be called the Normative Picture.

Dentistry: The Normative Picture

According to the Normative Picture, the dentist, like every health professional, has joined a group of persons who have made, both individually and collectively, a set of commitments to the community at large, commitments that entail important obligations for each dentist and for the dental profession as a whole. These obligations arise as a result of a complex relationship that exists between the profession as a whole, the individual professional, and the community at large. A brief examination of this relationship will therefore be helpful.

One of the most characteristic features of a profession, as has been noted, is expertise in a matter of great importance to the community at large. In this case it is oral health care. Professional expertise is not only a matter of knowledge; even more important is the profession's ability to dependably employ this knowledge to meet an important human need. In addition, the kind of expertise that we associate with a profession is exclusive in two ways. It is exclusive not only in the sense that within the division of labors that enables a society to function efficiently only certain persons will perform a given set of activities and hence become familiar with and efficient at performing them. Effective dental care also involves sufficiently esoteric knowledge and experience in applying it such that, as a prerequisite to dependably providing such care, extensive education is required, which can be provided only by persons who are already experts. For it is only those who are already expert who are able to train others in applying the relevant knowledge dependably, and only those who are expert are able to recognize if another person has become expert or not and to give dependable and timely (i.e., before irreparable damage has been done) judgments regarding the quality of particular instances of the profession's practice.

The second characteristic of a profession is professional authority. Because the larger community depends on this kind of expertise for effective dental care and at the same time values it greatly, the members of the community at large can see that it is in their interest, both individually and collectively, to place dental care decisions, to a significant extent, in the hands of those who have the expertise to provide it. Doing so, consequently, grants special social authority and, along with it, significant social power to these experts. Nevertheless, in the case of the dental profession, as of the health care professions generally, the community not only grants this decision-making authority regarding an important component of people's well-being to this exclusive group of experts but it also entrusts them with the task of self-supervising their use of this power.

Compare the authority and power granted to the dental profession with, for example, the authority and power granted to politicians in government. The community grants politicians authority and power over people's well-being without a sense of trust regarding its use, and it does not trust them at all to supervise their own exercise of the power granted them. Instead, the community supports a complex and seemingly inefficient system of checks and balances within government as well as the institution of periodic reelection, an aggressive and prying free press, and other costly structures aimed at maintaining close supervision on politicians' performances. But for the dental profession there has been little or no such close outside supervision, and there is relatively little distrust either.

Why does the community at large trust the members of the dental profession? What assurance does the community at large have that dentists will not abuse so much authority and power? The answer, as has already been noted, is what the Normative Picture of dentistry specifically focuses on—namely, that the dental profession and each of its members be committed to conducting themselves according to norms mutually acceptable to the community at large and to the expert group. For these norms, when conformed to, assure the community that the experts will primarily use their professional authority and power to address the oral health needs and secure the well-being of the people whom they serve and that they will work with society to preserve the trust between them that makes their response to people's health care needs possible. According to the Normative Picture of dentistry, when a person becomes a dental professional, he or she makes a commitment to ordinarily give priority to the patient's well-being and to act in accordance with the profession's ethical standards as he or she carries out the practice of dental care. A person entering the dental profession cannot legitimately say, "Dentistry may have an obligation of a certain sort, but *I* don't have that obligation because I didn't accept it." The relationship between the dental community and the larger community predates the entry of the individual student into dentistry, and acceptance of that relationship is a condition of entry. At the same time, it is because of the continuing pattern of acceptance of this relationship by each new dentist that it is reasonable for the larger community to continue trusting dentists to use their professional authority and power properly and to permit them so much autonomy, both in decision-making about their patients' well-being and in supervising themselves in how they do this.

The accuracy of the Normative Picture of dentistry is, as indicated earlier, a premise of this book. The Normative Picture of dentistry describes the ideals to which the vast majority of dentists and the dental profession as a whole strive to conform. It is the Normative Picture of dentistry that identifies the elements of professionalism that characterize the lives and professional practice of the most admired members of the profession. Although there are exceptions, a careful look at our society indicates that the dominant way in which dentists conduct themselves, and in which the larger community understands and expects them to conduct themselves, conforms to the Normative Picture rather than the Commercial Picture.

First of all, it is widely taken for granted that dentists *do* have obligations to their patients besides the marketplace obligations of not coercing, cheating, or defrauding. Dentists are widely understood to have a positive obligation to work for the patient's well-being by properly meeting his or her needs for dental care. Merely refraining from wrongdoing is not sufficient.

Second, dental care is not widely viewed simply as a commodity to be sold and bought solely on the basis of people's desire to buy it. Dental care is taken to have objective value, to be important to people's well-being, whether a given individual happens to value it or not. Oral health contributes importantly to people's ability to function in a proper and healthy way and to minimizing their pain and discomfort, neither of which is ordinarily considered merely a matter of consumer preference. This is also why the dentist has a positive responsibility to practice competently, because something of genuine value for the patient is at stake. In other words, caveat emptor, let the buyer beware, is not generally considered to be an adequate description of the proper relationship between dentist and patient.

Third, although each party to the dentist-patient relationship has interests at stake, this relationship is not ordinarily viewed, first and foremost, as a competitive one. Instead, the dentist has a primary obligation to the patient to act for the patient's well-being in relation to oral health and function and the dentist ought to ordinarily prioritize doing this rather than aiming solely to maximize the dentist's own interests. In addition, in an ordinary situation, the patient and the dentist need to work together, collaboratively, to achieve this end rather than treating each other as competitors. The Ideal Relationship between dental professional and patient will be examined in chapter 4, but the point for now is that this relationship is not primarily understood to be one of competing self-interests. As a result, the way a patient hears a dentist's recommendations for treatment is, generally, significantly different from the way he or she hears a shoe salesperson's evaluation of a particular pair of shoes. The dentist's recommendations are not only considered to be founded on expert knowledge and previous experience in practice but are also ordinarily trusted to be offered principally for the sake of the patient's greater well-being rather than for the dentist's self-interests.

Fourth, professional organizations play an essential and important role within dentistry. Although some dental organizations may share certain characteristics with trade organizations, the heart of professional dental organizations is to articulate, interpret, and supervise dentists' conduct in relation to the obligations that they have undertaken. The interest of such organizations in testing and approving various procedures and agents for use in dental practice, then, and in certifying educational programs in dental schools and designing and offering continuing education programs, is to secure proper dental care for patients and to support the well-being of the dentists themselves, who directly secure this care.

In each of these areas, as more detailed study of each of them would demonstrate further, it is the Normative Picture that describes the general situation of dentistry and of individual dentists, both in their own understanding of their role and in the larger community's understanding of it. Each of these areas could be subjected to careful sociological analysis to test more formally whether, granting that there are individual exceptions, the Normative Picture nevertheless accurately describes the situation of dentistry in contemporary American society. But this book will proceed on the premise that formal sociological study would only serve to confirm what is clear to any ordinary observer in this matter—namely, that the Normative Picture of dentistry is both factually accurate in general and describes the ideals to which the profession as a whole and the vast majority of practicing dentists ascribe. In other words, dentistry and dentists do make distinctive commitments to the larger society and therefore do have special obligations. This is precisely because they are professionals and because it is their adherence to dentistry's professional ethics that provides the solid basis for patients and the larger society to trust them to act accordingly.

PROFESSIONALISM AND SELF-FORMATION

Lived ethics is something concrete and practical. For the ethical dentist, it consists in having right relationships with patients, doing good work and responding effectively to patients' oral health needs, working effectively with staff, and managing a successful practice. This is why, when we consider someone we know to be an admirable dentist in some respect—and especially if we have been lucky enough to know a dentist who is admirable in many ways—what we admire in such a person is not usually how articulate he or she is about professional ethics but that the person's life and the way he or she practices embodies dentistry's ethics concretely and practically. This supports the definition of professionalism offered in chapter 1, that professionalism refers to conduct that exhibits the internalized and habitual ways of thinking and acting, along with the relevant skills, that characterize the life and practice of the most admirable members of the dental profession.

The importance of the word "habitually" in this definition of professionalism was already noted in chapter 1. Admirable people are not admirable because they occasionally do the right thing; they do the right thing routinely, dependably. That is possible, however, only because they have developed *habitual* ways of perceiving, evaluating, prioritizing, judging, and acting that take them in the right direction again and again, almost without their having to think about it (which is part of what we mean when we say something is habitual). Of course, even the most admirable of dentists encounter situations in which they have to stop and think carefully in order to act rightly. But even in these situations, their habitual ways of perceiving, evaluating, and prioritizing will most often make their path to judging rightly and acting rightly easier.

How does a person develop the right habits? It is not something mysterious or beyond an ordinary person's ability, but it does take ongoing, repeated effort. Consider for a moment the dental student learning technical skills. Compare the beginning learner's first uncertain efforts to manipulate an explorer or to excavate with a drill to the ease with which an experienced practicing dentist ordinarily performs these functions. What leads the learner from the one uncertain set of experiences to the other? It depends on knowledge, of course. But it is above all the formation of the right habits that brings about the change, and the key to forming right habits is practice, then self-assessment (to which others' constructive assessments can contribute), then repetition of what went well and avoidance of what did not, then more practice, more self-assessment, more practice, and so on.

The same learning process is needed to build the ethical habits of perception, evaluation, prioritization, judgment, and action that characterize the ethically admirable dentist. This self-formative learning process will be examined more fully in chapter 15, as will important barriers to dental professionalism at several points in the book, especially chapter 14. A person cannot develop the habits necessary for technical competence in the use of an explorer or a drill without having acquired the relevant knowledge, especially of what counts as competent use of an explorer or a drill to begin with. This is why professions emphasize lifelong learning, which is the heart of most continuing education programs sponsored by dentistry's professional organizations. But mastering the knowledge of what counts as professional ethical conduct in dentistry is just as necessary if one is going to acquire the habits needed for ethical dental practice. The aim of chapters 1 to 14 is to offer detailed surveys of the main components of that knowledge as well as descriptions of some of the most important skills needed to employ it.

THE BASIS OF PATIENT'S TRUST

Trust was introduced above as a patient's response to a dentist's commitment to primarily serve patients' needs and well-being. For most dentists, one of the hallmarks of a professional life worth living and one of the most satisfying features of professional life is that their patients *trust* in them. For most dentists, if one of their patients—even just one—seriously said, "I don't trust you," it would count as a significant loss to what being a dentist and being a professional means to them. It happens, of course, but when it happens the dentist sincerely hopes that, if he or she did something to bring this about, it is repairable and that the patient has, hopefully, simply misunderstood something that was in fact intended for the patient's benefit. (Some of the most important factors in dentist-patient relationships and in the larger society that can erode this trust will be examined in this and following chapters.)

There actually are three different kinds of trust that might occur in a patient's relationship with a dentist. The most important of these, from the point of view of dentistry's professional ethics, is what will here be called "Trusting the Person." The other two will be called "Trusting That" and "Trusting What."

One kind of trust that occurs within human relationships is only indirectly related to questions about professionalism or ethical conduct in general. This is the trust that is related to reliability. When we Trust That such-and-such a thing will happen or someone will act in the expected way, our trusting is, if well founded, an evidence-based judgment that we can reliably predict something about the future. This may be a prediction about a person based on evidence we have about the person, but this kind of trust is equally operative when we carry an umbrella because we Trust That it will rain today.

Dentists graduate from dental school and get licensed only after they can demonstrate to those who are already expert in dental practice that they have learned the relevant knowledge and have acquired the skills needed to safely and effectively provide dental services to patients. This is why a patient can ordinarily Trust That a degreed and licensed dentist has this knowledge and these skills and that this person can safely and effectively provide dental services and can rightly say he or she is a dentist. Moreover, the patient can reasonably Trust That this is the case even though the patient does not have the expertise needed to verify these things personally. Note, though, that the basis of the evidence for Trusting That this is the case is not evidence about the kind of person the dentist is or the kind of ethical commitments that the dentist has made. This category of trust is not, then, the essential kind of trust that is such an important part of the dentist-patient relationship.

A second kind of trust, Trusting What another person says, concerns truthfulness. To be sure, as chapter 4 will make clear, the relationship between dentist and patient would be far from ideal—in fact not even minimally ethical—if the patient is not truthfully told what the dentist believes is the case about the patient's oral health needs, possible treatments, and so on. But the patient who Trusts What a dentist says has no reason to conclude, just from this kind of trust, that the dentist's primary goal is to respond effectively to the patient's oral health needs rather than to the dentist's own interests. Trusting What the dentist says is part of what the dentist-patient relationship ought to be, but it is not the kind of trust that is central to the dentist's role as a professional.

The kind of trust that is a hallmark of a worthy professional life and is at the core of an ideal dentist-patient relationship is the patient's Trusting the Person of the dentist. This kind of trust is a response by the patient to the ethical character of the dentist—to the dentist's assurance that he or she is committed to the priority of the patient's well-being over the dentist's other interests and concerns and to the dentist's carrying out this commitment by adhering to the dental profession's ethical standards.

There are two ways in which a patient has good reason to Trust the Person of the dentist. The first is if our society's dental profession as a whole routinely (and with only rare exceptions) lives up to these commitments. When a dentist is in good standing with the profession and respected as an ethical practitioner by other dentists, a patient, though not yet knowing that dentist personally, can nevertheless reasonably Trust the Person of this dentist. Of course there is also a reliability judgment involved in this kind of situation—namely, a Trusting That the evidence of the dentist's being a member of this profession is predictive of the kind of person he or she is and the kind of professional commitments he or she lives by. But if there are any ways that the profession fails to communicate that the professional practice of its members is committed primarily to the well-being of its patients, every one of these failures erodes the basis for patients to Trust the Person of dentists whom they do not already know personally.

The second way in which a patient has good reason to Trust the Person of the dentist is, of course, through continued contact with him or her. This offers a continuous experience of witnessing a dentist adhere to the commitment of giving primary consideration to the patient's well-being and practicing according to dentistry's ethical standards. Few patients, of course, know dentistry's professional ethics in any detail. But every violation of its professional-ethical norms—unless the norms themselves are defective and need reform—will impact patients negatively and will therefore erode patients' foundation for Trusting the Person of the dentist. Even more obvious to the patient, however, will be actions by the dentist in which the needs and well-being of the patient are given second place to the dentist's own interests—that is, actions by which the relationship between dentist and patient is turned into one of competitors and thus conforms to the Commercial rather than the Normative Picture of dentistry.

How can a dentist work, then, to establish and then maintain this third kind of trust relationship in which patients Trust the Person of the dentist? The answer is, not surprisingly, found in the same process of growth in professionalism that was described in the previous section. Identify the ethical characteristics of the most admirable dentists, who will typically be the most Trusted as Persons by their patients as well, and then build these into habits of your own by practicing, self-assessing regularly, practicing more, self-assessing more, and so on.

THE CONTENT OF A PROFESSIONAL'S OBLIGATIONS

When a person becomes a dentist, then, he or she takes on a commitment to act in accordance with certain obligations in his or her practice of dentistry. But what determines the content of these obligations? It might appear that their content is principally determined by the published codes of ethics of the various dental organizations. But in fact the process is much more subtle than this.

The obligations of individual professionals arise because of the relationship between the profession as a whole and the larger community. Hence, the content of these obligations must be viewed as the product of an ongoing dialogue between the profession as a group and the larger community that the profession serves. This dialogue between the dental profession and the larger community is, to be sure, subtle and complex. It is ongoing in time, probably always somewhat incomplete, and rather slow to react to new circumstances. It is also only occasionally formally stated or made explicit in any detail. But this dialogue is nevertheless the source of the content of dentists' obligations specifically as professionals.

What role do dental organizations' published codes play? In each instance these codes should be considered to be, first, very important efforts to articulate certain elements of the content of dentists' professional obligations and, second, important teaching documents that inform the larger community of the profession's understanding of some important aspects of its commitments and also to assist in the education and formation of new dentists regarding the obligations of the profession.

The codes certainly do not legislate dentists' professional obligations, because the dental organizations do not have the authority to speak for both sides of the ongoing dialogue with the larger community. In fact, none of these organizations includes all members of the dental profession. But these codes are still important statements about the contents of a dentist's obligations because they are the work of thoughtful and active contributors to the public-professional dialogue who frequently examine a range of views before offering an opinion. For the same reason, and also because active participation in organized dentistry is itself a component of professional activity and may, thereby, further foster professionalism, these organizational codes are important teaching documents for young dentists. Using them for this purpose requires viewing them, though, as limited articulations by either dentists or experts employed by dentists; hopefully they are an accurate, though possibly flawed, articulation of the contents of the ongoing dialogue between dentistry and the larger community. In any case, students can always return to these codes as an important resource on the content of the ongoing dialogue.

The multiparty nature of the dialogue means that a dentist can never adequately determine what his or her professional obligations are simply by asking what he or she personally thinks would be best for dentists or the community nor only by asking what the dental community says about a situation or what its principal organizations say about it. The dental professional and the dental professions must also ask what the larger community currently understands about the profession's ethical commitments. This may seem a vague, even clumsy, and often frustrating test of one's professional obligations. But if these obligations are the fruit of an ongoing dialogue with the larger community—which in turn must constantly struggle to implement its understandings about many aspects of civic relationships at the local, state, national, and global level—then this is a test that may not be set aside.

What about the dental practice acts legislated by the various states? Can they be considered authoritative statements on the contents of the dialogue between the dental profession as a whole and the larger community about dentists' professional obligations? In one sense they cannot because it is unlikely that the contents of this dialogue would vary greatly from state to state, as the contents of dental practice acts could conceivably do. That is, it is not automatically the case that the products of a more localized political process will accurately articulate the contents of this dialogue.

On the other hand, the political process that leads to such legislation ordinarily includes participation by representatives of both the dental profession and the larger community, so a part of the larger dialogue is actually a component of this process. Moreover, when state-specific practice acts are compared, there are significant similarities. These patterns, it seems reasonable to say, do express some of the contents of the larger dialogue, and, in this respect, state-specific practice acts can be taken as useful statements of parts of that dialogue insofar as they are alike. But, finally, these patterns of similarity typically cover only the bare minimum of standards of professional practice and are, for the most part, mostly procedural, so very little substantive guidance about the positive contents of dentists' professional obligations can ordinarily be gleaned from them.

Dentists, and those studying to be dentists, are therefore obligated to reflect carefully on dental practice and to identify those aspects of conduct on which they can discern a broad consensus on the part of both the dental community and the community at large. On many matters this consensus will be obvious, although the application to the case at hand of what is widely accepted and agreed on may be more difficult to discern. On other matters the larger community and the dental community will not reach an obvious consensus, even after careful reflection and discussion. Whereas it is impossible to make this process any simpler, it is equally impossible and also undesirable to remove the need for thoughtful, conscientious judgment about professional conduct from the dentist's professional practice. Nor does either community want to transform living, conscientious (even if fallible) professionals into morally correct automatons—as if automatons were capable of moral judgment and free choice in the first place. Health care is too precious and the human beings who need it too uniquely situated for it to be placed in the hands of automatons. Only living, conscientious, fallible but committed professionals will do. This is why it is so important that committed professionals reflect carefully on the contents of their professional obligations. But these obligations are not simple, and it is best to follow the two most obvious paths in order to study them carefully: looking at them both in terms of general guidelines and in terms of particular sorts of ethical problems. Therefore, throughout this book, dentists' professional obligations will be examined from the point of view of the general guidelines they embody and the most important kinds of questions that need to be asked to address them. At the same time, the cases that begin each chapter and other examples will keep the discussion in touch with what happens at chairside.

USING THE INTRODUCTORY CASES

Each of the remaining chapters in this book will begin, as this one did, with a case, a story about someone who (1) must make a choice about how to act in some situation and who, therefore, (2) must come to a judgment about how he or she *ought* to act in that situation and who (3) must consider his or her professional obligations as a dentist to arrive at that judgment.

The purpose of these cases is not to inform the reader of the morally correct action in each of these situations so that the reader might then act accordingly when such situations happen to arise. That not only would exceed the authors' abilities and contradict our goals in writing this book but it would also be foolish because fourteen cases cannot possibly contain all the important ethical issues that arise in dental practice. Rather, the first purpose of each of these cases is to help the reader identify the kinds of questions they will need to ask themselves in order to determine what ought to be done. Some of these questions, as well as various possible answers to them, will be examined in the text of each chapter. Secondly, these cases are included to assist readers in applying what is proposed in the book to their chairside experience in the hopes that any learning achieved from reading this book will not be only at the level of theory and generality but will connect effectively with actual practice.

Consistent with these goals, there will not be a concerted effort to exhaustively analyze each case, much less to resolve any of the cases finally. At the conclusion of each chapter we will discuss certain themes from the case—namely those that accord with the subject matter of the chapter. But the *reader* should try to think the case through to a conclusion—in other words, to a judgment about what course of action the actor in the case ought to take and why. Eventually this will require the reader to consider all of the categories of professional obligation to be described in chapter 3 and possibly other moral categories as well. But even early in the book, when only a few general topic areas have been examined in detail, the reader should still make a point of going back to the case before reading the authors' concluding commentary in order to form his or her own judgment about what ethical issues arise in the case and what questions the dentist ought to be asking in order to act ethically in the case. That is, we hope the reader will stop and personally do his or her *own* thinking about each chapter's case *before* reading our commentary.

Finally, as was mentioned in chapter 1, there is an important oversimplification at work whenever a particular case is presented and examined. In actual real-life situations, especially when there is a patient waiting in the chair, few of us are likely to take time out to engage in a meticulous weighing of professional—or any other—obligations. Instead, most of our actions, professional and otherwise, are the product of trusted habits that we have formed and reinforced over the years.

But such habits can be subjected to reasoned examination as surely as the apparently spontaneous actions that they prompt. The skills needed for such reasoned examination of our habits are the same skills needed to examine specific alternative responses to a particular concrete situation. The principal focus of this book is the development of these skills, whether for application to our habits or application to individual actions. Therefore, even when the focus of discussion is on a particular case, with its specific details determining much of our reflection, the questions that must nevertheless be asked about it can, in each instance, be reformulated to read: Should a dental professional have a *habit* of acting in this way or that? In other words, reflecting on particular cases like those proposed in this book is a valuable way to examine and reshape our habits so we will act ethically in all those situations when we cannot or do not stop to reflect carefully. When students and dentists share these reflections together and make a habit of setting aside space and time to share their reflections both in small and larger groups, then the heart of professionalism will beat more freely.

THINKING ABOUT THE CASE

The case presented in this chapter clearly raises many important questions about dental professional ethics. One of these questions is whether Dr. Prentice views himself and his dentist employees according to the Normative Picture of dentistry or whether he sees dentistry as nothing but a commercial enterprise.

In posing this question, it is important to observe that the information given in the case about Dr. Prentice is quite limited. We have Jack's own observations of large numbers of patients and of dentists working hard and quickly, as well as his feeling that there is a lot of pressure on the dentists employed by Dr. Prentice. We have the words of one of Dr. Prentice's employed dentists, whose comments are suggestive of a very commercially oriented operation but who actually describes only Dr. Prentice's firmness in enforcing his expectations as an employer (in the form of "the target numbers") on his employees. This raises important questions about proper relationships between professionals when they are employer and employee: questions that will be addressed in some detail in chapter 10. But such questions arise under the Normative Picture of dentistry as well as the Commercial Picture and therefore don't tell us in themselves whether Dr. Prentice accepts the Normative or the Commercial Picture of dentistry.

Finally, we have Dr. Prentice's answers to Jack's questions. Does Dr. Prentice say anything that implies a rejection of the Normative Picture of dentistry? Are any of his answers inconsistent with the view that becoming a dentist entails accepting a set of significant obligations toward one's patients and the community at large and the commitment to ordinarily give priority to the patient's well-being?

On the one hand, Prentice clearly indicates that the dentists he employs are judged, and no doubt paid and retained, on the basis of the amount of income they produce for the practice. This suggests that they feel considerable pressure to do more work for each patient rather than less, which could lead to work being done that is unnecessary or is positively harmful. But Prentice explicitly rejects doing harm to healthy teeth. Also, the examples he gives of the kind of work that his dentists are expected to recommend in order to keep "the numbers high" could be defended as being still within the range of what is clinically acceptable, though optional and obviously not urgent, care. Prentice also stresses his unwillingness to employ dentists who are not technically capable; presumably this means hiring those who are not just minimally capable but are able to perform technically competent dentistry quickly and with a high volume of patients. He's also a realist about his community's needs, and his approach to doing something about it can provide good-quality dental care to a larger number of people.

To be sure, other dentists might not recommend or even mention replacing a slightly worn amalgam; they might not initiate a conversation about aesthetic interventions unless the patient mentioned aesthetics first. (Chapter 14 will examine some of the distinctive ethical issues that arise when patients seek aesthetic treatments that do not involve oral health goals as such.) But the question can at least be asked whether a more conservative "philosophy" of dentistry, which prefers to intervene in the least possible way and still is effective for the patient's oral health, is professionally *required*. If it is not professionally required, then the kinds of recommendations that Dr. Prentice requires of his employees, which produce greater income for the practice than a more conservative philosophy would yield, might be professionally acceptable. Determining this would require more data about how Dr. Prentice's dentists are required to function than has been provided in the case. But in the real world, asking this question and obtaining the data necessary to answer it would be extremely important.

In fact, there seems to be a range of dental "philosophies," from more conservative to more aggressive, that are acceptable guides to ethical dental practice. Therefore, another way to consider Dr. Prentice's approach is by asking whether it is within that range or not. But answering this question carefully, it seems clear, will require answers to a number of other questions—for example, about the hierarchy of values in Dr. Prentice's practice. (The Central Practice Values of dentistry will be examined in chapter 5.) Another question, already examined to some extent, concerns the relative priority of the patient's well-being as compared with profit in his offices. So, determining how Dr. Prentice stacks up against the Normative Picture of dentistry is, from this perspective, a task that would take considerably more study.

Another approach is suggested by Becky's question about patients' consent. Could it be argued that Dr. Prentice's style of practice is professionally defective because it deprives patients of the opportunity to give informed consent for the treatment they receive? Dr. Prentice claims that no treatments are given unless patients consent to them, but that answer does not tell us how well they understand the options available to them. However, the simple phrase "informed consent" is not a clear enough standard to help us answer this question. We need to explore the relationship between dentist and patient much more carefully, especially in regard to decisions about treatment, before a clear judgment can be made about the professional adequacy or inadequacy of the kind of decision-making process that Dr. Prentice counts on. (The Ideal Relationship between dentist and patient, especially from the point of view of decision-making, will be examined in chapters 4 and 7.)

Third, there is the question of motivation. Dr. Prentice seems to Jack, Becky, and Sandra to be motivated by the wrong reasons, practicing dentistry principally for the sake of money rather than the good of patients. But, as Len and Dr. Prentice both observe, a person cannot practice dentistry in US society without also being involved in a business, and if that business fails economically, the practice of dentistry and the good of patients it produces go with it. Are Dr. Prentice and Len to be credited with simply being genuinely "realistic," or are their values somehow inappropriate from the perspective of the Normative Picture of dentistry? Does the Normative Picture require everyone who becomes a dentist to have the same reasons for doing so, the same values that they hope to achieve? This seems most unlikely. The Normative Picture stresses that every member of the profession undertakes a certain set of obligations, the contents of which are the product of an ongoing dialogue between the profession as a whole and the larger community. But it does not seem to specify the reasons why a person would undertake these obligations. So why should Dr. Prentice's emphasis on making a good living strike Jack, Becky, and Sandra as professionally inappropriate, provided that he and his employed dentists are committed to fulfilling their professional obligations to their patients and the community?

The reason the students feel uneasy is the fact that fulfilling one's professional obligations will sometimes require the sacrifice of other things for the sake of one's patients; Dr. Prentice's way of speaking about dental practice may seem to imply that no such sacrifice is required or that it may justifiably be avoided—or even that sacrificing one's own interests, for patients or anyone else, ought to be avoided. That is, even though people become dentists for a variety of reasons, the well-being of patients must be among these reasons for the person's acceptance of the Normative Picture of the dental profession to be plausible or coherent. In this respect, it is interesting to examine Dr. Prentice's reason for hosting voluntary free clinics. Does he express concern for persons with unmet oral health needs or does he view it primarily as a useful marketing device?

In fact, we do not have enough information to judge Dr. Prentice conclusively on this matter. It would surely be unwise of Jack to join Dr. Prentice's practice without getting more information first. But what is clear is that judging whether a particular dentist or a particular group of dentists is practicing in a manner consistent with the Normative Picture of the dental profession requires a careful and detailed understanding of the obligations that, according to this view, dentists undertake. Most dentists practice in a professionally ethical manner without being able to fully articulate the professional obligations that they habitually fulfill. But when a set of harder questions arises, like Jack's questions about Dr. Prentice, it is important to be able to articulate the standards that ought to be applied. Facilitating reflection on the professional obligations of dentists and aiding in their more complete articulation is the aim of this book.

3

The Questions
of Professional Ethics

CASE: WHEN EVERYTHING WORKS RIGHT

George Anderson, a thirty-eight-year-old plumber, has diabetes and is under the care of his physician of seven years, Dr. Gannett. At his last visit Dr. Gannett told him that the on-and-off pain in his teeth could be related to his diabetes and that he should see a dentist. Dr. Orasony is the first dentist Mr. Anderson has seen since his "kid-dentist" referred him, in his early twenties, to an oral surgeon for his wisdom teeth. "I want all these teeth out," Mr. Anderson says to Dr. Orasony. "I need some plates to replace them. There's nothing I can do about this diabetes. I know myself. I'll never be able to follow the diet my doc says I have to for the diabetes.

"Dr. Gannett's always bawling me out," he adds, "so I don't go to see him; then he yells at me for that . . . or for not testing my blood sugar often enough or for something else. I do my insulin shot every day. I've got to or it'll kill me."

Dr. Orasony takes a quick look and notes several carious lesions, the upper-right second molar will likely need endodontics, and there is significant bleeding and swollen gums with mild localized recession and poor oral hygiene. When asked about his oral hygiene, Mr. Anderson says, "I brush a few times a week, when I think about it. I hate flossing . . . takes too much time. Makes 'em hurt and bleed and doesn't do any good."

"Despite what's in the news lately, flossing is important for anyone with teeth," says Dr. Orasony. "But for people with diabetes, I'm convinced it's absolutely necessary. Diabetes affects the body's natural repair system. It takes more self-care to help damaged gums stay healthy. I'll need to take X-rays and do a few measurements, but right now I'd say most of the pain in your teeth is probably from the damaged gums. Good brushing and flossing are critical for keeping down the plaque buildup on our teeth—the white fuzzy stuff we feel with our tongues. There are a few simple tricks to good daily mouth care. Careful instruction on how it's done and why it's so important takes a little time and some follow-up, but it's well worth it."

"My old dentist talked about that when I was a kid. That was when he said my wisdom teeth were causing my pain. Once they were out, I felt fine, so I didn't go back. Then he died."

"So you haven't seen a dentist since you learned you had diabetes?"

"Nah. After my wisdom teeth were pulled my teeth felt fine," says Mr. Anderson. "I've had dental insurance from work for a long time but never used it 'cause my teeth felt ok."

"Well, your diabetes really changes things, and the pain you're having is a sign of that. It's important that you start seeing a dentist regularly from now on. We'll help you learn how to take better care of your mouth, or you'll have a lot more problems than you have now. Your gums are already affected, but the damage seems only moderate and likely can still be fixed without major surgery. The most important part will be your changing the way you care for your mouth—and yourself."

"Yeah, but it's hard to do stuff like that, a lot harder than just taking a shot," Mr. Anderson says. "It sounds just like the diabetic diet. Don't you have a shot for the gums, too? I like things quick and dirty."

"It's hard," says Dr. Orasony. "Diabetes is a real bummer. You've got my sympathy."

"Well, what about just yanking them out and giving me the plates?" asks Mr. Anderson. "Won't that solve the problem and save us both a lot of grief?"

Dr. Orasony then carefully explains the long-term risks of this option and the reasons for keeping and maintaining natural dentition for as long as possible. "I hate taking such drastic action," he says, "I only consider taking teeth out in extreme cases—and rarely in someone as young as you.

"Still, your situation is a hard one," he says, "but it's not out of your control if you're willing to work at it. With the proper diet and oral hygiene that we can teach you, you really can manage the effects of the diabetes on your mouth. We'll work with you every step of the way."

"I'm not so sure," says Mr. Anderson. "I haven't done very well with the diet and the other stuff so far, only the shot 'cause it's simple and I know I need it."

"Well, why don't we try to change things now," says Dr. Orasony, "because you need these other things, too. I hate to be so blunt, but a bad diet will kill you just as surely as missing your shot will—it just takes longer. I'm not saying we're going to live forever, just that (speaking for myself) I'm more comfortable when I'm taking care of myself and feeling healthy than when I'm not. We all need to make a habit of good oral hygiene, especially in your situation, or your mouth will give you more trouble than it is now, and eventually that will lead to a lot worse problems."

"What should I do?" asks Mr. Anderson.

"To start with, after we get some measurements on your gums, you'll need several appointments to get your teeth properly cleaned, especially around the gums so they can start to heal. It doesn't look like it'll involve any surgery, though that is a minor possibility if it turns out that a good cleaning doesn't do the job. You also have several cavities that'll need attention once your gum situation is under control. There's one big tooth in the back that may need the tissue down inside it treated to save it—that's what's called a root canal. We'll need some X-rays before I can say what will actually be needed there. The most important, though, is the first step—the instructions and then the follow-up on your daily brushing and flossing. You'll have to make a habit of that. Now, I've said a lot and we still need to do the exams. But I want to be sure I'm not being confusing. Is what I've said clearing things up for you?"

"I'm not surprised I need some things done. I mean, it's hurting and all. My union health insurance is pretty good for dental work, so I'd say let's go ahead and see if it helps. Since I'm already here, can we start now?"

"I'd really like to. The first step is getting X-rays and the needed measurements before the dental hygienist, Miss Williams, starts the cleaning. Then she'll check with me, but she'll probably start the cleaning today, taking off that buildup on your teeth, especially around the gums. That'll help your gums feel better so you can brush and floss daily without the pain and bleeding. Miss Williams will go over some basic instructions about that before you leave today. She'll probably need a second appointment to finish the cleaning, though, so we can see whether other work might be needed to help your gums heal. Once that's under way I can start fixing the cavities. You mentioned on-and-off pain from your teeth. From what you're saying and from what I'm seeing, it's probably more from the gums than the cavities. But if you get more pain from any tooth or a throbbing anywhere, call me so we can fix it right away. Also, if your gums don't respond to the basic cleanings, we'll need to decide about gum surgery, so I need to mention that, and that may mean referring you to a specialist. There are several gum doctors—they're called periodontists—whom I work with here in town. But that's a bridge we don't have to cross now. Does this work for you?"

"It's fine. I'm just not sure I'm gonna do my part," says Mr. Anderson. "I wish you could just take care of it all. It's like the diet. I wish they just had a shot you could take instead of all that other stuff."

"When Miss Williams explains the brushing and flossing," says Dr. Orasony, "you can tell her all your doubts. She's very understanding and loves to help people fit good oral hygiene into their lives. I think you'll find the habits you need to build up easier to develop than you expect."

Dr. Orasony then asks permission to contact Mr. Anderson's physician so that they can keep each other informed of Mr. Anderson's progress. The hygienist, Sarah Williams, then completes Mr. Anderson's appointment and schedules him for a second one two weeks later.

During that time, Dr. Orasony calls Mr. Anderson's physician, Dr. Gannett, who, not surprisingly, is very frustrated with Mr. Anderson's health habits, given his medical condition. The two doctors agree that their support of each other's efforts could be the thing to trigger the needed changes. Dr. Orasony suggests that Dr. Gannett might be the best person to contact a nutritionist and a family counselor he knows at the local hospital to help both Mr. Anderson and his wife set up an appointment with their new program. Dr. Gannett isn't familiar with the program leaders' names or the program. "Those two women are phenomenal," says Dr. Orasony. "I was on a community education panel with them a couple of weeks ago. After their talk, a dozen people sur-rounded them with questions about changing the way their families talk about things and finding healthier ways for picking and fixing food so all of it could fit into their daily lives. I was very impressed."

At the second appointment, Miss Williams finishes the initial prophylaxis. She also talks with Mr. Anderson to determine how much he has retained from her instructions at his first appointment and then continues educating him. Dr. Orasony then explains the results of the X-rays and measurements to Mr. Anderson and confirms the treatment plan.

Mr. Anderson appears faithfully for a third and fourth appointment. The gingival tis-sue responds well. Both Miss Williams and Dr. Orasony see the effects of Mr. Anderson's brushing and flossing and strongly encourage him about it. Mr. Anderson then thanks Dr. Orasony for suggesting the meeting with the nutritionist and family counselor.

Restorative treatment, including endodontic therapy for one of his molars, is nearly complete by the sixth appointment. Mr. Anderson is clearly establishing a model daily routine of both oral and general hygiene, and he is even starting to take more pride in his dress. Dr. Gannett also calls Dr. Orasony out of the blue to thank him for putting him in touch with the nutritionist and family counselor because they have also helped three other diabetic patients of Dr. Gannett's to get their diets under control. At his sixth appointment, Mr. Anderson asks Dr. Orasony, "Is Miss Williams in the office? I'd like a moment with both of you before you numb me for these last fillings."

When Miss Williams walks in, Mr. Anderson says, "I'm glad you're both here today. Dr. Orasony says this'll be my last appointment for now. I'll just be coming in for checkups, and I just wanted to thank both of you for everything you've done for me and my wife. It was you and then the nutritionist and family counseling team at the hospital—Liz and Kim—who got us on the right track. We're sitting down to great meals all together now and the kids are getting to be little gourmet chefs. Our whole family seems to be working together and talking better with each other. I want you to know how grateful we are for everything you've done. If not for you two, none of this would've happened."

WHY THIS KIND OF CASE?

Some readers might find it puzzling to find a case like this in a book on professional ethics. There is a mistaken notion that the only cases useful for learning about ethics are either cases that describe some kind of unethical conduct or cases where the ethical issue is complex and difficult to sort out. Why have a case, then, as the title of this one indi-cates, where "everything works right"?

One reason for giving prominence to this kind of case is to remind us that observing appropriate behavior in someone else and trying to do the same is actually the main way we learn how we ought to act. There can be value in studying examples of unethical conduct, but only if we spend time carefully asking in what ways the action fell short, since this may point us in the proper direction. But simply avoiding inappropriate acts, obviously, is not the same as doing what we ought to do. Even focusing on an example of right conduct does not ensure we can act in the same way, though, if we do not carefully ask what it is about this example that made it professionally and ethically correct. Of course, this case where everything goes right is just a hypothetical example. A better source for learning how to act in accord with dentistry's professional ethics are examples of actual dentists acting in ethically correct ways and, then, asking ourselves what it is about these actions that makes them ethically correct. It is easy to overlook this resource for ethical growth; examples of dentists doing what they ought to do are so common that they may seem to have little instructional value. Yet every instance of ethical-professional conduct can be a learning opportunity if it prompts thoughtful analysis of the specific characteristics that make it ethical.

One thing that stands in the way of this kind of careful analysis of examples of dentists' ethical (or unethical) conduct is the assumption that ethical thinking is supposed to be simple and obvious. This assumption is false, although it is sometimes fostered by the way dental ethics is taught and by the way various codes of dental ethics articulate their content—in terms of straightforward dos and don'ts. As mentioned in chapter 1, the codes of ethics published by various dental professional organizations are intentionally brief. They are written to be, as our plumber friend would say, "quick and dirty." A code can only summarize the most obvious components of the profession's ethical standards. Of course, they can be useful educational documents because, in many situations, the action that is ethically required is obvious. But dental practice includes many situations in which what ought to be done is not simple and obvious and cannot be determined by referring to a list of simplified dos and don'ts.

Just as a lot of knowledge and skill must properly come together for a dentist's actions when treating a patient to be technically correct, so, too, are certain elements of knowledge and skill needed for a dentist's actions to be ethically correct. The difference between these two kinds of knowledge and skills is not that one is simple and the other is complex. The difference is that dental school faculty (as well as the dental researchers in the subfields that make up dental science) have identified and carefully differentiated the various components of knowledge and skill that go into technical proficiency in dental practice. As a result, teachers and students can then focus on them one by one and can then practice putting them together until they gradually become able to tell when they are doing all of them well or if they need more work on some of them in a particular practice setting.

There has been little comparable effort, however, to identify the knowledge and skill components of professional-ethical conduct. The dos and don'ts of codes are not enough. What is needed (and what is also needed by the authors and conservators of codes in order to be sure the dos and don'ts themselves are properly stated) is deeper understanding of dentistry's ethical norms. For the ethical norms of every profession, when they are fully stated, include at least nine kinds of ethical content, or, to say the same thing in different words, address nine sets of questions about how the members of that profession ought to conduct themselves.

The aim of this chapter is to identify the nine kinds of ethical content that are relevant to the ethics of every profession and then to describe the content of each of these categories of ethical norms as they apply to the dental profession. Then, the rest of this book can use these categories to unpack more concretely what is ethically at stake in different kinds of dental practice situations. After introducing the nine categories in very general language that applies to any profession, the opening case will be reviewed and the kinds of ethical questions identified that Dr. Orasony would have asked himself, or would at least have addressed without noticing it, in order to make "everything work right." This description of ethical thinking in the case will point out ways in which the nine sets of questions about professional ethics can guide a dentist's thinking in practice and, taken together, can provide dentists with a clear vision of what to aim for in practice. Note that, in addition to identifying the kinds of questions that dentists ought to ask and the kind of thinking dentists ought to regularly engage in as they practice their profession, the chapter is also providing the tools a dentist needs to analyze the ethical (and unethical) conduct of other dentists as well. Thus, it provides the reader with tools for asking about Dr. Orasony: What is it that makes his conduct professionally ethical?

Briefly stated—in question form—the nine categories of professional-ethical content to be discussed here are: (1) Who is the profession's Chief Client? (Dentistry and the other health professions have a special word, "patient," to name the people they serve, but most professions don't. The word "client" is used by many professions to name those they serve—for example, therapists, lawyers, and architects. It can make what professionals do sound too much like a market relationship, but other than "beneficiary," which already has a very specific meaning, there is no other generic English word that means "the person or group to be served," so this book will use "client" whenever professions, generally, are being discussed.) (2) What is the Ideal Relationship between a member of this profession and a client? (3) What are the Central Practice Values of this profession? (4) What are the norms of Competence for this profession? (5) In what respects do the obligations of this profession take Priority over other morally relevant considerations affecting its members, and what sorts of Sacrifices do they require? (6) What is the Ideal Relationship between the members of this profession and Other Professionals and those who assist the profession? (7) What is the Ideal Relationship between the members of this profession and the Larger Community? (8) What ought the members of this profession do to make Access to the Profession's Services available to all who need them? (9) What are the members of this profession obligated to do to preserve the Integrity of their commitment and to continue to grow in Professionalism?

NINE CATEGORIES OF PROFESSIONAL OBLIGATION

Now it is time to describe these nine categories of professional obligation more carefully. But it is worth explaining why they need to be carefully described—that is, how doing so can improve a dentist's professional-ethical thinking.

Back in chapter 2, the commentary on the case of Dr. Prentice identified two kinds of information that were lacking in that case. Because of this, a conclusive judgment could not be made about Dr. Prentice's conformity (or lack of conformity) to his professional obligations as a dentist. First, the case did not give enough information about how

Dr. Prentice actually practices, what he actually requires of his employees, and how he enforces those requirements. That is, important factual information about his practice of dentistry was missing from the case as presented. But one cannot do careful ethical thinking about a situation if crucial facts about the situation are missing (or the information one has about the situation is incorrect). On one hand, innumerable facts are available about any dentist's practice; on the other, however, only a certain number of those facts are important for making judgments about the dentists' conformity (or nonconformity) to professional obligations. In order to know which facts are relevant to doing good ethical thinking, though, one needs a detailed account of the contents of dentists' professional obligations, which is what this book aims to provide.

A second reason why a conclusive judgment could not be made about Dr. Prentice's conformity (or nonconformity) to dentistry's professional standards was that chapter 2 discussed dentistry's ethics only in very general terms. As mentioned earlier, doing good ethical thinking requires having a more detailed account of the contents of dentists' professional obligations. Therefore, the nine categories of professional obligations mentioned in the previous sections will now be explained in fuller detail. These nine categories will also be used throughout the book to determine which facts about the cases are most relevant to judgments about ethical or unethical conduct; they will help focus our inquiry on the most relevant components of dentistry's ethical norms and of the professionalism to which every dentist should aspire. In order to understand these categories and use them most profitably, it is best to continue thinking about each category as a set of questions. Each can be headed (for summary purposes) by a "master question"—one that identifies the main focus of each question in that set. Each of these sets of questions, when carefully answered in regard to a particular instance of professional practice or a particular policy or standard regarding practice, will reveal which facts are important for making a careful judgment about the situation (from the point of view of appropriate professional conduct). They will help identify, then, the most relevant elements of dentistry's ethical norms for coming to a judgment about what ought to be done in the situation. It is important to mention that some of the questions in each category address matters of importance to other categories—that is, these nine categories are not completely independent. Categorizing questions and data under these headings, however, is a useful way to keep moral reflections and judgments about professional conduct clear and on track. (If other ways of categorizing the contents of professional obligation also prove useful, more power to them, for the goal of this book is to offer tools for careful reasoning about professional obligation, not the preeminence of a particular set of categories or questions.) In the final section of this chapter, each of the nine categories will be described with direct reference to the dental case that opened the chapter.

The Chief Client

Every profession has a Chief Client or Clients. This is the person or set of persons whose needs and well-being the profession and its members, in their dialogue with the larger society, are chiefly committed to serving.

For some professions, including dentistry, identifying the Chief Client seems quite easy. There is even a special word, specific to the health professions, that seems to clearly identify dentistry's answer to this question. Surely, we might say, the Chief Client of the dentist is the patient. But this answer is too simple. To see this, look at a different profession for a moment. Who is the Chief Client of a lawyer? Is it simply the party whose case the lawyer represents or pleads or someone to whom the lawyer gives advice? Lawyers are instructed, however, and announce in their self-descriptions and codes of conduct that they have obligations to the whole justice system; therefore, there are things that they, as professionals, should not ethically do, even if doing these things would be advantageous to the party they represent or advise. So the answer to the question about the Chief Client of the legal profession is complex, involving both the person the lawyer represents or advises and the whole justice system—perhaps even the whole larger community served by that system. But once the complexity involved in identifying the Chief Client of the legal profession is understood, if we look again at dentistry we may find that determining its Chief Client is similarly more complex. For the dentist must not only attend to the patient in the chair but also to the patients in other operatories and those in the waiting room. The dentist also has some obligations to all of his or her patients of record. In addition, a dentist has some obligations to people who are not his or her patients (to the public as a whole, for example), because a dentist has an obligation to practice with caution so as not to spread infections from patients to other people and an obligation to assure that individuals seeking dental care in emergency situations do, in fact, find assistance, whether they become that dentist's patient or not. So it turns out that the question of who is dentistry's Chief Client is not as simple to answer as it first appears.

In addition, situations may arise in which persons from the different "subgroups" that a dentist serves may need care at the same time or care that requires the use of a limited supply of resources, especially time and effort but also material resources in some situations. In such cases, questions about which of these persons ought to be given priority—when all cannot be served simultaneously—also arise. In the health professions generally, for example, those who are in emergent, life-threatening situations ordinarily receive priority over patients whose care can be safely delayed, and patients with appointments ordinarily have priority over others, and so on. Within the dental profession, some of these priority questions are discussed in various dental organizations' codes and in the dental ethics literature; others deserve careful consideration but are often left to the individual dentist to sort out as best as he or she can.

The Ideal Relationship between Dentist and Patient

For every profession the point of the relationship between the professional and a client is to bring about certain values for the client, values that cannot be achieved for the client without the expertise of the professional. In order to achieve these values for the client, both the professional and the client need to make a number of judgments about what the professional could possibly do and ought to do to assist the client; they, then, must make a number of choices. The question addressed in this second category of professional obligation concerns the proper roles of the professional and the client as they make these judgments and choices.

At least four general models of the professional-client decision-making relationship can be identified. In chapter 4 these models will be examined in detail in relation to dentistry, and the chapter will propose that one of these models, the Interactive Model, is the ideal dentist-patient relationship. In addition, discussion of the professional-client relationship must include consideration of situations in which this Ideal Relationship is not possible. One example is identifying the proper relationship between a dentist and a patient who cannot fully participate in judgments and choices about the dentist's interventions. This fairly common situation will be the topic of chapter 7. The dentist's relationship with patients who are extremely uncooperative will be discussed in chapter 10.

The Central Practice Values of the Dental Profession

Every profession is focused only on certain aspects of the well-being of its clients. The rhetoric of many professions often speaks of caring for the whole person, but in fact, no professional group is expected by the larger community to be an expert in providing for their clients' entire well-being. Expertise is necessarily more narrowly focused. Therefore, no profession is committed to securing for its clients everything that is of value for them. Rather, there is a certain set of client-centered values that are the focus of each profession's expertise and that it is the job and obligation of that profession to try to secure for its clients. In this book these values are called the Central Practice Values of a profession because every judgment about what the professional ought to do to assist the client depends on them. The Central Practice Values of the dental profession will be examined in detail in chapter 5.

Competence

Every professional is obligated both to acquire and to maintain the expertise needed to undertake his or her professional tasks. This category of competence (i.e., technical knowledge and skill) is probably the most obvious category of professional obligation. It is also the easiest to describe in a general way. If a professional fails to apply his or her technical expertise or fails to obtain the expertise needed for undertaking some task, these failures directly contradict both the point of being an expert and the very foundation of the decision-making authority and power the larger community grants the professional in the first place.

But the determination of what counts as sufficient or minimally adequate technical competence on the part of a member of a given profession like dentistry, both in general and in relation to specific kinds of tasks, is a very complex question that is beyond the scope of this book. In practice, and almost of necessity, the working out of detailed judgments about requisite technical expertise in dentistry is left to the members of the expert group—that is, the dental profession itself. But the larger community usually requires of its professions that explanations be given regarding the general nature of the reasoning employed, especially regarding the inevitable values trade-offs involved in determining what counts as the norm of minimal professional-technical competence. Such determinations unavoidably include a risk-benefit judgment that balances the greater or lesser availability of expert assistance against the lesser or greater likelihood that the assistance of those who pass the profession's standards of competence might not serve those in need in the best possible way.

In addition to obtaining and maintaining the necessary technical expertise, every member of every profession is also obligated to undertake only those tasks that he or she is competent to perform and, when a patient's needs extend beyond the professional's level of expertise, to assist the patient in locating a practitioner who can assist them. In other words, a dentist always needs to be judging whether he or she has the expertise to handle a particular diagnosis or provide a particular form of therapy. The judgment about whether to treat a condition oneself, to refer to a more skilled specialist, or even to refrain from treating if no specialist is available is always an ethical question, not only a technical one. The delicate topic of incompetent dental work will be discussed in chapter 9.

Every profession's ethics also includes a reminder that professionals will experience conflicts between the benefits of their professional services to those they serve and the possible benefits they may receive from providing their services. These can obviously include possible financial benefits but also benefits in the form of prestige, career advancement, and so forth. Professionals are often instructed to avoid all conflict of interests, a directive that incorrectly implies that any interest of the professional other than the client's well-being is automatically unethical. A more correct view of the ethics of such situations is to ask if possible benefits to the professional are likely to interfere with that professional's expert judgment about the best ways to assist the client. This topic, along with guidelines for how dentists should proceed in these kinds of situations, will be examined in chapter 13.

Sacrifice and the Relative Priority of the Patient's Well-Being

Most sociologists who study professions mention "commitment to service" or "commitment to the public" as one of the characteristic features of a profession. Similarly, in the dental profession's published codes of ethics and other self-descriptions, the patient's well-being has always been identified as the dentist's primary goal. But these expressions admit of many different interpretations with significantly different implications for actual practice. It is important to ask just what measure of personal interest and of a dentist's other commitments a dentist is professionally obligated to give up.

The larger community surely does not understand the commitment of the dental professional to be absolute; nor does it aim to impose, in all circumstances, the utmost of sacrifices for the sake of one's patient. Such an interpretation of the prioritization issue would be extremely unrealistic—it would be unreasonable for the larger community to put itself at risk of having no dentists to meet its dental care needs. Therefore, while the well-being of the patient is to be given considerable priority, it is not reasonable to expect that this obligation entails giving it absolute priority. But how much priority is it to be given? When does the professional's commitment to the patient require significant sacrifice of other worthy concerns? This question will be examined in chapter 6 and will be referred to at other points in the book.

Ideal Relationships between Co-professionals and Others Assisting in Care

Each profession also has norms, usually mostly implicit and unexamined, concerning the proper relationship between members of the same profession and between members of different professions, especially when they are providing assistance to the same clients. But there is no widely accepted account of the ethics of such relationships, for example between *dentist and dentist* or between *dentists and other professionals*. Of course, there are many different kinds of such relationships. There are, for example, relationships to other dentists, both specialists and general practitioners, to dental hygienists, and to physicians and nurses. Relationships between dentists and other professionals as well as relationships between dentists and staff members or others who assist them in caring for patients will be examined more closely in chapters 8, 9, and 10.

The Relationship between Dentists and the Larger Community

In addition to relationships of professionals with their clients and professionals' relationships with one another, the activities of every profession also involve relationships between individual members of the profession and persons who are neither professionals nor clients. The kinds of relationships that ought to exist between the members of the profession collectively and the larger community as a whole or various significant subgroups of it must also be considered. Relationships involving the members of the profession considered collectively are typically carried out through the actions of professional organizations, although the degree to which a given professional organization represents all the members of the profession in a given society is itself a complex issue. Obviously, a wide range of diverse relationships is included in this category. One such relationship that is widely recognized is the obligation of the dentist to educate the larger community in matters relevant to oral health, both in regard to the importance of oral self-care for everyone and in advising the larger community when public health resources are being allocated. A number of relationships between dentists and various aspects of the larger community will be examined in various chapters of this book. Determining which of these relationships ought to be accorded the greatest attention by an individual dentist will necessarily depend on the particular details of the dentist's situation and abilities.

Availability of Services

Dentists are committed to responding to patients' needs; because of this they cannot be indifferent to the reality that a significant number of people in the larger society do not have access to adequate dental care. Individual dentists will fulfill their responsibilities regarding this aspect of their professional ethics in different ways. Some will provide charity care of one sort or another. Others will focus on advocacy for public dental programs or for a higher priority of oral health within society's health care policies. Others may focus on the design of social systems so that dental care will be provided most effectively and in just and equitable ways to those in need. In any case, the availability of the dental profession's services to those who need them deserves special notice and explicit attention in the articulation and practice of dentistry's ethics.

Integrity and Professionalism

Finally, there is that very subtle component of conduct by which a person communicates to others what he or she stands for, not only in the acts that the person chooses but also in how those acts are chosen and how the person presents himself or herself to others in carrying them out. The two words that seem to communicate the core of this concern are "integrity" and "professionalism," especially when the two words are paired together, for integrity is a characteristic of a person across time, and the habits of thinking and acting that constitute professionalism can be developed only through a process of self-formation over many years.

Dentistry as a profession stands for certain values and is committed to the well-being of those it serves. But a dentist's way of practicing may communicate a different set of commitments and priorities. This can be the case even for a dentist whose choices of treatments and efforts to secure each patient's informed consent or refusal, and so forth, conform to the profession's minimum ethical standards in these matters. If a dentist is concerned about ethical growth beyond the minimums, this should prompt the dentist to be observant of the ways in which other dentists conduct themselves and to seek to imitate those who demonstrate professional characteristics worth admiring even though this requires additional effort and a willingness to engage in regular self-assessment. So, a final set of questions about dentists' professional obligations asks what they are obligated to do and what they are obligated to refrain from doing to not only practice in a minimally adequate way but, more importantly, in order to increasingly grow as professionals in the habits of thought and attitude and action that characterize the most admirable members of the profession. This theme will be mentioned often throughout this book, and the skills needed to form oneself in professionalism—and some of the most important challenges to professionalism in today's world—will be specifically examined in chapters 13, 14, and 15.

THINKING ABOUT THE CASE

Before examining Dr. Orasony's actions to see how these nine categories of ethical content work in reaching the judgment that "everything worked right," a few words are needed about the term "obligation," which will be used often in the following analysis and throughout the book.

Obligation

Throughout this book, the oughts that apply to dentists' conduct by reason of their being professionals (where "profession" is understood according to the Normative Picture of dentistry explained in chapter 2) will often be expressed by calling them "obligations." Some people consider the term "obligation" to be too strong for the *oughts* of professional conduct or think this word has other meanings that are not appropriate for discussing a particular profession's ethics. But, like the terms "moral" and "ethical," the term "obligation" is used in so many different ways and with so many different meanings that it is impossible to claim that one particular set of ideas constitutes the word's only *true* sense so that all the other uses of it are defective. Nor can it be presumed that all those who read the word "obligation" in these pages will understand it as it is intended unless its sense—for the purposes of this book—is clearly stated.

In this book, then, to say that something is (or that someone has) an obligation is to say three things: (1) the person or persons ought to act, or refrain from acting, in some way; (2) there are defensible reasons to support the claim that one ought to act or refrain from acting in a particular way; and (3) these reasons make such actions or omissions relatively important in comparison with other possible actions in the situation. Because professional practice concerns things that are important to people, as was explained in chapter 2, the specifically professional *oughts* of the dental profession will always be, in a significant sense, *important*. Consequently, it is appropriate to call them, without further qualification, obligations.

Note, however, that the importance of obligations does not exclude the possibility of someone having *competing obligations* in a given situation. Several actions or omissions might be ethically important at the same time. Indeed, resolving conflicts between competing obligations is one of the principal tasks of moral reflection. Because this book is principally about *professional obligations*, however, other reasons why an *ought* might be important (such as family responsibilities or legal requirements) and hence may be properly termed an *obligation* will not receive much attention here. But the relative priority of a person's professional obligations when obligations compete with one another—or when they compete with obligations arising from other sources—will be considered in chapter 6.

Most practitioners have experienced cases similar to the one presented in this chapter, although the situation may or may not have worked out as well. One important factor is the patient. Although the patient in this case apparently did not exhibit such traits before meeting the dentist, he eventually interacts with Dr. Orasony as a reasonable, balanced, communicative man who values the assistance a dental professional can provide; trusts the dentist and the hygienist and respects their efforts to provide care; learns to understand his past failings; and is grateful for Dr. Orasony's and Miss Williams's help. Though he may have lacked it before, the courage and self-discipline he needs to respond to his situation in the best way possible comes to him during the time period considered in the case.

Most dentists are delighted to treat patients with such traits. But a dentist is obligated to act ethically whether or not the patient's behavior is ideal. Therefore, it is the characteristics of the dentist's actions in this case, not the characteristics of the patient, that most concern us. What makes Dr. Orasony's conduct in this case ethically appropriate?

One thing, surely, is his relationship with Mr. Anderson. Dr. Orasony clearly meets the standards of informed consent; he explains the patient's needs and the various available treatment options as well as the risks of not treating. But he does more. He tries to enhance the patient's own sense of well-being and the patient's ability to control his own health situation, which necessarily involves letting go of some control that he, the dentist, might retain. He works to help the patient choose on the basis of well-established professional facts as well as his own and the patient's values rather than attempting to frighten him or coerce him into doing what the dentist sees as best. Both the dentist and the hygienist treat Mr. Anderson with respect and communicate their confidence that he can control his life. Mr. Anderson learns from this and grows more able to respect himself and trust his own abilities as well as theirs.

In situations with patients who are less reasonable or less communicative, for example, the steps taken by the dentist to establish a constructive relationship with the patient will, necessarily, be different. But one point is clear: one key standard of professional conduct concerns striving for the best possible *relationship* between dentist and patient. This is, however, only one important category of professional obligation. It will be examined in greater detail in chapters 4 and 7.

Another feature that makes the outcome of this case work right is the match between what the dentist tries to achieve for the patient and what dentistry stands for. It is surely correct that Dr. Orasony attends to Mr. Anderson's overall health and not the health of his oral cavity alone. It is surely correct, as well, that he works to strengthen Mr. Anderson's self-discipline and Mr. Anderson's ability to take control of his own life (and in the process contributes to his family's ability to control their lives as well). These are all important values for dentists to foster in patients, along with the value of oral health itself.

In this particular case, with its happy outcome, it seems that many different values are fostered for the patient and that the often-repeated goal of benefiting the whole patient has been achieved to an unusually high degree. Is dentistry, though, really obligated to further every kind of well-being for its patients? Or is it only certain aspects of patients' well-being that are the principal ethical focus of dentists' interventions for their patients? The position being taken here is that the latter is the case, that dentistry—like every profession—is focused on a certain set of values that the profession is committed to securing above all for their patients and that the dental profession's expertise is specifically designed to bring about. We must ask, therefore, what are the values that are central to dental practice? Is dentistry committed to furthering just one central value or more than one? If more than one, is there some ranking or hierarchy among these values? Which should take priority when the values cannot all be maximized at the same time? Such questions about the central values that are to guide dentists' decisions for their patients are, clearly, questions about another category of professional obligation. In this book, these values will be called the dental profession's Central Practice Values because they are *central* (i.e., they take priority over other values) in every aspect of a dentist's *practice*. They will be discussed in detail in chapter 5 and will be referred to frequently throughout the book.

Dr. Orasony is also admirable for the extent of his commitment to Mr. Anderson. He does not hurry through the motions of giving information and receiving consent. Instead, he puts himself out: He calls the patient's physician, draws on experience in other situations, and so on. Dr. Orasony may not have been obligated to expend as significant an amount of time or effort as he did to treat Mr. Anderson, but in doing so he communicated to Mr. Anderson that the patient's well-being took priority over many other personal concerns and matters needing Dr. Orasony's attention.

This theme of putting a patient's needs first, as has already been noted, is one of the most important characteristics of a profession and of the ethical professional, and points to another set of questions that must be asked about a dentist's professional obligations. *How much priority* must patients be given in comparison with the dentist's other values and commitments? A dentist is also a person with needs, goals, and desires. Dentists have families, friends, and other commitments. How much priority must be given to the patient's well-being when other matters, such as a dentist's personal commitments, conflict with providing for it in practice? How much ought a dentist be prepared to set aside, or offer, for the sake of those whom the dental profession serves? This question will be a central topic in chapter 6 and will be raised again many times later in the book.

In addition, there is another question that must be carefully considered even before the preceding ones can be answered: Whose well-being—specifically in the case of dentistry, whose oral health and general health—is the dentist professionally committed to serving? Is it all persons with oral health needs? Or are some of these individuals not important to dentistry as a profession? Is it only the person in the chair at the moment or all of a dentist's patients of record—or everyone in the land? Would Dr. Orasony have been acting in a professionally ethical manner if he had taken less time to assist Mr. Anderson in order to spend more time with other patients in other operatories or serve more patients by scheduling more appointments each day? This is another set of questions about professional obligations that dentists need to ask.

What these questions are asking is this: Who (what group or category of people) is this profession socially assigned to serve above all? In an important way, this is a more fundamental question than the questions about professional obligations already described, for none of them can be answered meaningfully until we know who this profession is obligated to serve—that is, what category of human needs it is authorized to address. For this reason, in the list of nine questions that were identified in the previous section as describing the obligations of any profession, this question—who is this profession's Chief Client?—was listed first.

The obligation to practice in a technically *competent* manner, according to the profession's accepted norms for practice in each kind of clinical situation, is surely the most obvious professional obligation of a dentist. It is unlikely that the happy results of this case could have come about without the competent practices of the dentist and the hygienist, as well as the physician, the nutritionist, and the family counselor who were also involved.

Dr. Orasony did not, furthermore, rely only on his own judgment about the possible connections between Mr. Anderson's oral condition and his diabetes. Instead, he contacted Mr. Anderson's physician and learned from him about what was medically important in this case. In a similar way, Dr. Orasony—by way of a recommendation to the physician—guided Mr. Anderson to a nutritionist and family counselor so that the patient and his family could benefit from expertise that Dr. Orasony did not have himself. Dr. Orasony also prepared Mr. Anderson for the possibility that his periodontal needs might require a referral to a specialist. One of the most important components of ethical practice is that a dentist routinely evaluate his or her competence to provide the services that the patient needs; he or she must be prepared either to consult those with the needed information and/or skills or refer the patient to them—whichever is going to best serve the patient's needs and the situation at hand.

In connection with these judgments, Dr. Orasony interacts effectively with the patient's physician and, indirectly but also effectively, with a nutritionist and family counselor. Dr. Orasony also seems to have an excellent working relationship with Sarah Williams, the hygienist. The patient then views the expertise of the hygienist and the assistance she offers with respect, and benefits accordingly. The relationships between dentists and *other professionals*, especially professionals who are attending to the same patient, are often overlooked in discussions of the ethics of dentistry. But fostering these relationships properly, along with dentists' relationships with office staff and others who interact with their patients, is obviously an important component of a dentist's ethical conduct in practice. Therefore, this is another set of questions to ask about ethical dental practice. It will receive special attention in chapters 8, 9, and 10.

As a profession, dentistry is involved with the larger community in many ways, but every dentist has *relationships with the larger community* beyond the people who are in need of dental care—whether they are actively under the care of professionals or not. In the case at hand, for example, we know that Dr. Orasony has spoken at a public education event. Every profession has obligations to educate the larger community about the values it seeks to secure for those it serves and about the importance of these values to people's overall well-being. Dentists can also contribute to the larger community by contributing their time and effort to the activities of organized dentistry—for example, by promoting and helping systematize professional collegiality and professional obligations or working in such organizations' various community outreach activities. These points suggest that there is another set of questions to ask—namely, what makes a dentist's professional acts ethical in relation to the larger community? Chapters 10, 13, and 14 will address various aspects of these issues.

One particular set of issues relating to the larger community concerns access to dental care. In this case, the patient has dental insurance; his ability to pay the costs of the dental and other health care he needs is not a central consideration of the case. For many, if not for most people in our society, paying for dental care and even having access to dental care within a reasonable distance is a more complex matter. Because dental care aims to be responsive to patients' oral health needs rather than commercial wants, part of dentistry's commitment is being attentive to those whose basic oral health needs are not being met. But a dentist's accessibility to patients needing care depends in part on a complex system of economic, legal, and social structures and in part on the dentist's willingness and ability to practice in ways that are independent of those structures—for example, by providing some care for free or at cost, by being available outside of office hours, or by otherwise addressing the needs of those who do not have easy access to oral health care. Dentists in different circumstances, though, will respond to this obligation in different ways. But indifference to the issues of *access to dental care* and unmet dental needs within the community is not consistent with a dentist's professional commitment. So this is another category of dentists' professional obligations. This topic will be addressed in chapters 11 and 12.

Finally, it is important to ask why a patient like Mr. Anderson would trust Dr. Orasony—not simply to practice competently and not simply to speak the truth as he understands it but also to offer reliable evidence of the importance of certain human values and virtues. Dr. Orasony isn't only looking for an opportunity to do technical procedures or pass on information. His work, in this case, includes having a significant impact on Mr. Anderson's conduct and indirectly on the conduct of his family. What characteristics does Dr. Orasony possess, then, that are relevant to Mr. Anderson's positive response to the dentist in this regard?

It seems doubtful that Mr. Anderson would accept the challenges of placing his health ahead of his fear, disturbing the ease of continuing his old habits, or strongly committing to working on more self-control if he did not trust Dr. Orasony not only to speak truthfully and be a reliable resource on how Mr. Anderson can best improve his oral and general health but to be a certain kind of person. Few people are moved to make sacrifices by people who do not demonstrate that they themselves live by long-time commitments and have worked hard and made genuine sacrifices in order to do so. This is a subtle area of character traits, not one that can be described in a brief case. It involves the long-term, indeed the lifelong, effort needed to build the relevant habits of perceiving, evaluating, prioritizing, judging, and acting. In the case, evidence that Dr. Orasony is admirable in this respect is the fact that Mr. Anderson responds with an energy and commitment of his own to Dr. Orasony's recommendations. This might be solely to Mr. Anderson's credit, of course, but this much effort is most often motivated by admirable characteristics observed in others. The case, therefore, strongly suggests that Dr. Orasony's *integrity* and his commitment to grow continually in *professionalism* contributes significantly to this situation being one in which everything works out right.

So there is a ninth set of questions to ask about dentists' professional obligations. What are dentists required to do, and what are they obligated to avoid in order to grow in integrity and professionalism? It is one thing to perform ethically correct behaviors, both technical and relational, so that one does not fall short of the simplest dos and don'ts of the dental profession's codes. It is another thing to view being a professional as something in which one continues to grow and does not stop growing, continues to look for the characteristics that make some dentists particularly admirable and to strive to imitate these, to practice them, to self-assess, and, through this process, to keeping growing in professionalism throughout one's life.

On this view, the dentist graduating from dental school and beginning to practice is indeed a professional in the sense of being a member of the profession. But he or she is only just beginning to form the kinds of habits and ways of thinking and acting that characterize the most admirable members of the profession. Accomplishing that in one's life will take not only a lot of experience in practice but observation of dentists who are admirable in various aspects of professionalism and who regularly, even daily, self-assess, self-correct, and, when appropriate, self-commend, followed by more practice, more self-assessment, and so on. The Mr. Andersons of the world are unlikely to act on a dentist's recommendations as responsively as the Mr. Anderson in this case unless they can see that the dentist is fully committed to growing steadily in his or her own professionalism. This topic will be the focus of chapter 15 but will also be relevant to many other issues discussed in this book.

These nine categories, or nine sets of questions, can now be used to make the study of dentistry's professional obligations more specific and concrete. If one's goal was to formulate a definition of a particular profession, the first two categories would be the ones to examine first. But when the goal is to shed light on the ethics of dentistry as it is practiced, it is more useful to focus on the third category, the Ideal Relationship between dentist and patient. So that is the topic of the next chapter.

4

XXXXXX

The Relationship between Patient and Professional

CASE: THE DREADED ROOT CANAL

Roger Vianni is one of Dr. Clarke's patients. For the past seven years he has constantly talked about his anxieties, the condition of his teeth, and what might need to be done about them. Dr. Clarke always responds calmly and sympathetically; she has learned that gentle words, however, are rarely enough to calm Mr. Vianni's churning anxieties. His fear also heightens his sensitivity to pain and pressure, so local anesthetic has been needed for even superficial procedures. At each visit, he invariably tells a new story about an acquaintance who recently suffered some oral tragedy. He tells her at each visit how grateful he is that he has never suffered such a tragedy, especially the dreaded root canal.

Luckily, Mr. Vianni has not needed much dental work. But Mr. Vianni's last visit was nearly a year ago, and this time he complains of severe pain in his upper-right jaw. On examination, Dr. Clarke first notices a fractured shallow amalgam in the upper-right second premolar; it simply needs replacement. More importantly, she also sees the likely cause of Mr. Vianni's pain—a more sizable carious lesion in the adjacent first molar next to and under a large amalgam restoration placed before Mr. Vianni came to Dr. Clarke. There is, in fact, little sound enamel remaining. Examination of the radiographs confirms apparent pulpal involvement, with the treatment of choice being endodontic therapy and eventual full-coverage restoration.

Dr. Clarke is certain, however, that if she describes the root canal procedure and the drilling necessary for the crown preparation, Mr. Vianni will simply refuse. It's not that he would rather lose the tooth or that he has financial or other reasons for not wanting a root canal and crown; he has often said he values his teeth greatly and is willing to spend whatever it takes to keep them healthy as long as possible. Yet he consistently reacts strongly to the thought of a drill and especially to the prospect of endodontic therapy. The fact that the procedure will resolve, rather than cause, pain and can ordinarily be completed without significant pain or discomfort will not change Mr. Vianni's reaction. From her previous experiences with this patient, Dr. Clarke is certain that if she explains the situation he will either demand to have the tooth extracted or simply leave the office.

Luckily, Dr. Clarke mentions the simple problem with the premolar to Mr. Vianni as soon as she notes it, before looking closer at the first molar. He musters up his courage and agrees to its repair, "provided you freeze it up real good." The first molar would easily be anesthetized with the premolar without Mr. Vianni knowing the difference. She could then proceed with the pulpectomy on the molar without Mr. Vianni having to suffer from the knowledge of what is going on until the parts he utterly dreaded are complete. She could also avoid lying to him since she could truthfully say that she is doing some superficial drilling on the premolar. She would, of course, tell Mr. Vianni the whole story of what she did to save him from anxiety and suffering as soon as the molar work is completed. At that point she could ask about his choice either to complete the root canal treatment and start a porcelain-fused-to-metal restoration (including the need of an interim temporary crown until the permanent crown is fabricated) or of a transitional amalgam buildup or even a tooth extraction (with or without various kinds of replacements) according to his preference. But that way he will not have to face the anticipation of starting a root canal procedure that he so much fears.

Dr. Clarke is almost certain that if she could describe the situation to Mr. Vianni—without him knowing it is in reference to his own mouth—he would understand and agree that endodontic therapy, along with proper restoration of the tooth, is the most reasonable and appropriate treatment and that he would be happy to pay the fees involved. The problem is that, in his own case, his judgment may be clouded by his anxiety about the idea of drilling and receiving root canal therapy in his own mouth. (While slightly anxious about the risks of being sued, Dr. Clarke is actually quite certain that Mr. Vianni would understand her judgment on his behalf and that the risk of a lawsuit in his case is merely hypothetical.)

Dr. Clarke is certain that Mr. Vianni trusts her to do whatever is best for him. She is also sure that if he could judge the matter objectively, Mr. Vianni would not want to suffer the anxiety of deciding about this treatment for himself. What good reason is there, then, for putting him through the pain of including him in this part of Dr. Clarke's decision?

What should Dr. Clarke do and why?

THE DENTIST-PATIENT RELATIONSHIP

At the center of most issues in dental ethics we find a patient, a dentist, and a relationship between them, and we find a decision needing to be made about treatment or some other kind of professional action or intervention on the patient's behalf. The previous chapter proposed that for every profession there is an Ideal Relationship between professional and client and that it is one of the most important norms of ethical conduct for members of that profession. What is the Ideal Relationship between dentist and patient? What are the proper roles of the patient and the dentist in the decision-making process that is so central to their dealings with one another? This is the topic of the present chapter.

Not all patients, though, are *capable* of making or participating in decisions about their treatment or other aspects of their health care. Some patients are young children or are severely disabled developmentally. Other patients suffer from other deficits that impair their capacity for decision-making. It will be important to carefully examine what a person needs in order to participate effectively in a decision-making process and what sorts of deficits justify a doubt about someone's capacity to do this. These matters will be addressed in detail in chapter 7 along with the question of how a dentist ought to relate to patients who exhibit such deficits, whether their capacity for decision-making is only partially diminished or whether they cannot participate at all in decision-making about their dental care. The focus of this chapter, however, is on the dentist-patient relationship in situations where the patient *is* capable of making an autonomous choice in the decision-making process with the dentist.

There is no single English word that means the same thing as "capable of making an autonomous choice." But this is a cumbersome phrase to repeat over and over. There is a word in ordinary usage that expresses this idea: "competent," along with its noun, "competence." Unfortunately, this term has an important technical meaning in the law that is quite different from its commonsense meaning. In the law, anyone who has reached the age of an adult (as defined or stated by law) is competent; that is, a person who has reached the legally determined age can make decisions and take actions that have legal standing and can do so unless a judge in court rules that this person is no longer able to do so. Thus, a person who is permanently comatose is still legally competent until the person is declared incompetent by a judge, or other designated legal authority, after an appropriate hearing and not before then. Similarly, with a few exceptions, a highly intelligent, thoughtful, sensitive seventeen-year-old is, in the eyes of most state laws in the United States, as incompetent to make health care decisions as an infant. So using the word "competent" can lead to some confusion.

It seems best, therefore, to reserve the terms "competent" and "competence" as well as "incompetent" and "incompetence" for legal contexts and to use them only in their technical legal sense. Therefore, the word that will be used throughout this book as shorthand for the phrase "capable of making an autonomous choice" will be "capable," and the noun "capacity" will be used for the phrase "capacity for autonomous choice."

In this chapter, decision-making by dentists and capable patients will be examined under three headings. First, four possible models of the patient-dentist relationship will be examined and an account of the ethical implications of each in the decision-making of a patient and a dentist will be compared.

Second, the principle of respecting autonomy will be examined. The notion of autonomy is particularly relevant to decision-making and is a central moral principle in the culture of the United States as well as in many systems of moral philosophy. In the course of examining this principle, we will also ask whether circumstances ever justify violating someone's autonomy precisely for that person's benefit, a pattern of thinking and acting that is sometimes called paternalism. That is, could a dentist ever be morally justified in violating a patient's autonomy for the sake of the patient's oral health? (Admittedly, doing so could put the dentist at legal risk. But even so, avoiding legal risk is no guarantee that moral error will be avoided. Sometimes morality requires a person to take a serious legal risk, so the question of whether paternalism is ever morally justifiable still needs to be asked.)

The third way of addressing the issue of the proper relationship between dentist and patient will focus on the moral norm of telling the truth and the principle of Informed Consent/Refusal that currently describes the legal minimum for the dentist-patient relationship. This will also be the place to talk about patients' trust. For the kind of relationship that a dentist should strive for in order to earn and maintain their patients' trust is, as will be explained, an Interactive Relationship.

FOUR POSSIBLE MODELS OF THE DENTIST-PATIENT RELATIONSHIP

The dentist-patient relationship can be conceived according to many different models, of which four seem the most important. These will be explained and compared, and the case will be made that one of these, the Interactive Model, describes the Ideal Relationship between a dentist and a capable patient. The four models to be examined are the Guild Model, the Agent Model, the Commercial Model, and the Interactive Model.

It is obvious that a dentist's ability to establish an Ideal Relationship with a given patient will depend on how the patient responds to the dentist's efforts. Actual relationships will vary, but the Ideal Relationship that the dentist strives for should not. The four models described here present very different pictures of the relationship that the dentist ought to be striving to bring about, and only one of them can properly be thought of as the Ideal Relationship from the point of view of dentistry's professional ethics.

The Guild Model

In the Guild Model, the dentist is the only active party in decision-making, and the proper role of the patient is to be completely passive and to accept whatever decisions the dentist makes. This model focuses exclusively on the dentist's expertise and the patient's utter lack of it. The dentist obviously has the ability to understand and explain the patient's condition (diagnosis), to predict various future paths that might be taken under various circumstances (prognosis), and to intervene with treatments and other forms of care in order to maximize various aspects of the patient's well-being in the outcomes (therapy). But in the Guild Model the dentist is also considered to know everything else relevant to determining what is best for the patient. The patient not only lacks the theoretical knowledge, skills, and experience that enable the professional to apply his or her expertise effectively in each particular set of clinical circumstances, but, in addition, in the Guild Model the patient is viewed as having nothing at all to contribute to judgments about what is best for him or her. What the patient values and how the patient would prioritize possible treatments or other interventions the dentist might undertake is deliberately excluded from consideration in the Guild Model. In the Guild Model, the dentist makes all of the value judgments and determinations of need.

Therefore, in the Guild Model, the proper role for the patient in all important aspects of dental decision-making is that of being one to whom things *are done*. For the patient in this model is considered to be simply unable to understand what would contribute to his or her well-being and is, therefore, unable to make any important contribution to dental decisions about his or her situation.

But the Guild Model does not see the dentist as an independent expert. In the Guild Model, the source of the dentist's technical expertise and value judgments about patients' well-being is the dental profession—that is, the community of dentists who preserve and advance dental knowledge and practice and are committed to the central values of oral health care. It is the profession that trains and then certifies that the individual practitioner is qualified to assist patients and make dependable judgments about what is best for them. It is the profession that determines the fundamentals of how individual dentists should act toward patients, both therapeutically and ethically. In addition, in the Guild Model it is the profession and the profession alone that determines the specifics of a dentist's obligations to patients. Since those who are not dentists are viewed as having no understanding of oral health or their need for it, the Guild Model has no role for the larger community either in the creation of a profession to begin with or in determining the contents of a profession's ethics. Similarly, in the Guild Model, the individual dentist undertakes his or her professional obligations not by making a commitment to the larger society but solely by a commitment to the profession.

There is a serious moral problem with the Guild Model in the eyes of many people, including many dentists. One way to state this problem is to point to the Guild Model's failure to respect the autonomy of patients who are capable of autonomous decision-making. For, according to the Guild Model, a dentist is to treat patients as if they were not capable of autonomous decision-making when they are. Doing so is obviously a violation of the patient's autonomy.

The principle of respecting autonomy and the question regarding whether it may ever be justifiably violated for the sake of the patient will be examined more fully in the next section. But there is one response to this objection to the Guild Model that deserves immediate consideration. Even if these patients are capable of autonomous decision-making in other respects, the defender of the Guild Model would respond that they still do not have the dentist's knowledge and skills in regard to oral health, which are precisely what they will need if they are to be capable of making decisions about their dental care. In addition, patients are often in pain or in considerable distress as well. Therefore, the defender of the Guild Model concludes that it is the dentist who should be making all the decisions because the relationship is inherently asymmetrical or unbalanced in this way.

What the Guild Model fails to account for is that there are important components of every dental decision that are not included in the expertise of even the most acutely trained and extensively experienced dentist. The reason for this is that therapeutic alternatives are never value neutral. All therapeutic choices involve selecting one set of life experiences for the patient over another set, and the knowledge and skills that the dentist brings to the situation are not adequate tools for comparing the value of these possible experiences within the *patient's* life. Instead, the patient's own values must also be brought to bear in the choice of dental interventions. But only with the patient's participation in the dental decision will the patient's values dependably direct that decision.

Therefore, the Guild Model's picture of the patient as the passive recipient of expert dental interventions does not fit the ethical reality of patients and dentists in their actual relationships. In fact, as will be explained in chapter 7, the Guild Model does not even adequately portray the dentist's proper role in treating patients who are not capable of autonomous choice. For these reasons, the Guild Model should not be considered to be the Ideal Relationship for ethical dentist-patient relationships.

The Agent Model

A second model of the dentist-patient relationship reverses the dentist's and patient's roles from the Guild Model. In this second model, the most important aspect of the decision-making activity in dental care—determining what values should shape and control the decisions—is assigned entirely to the patient. Here, the professional simply puts his or her expertise at the service of the patient's aims and values. The dentist's task is only to give effect to the patient's values and the patient's choices made on the basis of those values, responding as efficiently as possible to fulfill the patient's choices based entirely on the patient's goals and values. The dentist is to act, in other words, only as an *agent* for the patient. Hence, this is called the Agent Model.

This model is not often discussed in regard to dentistry or the other health professions—probably because it severely misrepresents our ordinary understandings of a health professional's ethical commitments. The professional example most commonly discussed in terms of the Agent Model is probably the image of the lawyer as a "hired gun," but the Agent Model is no more defensible as a description of the lawyer's ethical commitments than it is of the health professional's commitments. As an example from health care, imagine a dentist, physician, or nurse who agrees to use his or her access to controlled substances to meet the desires or needs of a patient's addiction simply to serve the patient's choices more completely, without asking how that action connects to the other elements of that patient's well-being that the society believes the health professional is committed to fostering.

The failure of the Agent Model is that it simply sets aside the idea that each profession has certain values that it is committed to fostering for those it serves through the use of its expertise. These values, which are called Central Practice Values in this book, will be examined in detail in the next chapter, where the role of these values in the dentist's professional-ethical decision-making will be explained. The Agent Model simply ignores the values to which the dental profession is committed even though these are central elements of how the dental profession functions ethically in our society.

A patient's own values and conception of his or her well-being certainly does have an important role to play in decisions concerning the dental care he or she receives. But these are not the sole determinants of how dentists, striving as committed professionals to bring about the Central Practice Values of their profession for their patients, are to act. Therefore, the Agent Model must be rejected as a candidate for being the Ideal Relationship between dentist and patient.

The Commercial Model

The weaknesses of the Guild Model and the Agent Model have prompted a number of people to turn to the Commercial Model to replace them. The consumer movement in health care, as well as proponents of a still-wider role for free enterprise in our health care system, claim that the Commercial Model is the best guide for health professionals, including dentists, to follow in their relationships with patients.

According to the Commercial Model, in contrast to the Guild Model, the patient is indeed a decision-maker about his or her health care and, in contrast to the Agent Model, the dentist is also a decision-maker with his or her own professional values to pursue rather than functioning as a mere agent of the patient. In these respects, the Commercial Model may appear preferable to each of the others. Yet other features of the Commercial Model make its claim to be the Ideal Relationship problematic.

According to the Commercial Model, a member of a profession is simply another producer selling his or her wares in the marketplace. Thus, a dentist has a product to sell, and patients may want to buy it. The two parties may make whatever agreements with one another that they are willing to make. By the same token, both the dentist and the patient may refuse any arrangements that either one chooses to refuse. In other words, according to the Commercial Model, the only moral norms that apply to dentistry are those that apply to every other bargainer in the marketplace. These norms require that marketplace bargainers not coerce, cheat, or defraud one another, and they are obligated to keep the contractual commitments they freely make with others. Beyond these obligations, according to the Commercial Model, the dentist has no other obligations to any patient except such obligations as the dentist and the patient voluntarily undertake. According to the Commercial Model, in other words, there are no specifically professional values or obligations on the part of the dentist; there is nothing to which a dentist is obligated *because* he or she is a professional.

In addition, as in all market relationships, in the Commercial Model the dentist and the patient are first and foremost competitors. That is, each is trying to obtain from the other the greatest amount of what he or she wants (money, satisfaction, effort, time, and other aspects of well-being) while giving up in the exchange as little as possible of these things. The dentist is concerned about the patient's well-being only as a means of improving his or her own interests and fulfilling his or her desires. Thus, the dentist has no obligation to any patient to preserve or foster the patient's oral health or any other aspect of the patient's well-being until the dentist specifically contracts to have such an obligation. For this reason, no patient should presume that a dentist has such an obligation or commitment in advance of a specific contract to this effect between the dentist and that patient. At the point when the patient is seated in the operatory chair, then, the patient and dentist are first and foremost competitors.

In the Commercial Model, furthermore, the patient's need for care is not a direct determinant of a dentist's actions. The patient's need has no special ethical import for the dentist, and there is certainly no antecedent obligation to meet a patient's needs; there are only whatever obligations the dentist and patient subsequently negotiate regarding their relationship. Need does function, of course, as a potent motivator for patients to seek and contract for dental care. As such, the dentist can effectively use the patient's needs to market his or her services to the patient. But in the Commercial Model, when a dentist says to a patient, "this procedure will answer your need for . . ." these words should not be received by the patient with any special degree of trust, no more so than would the comments of a person selling anything else. That is, trust that the dentist has the patient's oral health or any other aspect of the patient's well-being as a primary goal has no place in the Commercial Model's view of their relationship.

Obviously, in this model the patient is not a *passive* recipient of expert professional services, as in the Guild Model. The patient first judges the value of the information that the dentist can supply and then chooses whether or not to be guided by it. Then, after judging alternative courses of action on the basis of this information, the patient judges the value of various therapeutic interventions by the dentist, or others, and chooses either to purchase them or not. The patient in the Commercial Model is regarded as an example of *Homo economicus*, the rational consumer, who weighs all the elements of cost and benefit relevant to a given exchange and chooses the available product or service that yields the best combination of these or else chooses not to purchase anything at that time.

The Commercial Picture of dentistry as a profession was rejected in chapter 2. But it might be possible, or at least not simply contradictory, for the members of a normative profession to have a commercial relationship as their Ideal Relationship with those they serve. Because a number of authors, including a number of dentists, propose that this model describes the Ideal Relationship, this proposal deserves careful examination. First, is the Commercial Model a realistic possibility for the relationship between patient and dentist? Second, if dentists and patients could realistically function in this way, does the Commercial Model describe the Ideal Relationship between them?

The extent to which patients not comprehensively trained in dental science can understand the subtle differences between alternative oral conditions and alternative interventions to address them is very limited—even if they have obtained a great deal of accurate dental information from reliable sources. The key point, here, is that dentistry's patients have not had the benefit of dental practice—that is, using expert information to respond dependably and effectively to patients' oral health needs. For practice experience is every bit as important in forming good dental judgments at chairside as scientific theory and familiarity with the current literature. It is therefore a legitimate question to ask whether the average patient can realistically play the rational consumer's role in comparing alternative therapies.

Another consideration is that many patients in our health care system do not contact a dentist until they believe refusing dental care is no longer an option. But it seems clear that one cannot function as a rational consumer, comparing all alternatives in terms of cost and benefit, if one has already set aside the option not to buy at all. The rational consumer must be able to leave the relationship if none of the products offered is on his or her list of optimal cost-quality exchanges.

One response to these arguments is that dentists ought to be more effective at communicating with patients; that is, dentists should give more attention to patient education (which is not the same as sales information). But this response, in fact, already begins to view the patient-dentist relationship as having the patient's oral health as a primary goal, and that is not how the patient-dentist relationship is viewed in the Commercial Model. The most that the Commercial Model can say is that the dentist who communicates and educates better has a better information product to sell and will ordinarily sell more of it for a better price. But that is very different from saying that the dentist has an obligation to communicate and educate effectively because of the ethical importance of effective patient decision-making for the patients' oral health. If one says that dentists *ought* to be more effective at educating and communicating with patients, this points to a different picture of the patient-dentist relationship from the picture offered in the Commercial Model. This other picture sees the dentist and the patient working out their judgments and choices about the patient's oral health together, to the extent that this is possible under the circumstances, rather than competing so each is trying to maximize only his or her own gain.

Another negative aspect of the Commercial Model is that patients ordinarily view life and health as values much too important to put them into the hands of someone who is simply a competitor. The actual reality of the patient-dentist relationship is therefore unavoidably more than one of competition. Even if the dentist tried to be simply a competitor and the patient was intensely competitive, it is doubtful—with the patient's health at stake—that they could maintain a relationship on these terms for long or that patients' trust in their dentists would be fostered under such circumstances. When looked at carefully, the Commercial Model clearly does not describe the Ideal Relationship between dentist and patient.

At the same time, this should not drive us back to the Guild Model, because what counts as the patient's well-being is not something fully known by the dentist, either by training or by experience. The dentist's commitment to the goal of fostering important aspects of the patient's well-being can only be carried out through empathetic communication and a shared judgment and a shared choice with the patient. The point, then, is not only that the Commercial Model and the Guild Model each falls short; it is that some sort of shared judgment and choice between dentist and patient is what ought to characterize the dentist-patient relationship, and the question is what kind of relationship is most likely to lead to this shared decision-making most effectively.

Another weakness of the Commercial Model is this: When a person's body is not doing what the person wants, this is almost always experienced as a lessening of the person's ability to direct and control not only their bodies but their lives. The reality is not just that illness and other physical deficits involve deficits of function, pain, and other symptoms—although all of these occur to varying degrees in most cases. More importantly, illness and physical deficits, including oral pain and deficits in oral functioning, are experiences of not being in control. One's goals, one's plans, and one's capacity to achieve anything at all are actually or potentially compromised. Even patients who are not presently in pain or aware of some oral deficit still come to dentists in large part to prevent such loss of control from occurring in the future.

In other words, one important reason why patients come to dentists is to recover their lost autonomy in controlling their bodies (or to secure it from being lost), even as they are also trying to exercise their autonomy in choosing particular dental treatments while in a dentist's care. They come to dentists hoping that the dentist's expertise will restore their lost control and their full ability to direct their lives. In this respect, they do not come simply as bargainers, coequals with dentists in the marketplace. Instead, their sense of themselves is, in part, that they have lost or are at risk of losing the ability to fully control an important aspect of their lives, and they need the dentist's assistance to recover or retain it. (But at the same time, they also do not come incapable of autonomous choice; they can still play their appropriate role in making the decisions and choices necessary to restore their control over their bodies and lives.) In other words, the Commercial Model's picture of the dental patient—as someone in full control of his or her life—is incomplete at best and often simply false.

For all these reasons, the Commercial Model should not be accepted as the ethical ideal that dentists ought to be striving for in their relationships and their decision-making with their patients. It is not the Ideal Relationship between dentist and patient.

The Interactive Model

The reasons for rejecting each of the first three models can now be brought together to formulate a fourth model of the patient-dentist relationship, the Interactive Model. In this model, the dentist and patient are equal partners in three important respects. They are equal, first, in that each has standing in the relationship as a distinct chooser who deserves the other party's respect as such. Second, each is someone who has, by life-choices and commitments of many sorts, a set of values that he or she is trying to live by and secure in the choices he or she makes regarding dental care, and each is, therefore, obligated to respect the other as a *valuer* as well as a *chooser*. Third, each comes to the decision-making process about the patient's oral health possessed of understanding about the decision that the other lacks and that can be made up for only by communication and mutual cooperation. On one hand, the dentist has the expertise on which the patient's oral health and the patient's retention or recovery of oral function and lost autonomy depend, and the dentist is committed to supporting the values—dentistry's Central Practice Values—that are the reasons behind society's establishment of dentistry as a profession in the first place. On the other hand, the patient has the understanding of his or her own values, goals, and priorities, without which the decision to accept the professional's interventions cannot be coherently justified. In the Interactive Model the patient and dentist are equally respected contributors to the decisions to be made, though their contributions are different and, in important ways, asymmetrical. Their respective contributions cannot, furthermore, be put together without careful communication on both sides and effective dialogue between them. This is why this fourth model is here called the *Interactive* Model. It is this model that describes the Ideal Relationship that dentists ought to be striving to achieve with every capable patient.

Unlike the Guild Model, the Interactive Model stresses the value of the patient's autonomy to the maximum degree that a patient can exercise it. It views the preservation and maximization of the patient's autonomy as one of the principal goals of dentists. Unlike the Commercial Model, the Interactive Model does not simply assume that patients are effective market decision makers about oral health care. Though most patients lack the dentist's expertise, they are aware of an oral health need, either manifested now in the form of oral pain or other symptoms or else foreseen in the future unless preventive measures are taken. But that means they see themselves as not fully able to control the circumstances of their lives without the dentist's assistance. Rather than granting the dentist a competitive edge in these respects, as the Commercial Model would if it were taken seriously as an ideal model of the dentist-patient relationship, the Interactive Model sets aside competition in favor of collaboration, a very specific form of collaboration that is unique to professionalism. The dentist, to the extent that he or she is able, is therefore committed to enhancing the patient's control over his or her life, both in terms of the patient's oral health and also in supporting and enhancing the patient's autonomous decision-making capacity.

The Interactive Model can be summarized as the dentist and patient having equal moral standing within their relationship. But their equality—their equal claim to voice and vote within their relationship—derives from different grounds (i.e., asymmetrically) on the two sides. For the patient, it derives from the importance of the patient's own values, from the patient's autonomy, and from the fact that it is the patient's body and life that are being affected. For the dentist it comes from the dentist's expertise regarding the patient's health needs, from the dentist's ability to enable the patient to regain or maximize control over his or her body and life, and from the centrality of dentistry's Central Practice Values in the life of a dentist as an ethical professional. Thus, in the Interactive Model, both parties have unique and irreplaceable contributions to make toward their judgments and choices together and both the patient's and the dentist's values serve as determinants of what they do together.

It is common in many people's thinking to look on all choices as the work of individuals alone. But a little reflection suggests that spouses, families, friendships of two or three persons or more, and many other kinds of groups do in fact make choices together, as a unit. The Interactive Model of the patient-dentist relationship proposes that the choices that issue from their transactions are, in the ideal situation, made by both parties together in this way. To be sure, this ideal situation is often not realized in practice, either because of limits on the patient's ability to contribute to their collaboration or other circumstances or because one or both parties do not have the achievement of an Interactive Relationship as a goal to work toward. As a first step in understanding the fundamental elements of the patient-dentist relationship, however, it is important to realize that such a relationship is possible and that, when it occurs, it overcomes the clear limits of the Guild, Agent, and Commercial models of this relationship. For these reasons, the authors propose that the Interactive Model is the best articulation of the Ideal Relationship that every dentist ought to be striving to achieve with every capable patient.

AUTONOMY AND THE QUESTION OF JUSTIFIABLE PATERNALISM

Both in contemporary Western culture and in most theories of moral reflection developed in the West, respecting a person's autonomy when the person is capable of autonomous decision-making is a very important moral principle. The several capacities that, taken together, make a person fully capable of autonomous choice and action will be examined in chapter 7. For the present, a shorter description of autonomy will suffice. *Autonomy* will be taken here to refer to a person's choosing and acting on the basis of his or her own values, principles, goals, purposes, or ideals of conduct. The wording of this description is deliberately open-ended to include a wide variety of bases of action that a person might choose from. The central point is that the person chooses and acts from his or her *own* base of action. In fact, this is exactly what the root ideas behind the word "autonomy" convey. In ancient Greek, *auto* stands for "one's own," and *nomos* stands for "rule, principle, or law." Thus, *autonomy* consists in "living or acting according to one's own rule, principle, or law."

A number of philosophical arguments aim at showing why the principle of *respect for autonomy* is such an important principle for moral reflection and action. One set of these employs a consequentialist or outcome-focused mode of moral reasoning. That is, these arguments defend the importance of this principle by trying to show that actions that are respectful of autonomy are ordinarily more beneficial for the parties involved than alternative courses of action would be.

There are three consequentialist arguments that support a principle to respect people's autonomy. The first of these can be called the "short-term efficiency argument" for respecting autonomy. It points out that, in most circumstances, capable adults are the best judges of what will maximize their own well-being. Of course, people sometimes misjudge what is best for themselves, but in the vast majority of such cases, when this happens, it is because their capacity for autonomous choice is partially compromised at the time—either through lack of correct information or for other reasons. When people are genuinely capable, however, their choices about matters that affect them will almost always be more efficient producers of their maximal well-being than if someone else had chosen in their stead.

Consequentialist arguments focus on identifying the course of action that will maximize values or well-being for everyone affected by what is done. In this case, we are comparing two principles of conduct that could be adopted by people generally in all the actions they undertake. The argument is that far more well-being will be realized by those persons affected if people, when they are capable, are not interfered with by others and are allowed to make their own choices about the things affecting them than will be realized if others make these choices instead. In sum, to maximize well-being, don't interfere with capable people's choices.

The second consequentialist argument for respecting autonomy calls our attention to how painful we find it when someone interferes with our chosen actions and to the fact that the more we consider our actions to be based on our *own* values, goals, principles, and ideals the more painful it is if others interfere. By contrast, when we choose a course of action and carry it out without interference, we often experience a very special kind of satisfaction from being the ones who chose the action and carried it out in accord with our *own* values, goals, principles, and ideals. The positive value associated with choosing and acting autonomously and the negative value associated with being interfered with are considered by some people to be among the strongest positive and negative experiences of value in human life. And, in any case, these are important matters for almost everyone capable of autonomous choice.

Consequently, respecting someone's autonomy yields satisfaction for that person directly; interfering yields a form of pain or suffering. So this consequentialist argument's conclusion is that, to maximize values and well-being, the best principle to follow is *don't interfere with capable people's choices.*

The third consequentialist argument is a "long-term efficiency" argument. Consider those persons, perhaps young men and women, who have been brought up in households or other circumstances in which they have had little or no opportunity to make choices for themselves on the basis of their own values, goals, principles, and ideals because someone else made all of their choices for them. Almost always, when they first encounter the need to make choices for themselves, they find this distressing. In addition, they are not very good at it at first and are prone to make errors of judgment that do not in fact maximize well-being for themselves or for others. Therefore, those who have had greater opportunity to take actions that were based on autonomous choices and were not interfered with will grow increasingly efficient in their choosing, and those with less opportunity for such choices and who have been interfered with more will not. The same is true of whole communities of people. Where opportunities for the exercise of choice are newly won, for example, it takes time and experience to make the collective choice-making process reasonably efficient. So both for individuals and for groups, and even for whole nations, respecting people's autonomy is far more likely to produce far greater benefits for people's well-being over time than interfering with their autonomy would. Again, the lesson for one aiming to maximize values is to respect people's autonomy.

Do these three arguments mean that it is always simply wrong to interfere with a capable person's autonomy? Consequentialists are rarely willing to claim that they can imagine every possible set of circumstances in which even a quite general principle like *respect people's autonomy* might be challenged. Thus, they are not in the habit of saying "always" when such principles are being discussed. There are ethical theorists from other traditions of moral philosophy, however, who would say that the principle of respecting autonomy is so fundamental to morality that it may never be morally violated. They will be considered shortly.

But more specifically, there is at least one kind of situation in which, in most consequentialists' judgment, interfering with an autonomously chosen action will lead to better outcomes for the people affected than not interfering will. This is the circumstance in which one party, A, is autonomously acting to harm or to threaten harm to another party, B, who does not choose to be so harmed. In such a case, interfering with A's autonomy preserves B's autonomy from interference and also preserves B from harm; that is, it is very possible that the negative outcomes will be lessened if A is interfered with rather than if not. In actual life, it will always be necessary to carefully weigh what is needed to interfere with A's contemplated action and also to weigh the precise nature of interference with B's autonomy and the harm it poses to B—for consequentialist moral reasoning is always of the form "such-and-such action is justifiable if, among the actions available, it produces, for the persons affected, the greatest benefits and/or the least harms possible under the circumstances." But it is clear even from this brief argument that, from a consequentialist's perspective, the general principle of respecting capable people's autonomy must be supplemented with another principle, often called the Harm Principle. It holds that it may be justifiable to interfere in the actions of someone who is interfering with and harming or threatening harm to someone else.

As was mentioned, some moral theorists consider the principle of respecting autonomy to be absolute and without exceptions. For example, the late eighteenth-century German philosopher Immanuel Kant claimed that violation of another person's autonomy is, in effect, contradictory. The other person's autonomy, he argued, is no different in kind or worth from one's own. So how could we consistently refuse to permit anyone else to choose our actions for us while simultaneously preventing someone from choosing his or her own action through our interference? The contradiction here demonstrates, Kant held, that violating autonomy is always not only irrational but profoundly immoral. Other moral theorists defend the same conclusion by arguing that every capable human being has a fundamental right to respect for his or her autonomous decisions. Because no violation of this right can ever be justified, they argue, there are no exceptions to the principle that autonomous decisions of a capable person must always be respected. However, both camps that defend the idea that the principle of respecting autonomy has no exceptions recognize that situations can arise in which a person who is violating or threatening to violate another's autonomy must be confronted. They acknowledge that it would certainly be strange to consider interfering with such a person in order to protect the autonomy of his or her victim to be an immoral act. Such thinkers address the question of whether such reasoning, in fact, counts as an exception to the principle by proposing, for example, that acts that violate the principle of respecting autonomy have already been proven irrational (because they violate that principle) and therefore that such acts are not truly autonomous (since thinking rationally is one of the components of autonomous decision-making), so interfering with a harm doer is not a violation of his or her autonomy. A harder question for both consequentialist thinkers and those who defend the principle of respecting autonomy as having no exceptions is whether it is ever justifiable to interfere with a person's autonomously chosen action when that action is harming or is very likely to harm only *the chooser*. Such interference is often called *paternalistic* in the literature of moral philosophy, and the view that it is sometimes morally justifiable to interfere in order to benefit or to prevent harm to the one interfered with is often called *paternalism*.

The term "paternalism"—and its less sexist equivalent, "parentalism"—are not literally appropriate to the issue here. Taken literally, they refer to interfering with the actions of a small child, and small children are not capable of autonomous choice. In addition, the word "paternalistic" is sometimes applied to interventions with a person who does not know or is assumed not to know, that his or her action will be harmful and who is, in that respect, not a capable decision maker. These usages of the term make for considerable confusion in discussions of paternalism. For the sake of clarity, interventions with someone who is known to be or is presumed to be unaware of some likely harm will not be called paternalistic here. Instead, an act will be called paternalistic in this book only when it interferes with the choice or action of a person presumed to be acting autonomously, and therefore knowingly, in a manner that is harmful to or prevents a benefit to that person.

Terminology aside, the question remains whether it is ever justifiable to interfere with someone's autonomously chosen action in order to prevent him or her from self-harm or to provide a benefit. At the heart of this question is a question about the relative importance of the value of autonomy or of the moral principle of respecting autonomy or of the moral right that autonomy be respected. Is autonomy the most important norm of morality so that, if both autonomy and some other moral value were at stake in some action, choice of the other value over autonomy would always be wrong? Or are there other values that are equal to autonomy—or of even greater importance than autonomy—such that these other values could be morally chosen over autonomy when both could not be maximized or respected at the same time? In that case, some paternalistic actions would be morally justifiable. Moreover, even if autonomy is held to rank higher than any other moral consideration, is it also so supreme that even a potent combination of all the other lower-ranking values could still not justify an act that fails to respect someone's autonomy to prevent that person's own harm? If this were the case, then no paternalistic act could ever be morally justified.

Philosophers and other moral theorists have wrestled with these difficult questions for centuries, and, as yet, no final answers about the relative importance of autonomy and other moral standards in human morality exist. Still, the specific commitments dentists make when they become members of this profession, it has been argued, do require them to respect and support their patients' autonomy by striving to actualize the ideal of an Interactive Relationship with each patient. This much clarity about dentists' professional commitments, though, still does not resolve the question about the *relative* importance of patients' autonomy for a dentist—that is, in comparison with dentistry's other Central Practice Values when circumstances arise in which they cannot all be maximized or respected at once. The proper ranking of dentistry's Central Practice Values when they cannot all be respected at once will be discussed in the next chapter.

TRUTH TELLING AND INFORMED CONSENT

A series of important court cases—for example, *Schloendorff v. Society of New York* (1914), *Salgo v. Leland Stanford University Hospital* (1957), and *Canterbury v. Spence* (1972)—and legislative acts in many jurisdictions have made Informed Consent the legal standard for judging the relationship between a patient and a health care provider. Very briefly, the law requires that this relationship include a choice by the patient, if he or she is legally capable of choice (legally *competent*), and that this choice be *informed* by the provider, who must explain to the patient each of the courses of action that are available to the patient in the professional's expert judgment (including taking no action), as well as the likely outcomes of each.

The phrase "Informed Consent/Refusal" is also often used to name the *ethical* norm for judging the relationship between a patient and a health care provider. Certainly in dentistry Informed Consent is a very common description of a professionally correct relationship with a patient. But it is worth asking whether this notion really is adequate for the job or whether the Ideal Relationship between dentist and patient involves more than this.

One component of the dentist-patient relationship that has not been stressed so far in this chapter is telling the patient the truth. Truthfulness is an important component of an ethical life, and it has a special importance in the relationship between a health professional and patient because they depend on each other for the information they need to play their respective roles in the relationship. The dentist depends on the patient for important information about the patient's general health, medical condition, medications being taken, and patterns of oral hygiene and self-care. The patient depends on the dentist for an understanding of the condition of his or her mouth, the need for intervention by the dentist, and the likely outcome of alternative treatments. Neither party could function effectively, and dental care would be of far lower quality if patient and dentist alike could not count on truthfulness in their relationship.

For many dentists, the word "informed" in the phrase "Informed Consent" is a reminder of this obligation to truthfulness on their part. But the phrase "Informed Consent" actually speaks directly to only the *patient* being informed and implies, on the part of the dentist, only an obligation to communicate truthfully and effectively. These two components of the dentist-patient relationship are also what are emphasized in the legal cases that have given us this phrase. But in actual practice, *both* parties must be informed and *both* parties must communicate truthfully and effectively. The Interactive Relationship requires *two-way* communication and shared understanding and is in fact a shared process and a shared judgment about what ought to be done and then a shared choice to do it. Our ordinary understanding of Informed Consent as a documented, signed contract, however, does not point us clearly enough in this direction. In this respect, the Interactive Relationship, which includes this two-way collaborative effort, describes the Ideal Relationship between dentist and patient far better than Informed Consent.

In addition, the word "consent" is really not a good description of what the patient does when the dentist-patient relationship is at its best, for "consent" means agreeing with what someone else has determined to do. But in the Ideal Relationship, *both* parties contribute to the determination about what ought to be done. Furthermore, the phrase "Informed Consent" directly mentions only the *patient's* choosing and implies, on the doctor's part, only an obligation to respect the patient's choice in the situation. But again, when the relationship is at its best, *both* parties to the relationship have choices to make and an obligation to respect the other as a chooser. The Ideal Relationship involves more than this. It is an Interactive Relationship that is the ideal to be striven for, for it consists in choosing on both sides and mutual respect for autonomy on both sides as well.

To be sure, the Ideal Relationship asks much more of the dentist (and ideally of the patient) than Informed Consent does. As already noted, whether they are currently experiencing oral pain or dysfunction—or are only aware of its possibility and hope to forestall it by preventive care—dental patients seek the dentist's help because they cannot fully control this important part of their bodies without it. They come to the dentist aware that they are not in complete control of their bodies and aware that the dentist's expertise can significantly restore or prevent their loss of control. This fact, plus the more variable factors of actual pain, fear, and inequalities of education and social position, mean that even when the patient is trying to contribute as much as he or she can to the relationship, most of the initiative in controlling the situation and bringing it as close as possible to being an Interactive Relationship rests with the dentist.

In other words, it is not enough (it falls far short of the ideal) for the dentist merely to initiate the provision of information, however truthful, and ask the patient to consent—or not—to a recommended course of action. The achievement of mutually effective communication and a shared judgment about what ought to be done and a shared choice to do it together depends on the dentist taking the initiative, not only doing his or her own part in this interaction but also prompting and assisting the patient to also do his or her part. In the Guild Model, the patient's tendency to passiveness in the relationship is viewed as completely appropriate. But in the Interactive Model, the patient's tendency to passiveness—to merely being informed and consenting to the actions recommended, or to even less of a role than this—is viewed as something for the dentist to work to overcome if possible. It is to be overcome gently, with prompts, support, and assistance, rather than with pressure or negative judgments, because only in this way is the dentist genuinely respectful of the patient's actual choices—about the relationship as well as about treatment—as they are being made. But every response by the patient in the direction of sharing in the process of communication and mutual decision-making is to be valued as progress toward the dentist's professional ideal and certainly not as a mistaken intrusion into the dentist's area of control.

A dentist must certainly pay attention to the standard of Informed Consent because it defines the minimum standard of legally acceptable relations between the dentist and his or her legally competent patients. Moreover, insofar as the phrase "Informed Consent" has come to express for many dentists their professional commitment to ethical norms of truthfulness and respect for patients' autonomy, it expresses a worthy ethical standard as well. But dentists must also ask themselves if Informed Consent is a full statement of the Ideal Relationship between dentist and patient. The proposal defended here is that it falls far short because the Ideal Relationship is a relationship of *mutual* communication and *shared* understanding and *shared* choice, even though the initiative for bringing the relationship with a particular patient as close as possible to this ideal most often rests principally with the dentist.

THE IDEAL RELATIONSHIP AND PATIENT TRUST

The discussion of trust in chapter 2 distinguished between Trusting That, which is essentially a matter of predictability; Trusting What, which is about truthfulness; and Trusting the Person. While Trusting What the dentist says is a part of what the dentist-patient relationship ought to be, it is such because of the kind of relationship that ought to exist between the patient and the dentist. That is, it cannot be the case that the patient and dentist are really engaged in seeking a shared judgment about what ought to be done and a shared choice to do it—that is, an Interactive Relationship—if they are not being truthful with one another.

But a dentist cannot make any headway in trying to achieve an Interactive Relationship with a patient if he or she does not communicate clearly (and honestly) a commitment to having the patient's well-being as the primary goal of his or her contributions as a professional to that relationship. But it is this commitment to the priority of the patient's well-being over the dentist's other interests and concerns—and the dentist living out this commitment in practice—that was identified in chapter 2 as the foundation of patients' trust in the dentist in the first place.

The kinds of relationship skills and the habits of perceiving, valuing, prioritizing, thinking, and acting that are needed to become skilled at guiding patients toward and actually achieving the Ideal Relationship are the very elements of professionalism that, because they shape the dentist into becoming a certain kind of professional and a certain kind of person, most effectively prompt patients to Trust the Person of the dentist. In other words, striving to achieve an Interactive Relationship with every patient to the degree that this is possible is intimately connected with patients trusting the dentist as a person in this third and most important sense of trust.

CHALLENGES TO COMMUNICATING INTERACTIVELY

A dentist who reviewed the cases in this book commented on "how civil" the conversations are in these cases. "The patients in them are nice and thoughtful. . . . In reality, some of the people a dentist cares for are definitely less than civil." In giving priority to their patients' well-being, dentists and all health professionals accept that they will have to care for people who are not very nice in terms of their words, their tone, or their attitude—not to mention their manners and dress and ordinary hygiene. Overlooking such things—or working past them when overlooking them is impossible—is part of the dental professional's effort to focus on communicating as interactively as possible with the patient. In addition, dentists' practices include children who are not fully capable of participating in decision-making, patients who have developmental disabilities, or older persons whose ability to make dental care decisions have become compromised. Chapter 7 will examine the special ethical questions that arise regarding patients whose capacity for full participation in an Interactive Relationship is compromised. But the goal of educating such patients about their oral health and engaging them collaboratively as much as possible is still the same.

In addition, however, there are several kinds of patients whose view of their relationship to the dentist directly conflicts with developing an Interactive Relationship with them. The dentist's goal needs to remain the same: to communicate and reach a treatment decision with these patients as interactively as possible. Because what they bring to the situation and have in mind appears to be a different goal, however, learning how to work toward an Interactive Relationship with them takes special effort and, for most dentists, developing skill at doing this takes time and experience in practice. For the ethical dentist, though, it is always worth trying.

Among these are patients who are capable decision makers but who apparently want the dentist to make all the decisions about treatment for them. It is as if they believe in the Guild Model—even though the fact is that *they are choosing* this position and that, therefore, *they have values* that they want to prioritize. For these facts mean that they are not wholly passive, as the Guild Model demands. Such patients will often explain their taking this position because they trust (Trust That) the dentist's expertise or, perhaps, because they trust (Trust the Person) the dentist to be committed to their well-being.

But in both cases, the question they need to answer is whether they are as committed to their Oral and General Health—in comparison with other values in their lives—as the dentist is (see chapter 5 on dentistry's Central Practice Values). They need to answer this question because the dentist cannot possibly answer it for them. And even if their answer is genuinely a yes, then they ought to learn more about what prioritizing their oral health means practically rather than pretending that it is enough for the dentist to know these things.

It may be difficult to have a conversation about the patient's values that are relevant to a thoughtful decision about treatment when the patient prefers passivity to communication. Understanding what the conversation is missing, though, is the first step in rectifying it. So the dentist who aims to make the relationship as interactive as possible will, therefore, try to shape a conversation that not only allows but also draws the patient to answer these questions. Ideally, this will prompt the patient to start asking further questions about diagnosis, possible interventions, costs and benefits, how and who pays, and so forth that are required for answering the value questions. Ideally, asking these questions will lead the patient to take a more active role in the actual decision-making. If these efforts fail, however, there is an ethically proper default response, which will be described below.

Another group is the internet-savvy patients who have learned something they think is relevant to their own oral health needs and who consider their knowledge of what they need to be just as valid as that of the dentist. The equality of patient and dentist in the Interactive Relationship is moral equality; it is the equality of each party as a judge of value and chooser of the next steps that the two will take together. It is not equality of expertise. So successfully educating such patients about the condition of their mouths, their treatment needs, the possible costs and outcomes of available treatments, and how it might be paid for can be seriously hindered when patients think they already know all they need to know about these matters. And it is especially so when the information they have is mistaken.

It is easy for a dentist to be insulted by such patients' naïve confidence in their knowledge. For one thing, the dentist's expertise has been achieved through years of committed hard work and practice experience. More importantly, however, *factual knowledge* about oral health—whether learned in dental school or on the internet—is of little value by itself. What is crucial to dependably helping patients, and is at the heart of dental expertise, are the *skills of responding effectively* to actual people's oral health needs. But responding to the implied insult to the dentist's expertise will be of little help in achieving an Interactive Relationship.

There are, however, two positive aspects of such patients' positions that offer a place to try building a proper relationship with them. First of all, such patients desire to manage their own oral health. This is something the dentist can build on, not only by commending it but by making it clear that the relationship the dentist is hoping for is a collaborative one that aims at a shared judgment about what ought to be done and a shared choice to do it. Many such patients educate themselves in these ways precisely as a defense against being offered no active role in the decisions about their care.

Second, such patients do understand that the decisions needing to be made depend on knowledge about the oral cavity and possible interventions. This, too, is something the dentist committed to an Interactive Relationship can enthusiastically support. Of course, the dentist will need to fill the gaps in what the patient has learned. It is not necessary for the dentist to challenge whatever the patient has learned correctly, though, only to add to it. So what is missing can, if offered carefully, be supportive of the patient's efforts at self-education. There will often be factual gaps about the oral cavity, especially about the patient's own mouth, that will need to be added to what the patient has learned. Moreover, even if the patient has learned correctly about possible interventions, it is unlikely that the patient will know the full range of possible treatments; their benefits and risks for the presenting conditions; and the likely cost of each and how such treatment might be paid for. (As dentists observe more internet-savvy patients coming into their offices, it would very helpful if they were able to recommend dependable and accurate internet sources for oral health education. The dentist who is internet savvy will obviously have an advantage in guiding this group of patients toward an Interactive Relationship.)

The key is trying to communicate these matters so that the value of the patient's effort—to become educated—is affirmed while completing what the patient needs to know to make a good judgment about what ought to be done, along with stressing that the patient's values are essential components to the kind of collaborative decision-making that the dentist's goal of an Interactive Relationship calls for. (We take it for granted that the dentist might never use the phrase "Interactive Relationship" in working toward this goal. The actual words are not what is important here; the goal is the kind of collaboration that they refer to.)

The more difficult situations are those where what the patient has learned is incorrect—either inaccurate information about the oral cavity, about possible diagnoses, possible treatments, potential costs and risks, how the situation is being paid for, or some combination of these. Helping the patient realize that the topic area is in fact complex (i.e., has aspects that the patient would not be expected to have been aware of and that the internet source failed to explain) may help the dentist locate the responsibility for the error in the internet source or in the complexity of the topic rather than in the patient. For here, too, the most effective starting point will be to affirm the value of the patient seeking education and trying to manage his or her own oral health, since informed self-care and active participation in decision-making with the dentist are commendable characteristics in every patient. If these efforts fail, however, there is an ethically proper default response, which will be described below.

A third group presenting special challenges to developing an Interactive Relationship are patients who assume that this is a competitive market relationship to begin with rather than a collaborative relationship. Such patients may have no understanding of what a profession and professionals are committed to. In such cases, some education about this matter may actually be useful, especially if made personal by the dentist's identification of himself or herself as a professional. But when there is no time for this or it is not possible for some other reason (or it is ineffective), there is an ethically proper default response, which will be described below.

In some cases, while the patient may be familiar with how professionals ought to deal with those they serve, he or she may now view dentists as no longer being committed professionals in this way. As in the previous paragraph, a dentist can only learn that this is how the patient views dentists by addressing the difference between the patient's stance toward their relationship and the dentist's own. It is likely that a forthright statement of professional commitment by the dentist will surprise such a patient. But whether it will prompt a conversation that would redirect their relationship will depend on how "hardened" the patient is in his or her views of dentistry and dentists. (An important ethical issue that is relevant here is whether there are ways dentists send a commercial—rather than a professional—message about dentistry to the larger community. This will be discussed at several points in the following chapters and especially in chapter 13. In addition, chapter 11 will discuss the patterns in US health policies and in the views of most people in our society that accord oral health and oral health care considerably less priority than other aspects of health and health care.) If this conversation does not redirect the relationship toward one that is noncompetitive and more interactive—if the patient hears the dentist's explanation that he or she is a committed professional but, in effect, does not believe it—then there is an ethically proper default response, which will be described below.

In other cases, the patient may in fact understand that dentists are professionals who have made ethical commitments that will shape how they communicate and care for their patients. However, the patient may be so used to thinking, valuing, and dealing with people according to marketplace standards that the patient, so to speak, "forgets" to switch gears now that he or she is dealing with a professional. Here, ideally at least, calling attention to the mismatch of relationships will "remind" the patient that this relationship can and ought to have different qualities from that of a marketplace relationship. Ideally, the patient will then begin to work with the dentist to make their relationship as interactive as possible. Here, as in the above cases, the dentist may feel insulted by the stance the patient is taking. But again, reacting to the implied insult will do little to move the relationship toward more interactive collaboration. If the dentist's efforts to draw the patient into the task of working toward an Interactive Relationship fall short, however, there is an ethically proper default response, which will be described below.

Finally, there are patients who present themselves as "entitled" to a certain level of dental services, patients who, if their sense of what they are entitled to cannot be honored, begin to treat the relationship as a competitive marketplace relationship. What they are actually entitled to, though, may be limited because of restrictions on their insurance coverage, justifiable limits on the dentist's ability to offer charity care, our society's failure to provide a dependable means for them to meet their legitimate needs, or for other reasons. Under such circumstances, the dentist should try to explain what the patient is actually entitled to and why it is different from what they were expecting and, if possible, offer to provide what they are entitled to.

Regarding such explanations, chapter 12 will examine the ethical questions that can arise as dentists deal with the complexities of patients' dental insurance policies and patients' common misunderstandings of them. Chapter 6 will examine the justifiable limits of the obligation that professionals have to give priority to and make certain kinds of sacrifices for the well-being of the persons they serve. Chapter 11 will examine ethical arguments in support of an obligation on the part of the larger society to be responsive to people's unmet basic health care needs, including certain oral health needs, and the de facto limits of our society's current responses to these needs.

Such explanations, though, will often be about complex matters. These may well be beyond some patients' abilities to make sense of them or patients' willingness to process them. Furthermore, these explanations will rarely respond to the emotional force of the patient's sense of injustice. If the patient is able to appreciate that the dentist is not unconcerned about the patient's need, however, then a sincere expression of empathy and concern by the dentist may be beneficial.

In any case, as mentioned above, there is an ethically proper default response for a dentist to use when the suggested avenues of improving the relationship—and others that a dentist may learn—fall short. This is to continue engaging the patient in ways that affirm the importance of collaboration and the moral equality of dentist and patient and—because the goal does not change—to remain working toward as interactive a relationship as is possible under the circumstances but without pressuring or manipulating the patient to participate in these efforts. For no matter how remote an actual relationship is from the ideal dentist-patient relationship, the dignity of the patient and the priority of this aspect of the patient's well-being—along with his or her Oral and General Health—remain the essential ethical focus of the dentist's efforts.

THINKING ABOUT THE CASE

Determining what ought to be done in the case of the dreaded root canal would first require determining whether Mr. Vianni is capable of autonomous decision-making regarding the decision at hand. A fuller description of what is involved in autonomous decision-making will be given in chapter 7, but two of its elements have been described here. First, the autonomous decision maker can understand the alternative treatments that the dentist explains and their likely outcomes, as well as the likely outcome of no treatment at all. Second, the autonomous decision maker can act on the basis of his or her own values, goals, purposes, and principles of conduct.

The case gives no reason to doubt that Mr. Vianni can understand simple concepts such as the structure of a tooth and the various steps involved in a root canal procedure. Nor does he exhibit any deficit in general intelligence. So the question regarding his ability to make autonomous decisions about his dental treatment rests more on the question of whether his likely refusal of endodontic therapy, if he is presented with this treatment option up front and asked whether he will choose it, would be in accord with his own values, goals, or purposes. Mr. Vianni is highly fearful of endodontic therapy and is so anxious about use of the drill that it sharply heightens his sensitivity to pain and discomfort. That is why Dr. Clarke expects that he would refuse the root canal.

Although Dr. Clarke might judge a refusal of endodontic therapy by Mr. Vianni to be a serious error on his part, the case could be made that this move would be consistent with his genuine and frequently expressed desire to avoid this procedure and other procedures involving extensive drilling. The case might be made, then, that Mr. Vianni is a capable decision maker in this matter and that any move by Dr. Clarke to withhold information about his treatment alternatives until one set of them has been completed would be a violation of the principle of respecting autonomy.

On the other hand, if autonomy is choosing and acting on the basis of one's own values, Dr. Clarke is certain that the treatment most in accord with Mr. Vianni's repeatedly expressed valuation of his oral health is endodontic therapy and a crown. In fact, she could argue that failure to perform this procedure would violate the principle of respecting Mr. Vianni's own values. In temporarily screening him from certain facts, she might argue, she would only be assuring that he actually would evaluate those facts according to his own values, rather than on the basis of fears and anxieties that are not only unreasonable from an observer's point of view but are in fact inconsistent with Mr. Vianni's own values.

But if Dr. Clarke genuinely believes that Mr. Vianni is psychologically incapable of choosing in accord with his autonomy in this matter, then Dr. Clarke must act on the basis of some principle other than respect for autonomy. For on *this* interpretation of Mr. Vianni's situation, he is not a capable decision maker about endodontic therapy and there is no autonomous decision on the part of Mr. Vianni for her to respect. Determination of a patient's capacity for autonomous decision-making ultimately requires a more detailed understanding of autonomy than this chapter has offered. In addition, the guidelines that a dentist should follow in determining treatment and other interventions for patients who are incapable of autonomous decisions require careful study. These tasks will be undertaken in chapter 7. For present purposes, let us presume that Mr. Vianni *is*, in fact, *capable* of autonomous decision-making in the matter of his first molar, although he is moved by powerful fears and anxieties regarding the ideal treatment available to him (endodontic therapy). Let us ask whether, if we make this assumption and assume it is Dr. Clarke's view on the matter, Dr. Clarke could still be ethically justified in violating the principle of respecting autonomy in order to provide Mr. Vianni with the best possible treatment for his situation. Are there any other features of the case that would justify such a violation, anything about the case that is of greater moral significance than respecting Mr. Vianni's autonomy?

Before proceeding, it is important to note that if Dr. Clarke were to do this, she would be engaging in legally risky action because Mr. Vianni is certainly legally competent and therefore has a legal right to either consent to or refuse endodontic therapy. But the present task is not to ask if such an action would be legally correct or legally risky but to ask whether it would be professionally unethical. Is the dentist's commitment to the patient's autonomy such that, for a patient capable of autonomous decision-making, the dentist may never place any value for the patient ahead of the patient's autonomy?

It is also important to avoid any false position that would hold that a patient is automatically and certainly incapable of autonomous decision-making simply and solely because he or she disagrees with the dentist about the treatment to be chosen. The determination of a patient's incapacity must depend on evidence about his or her capacity, not simply on whether the patient agrees or disagrees with the dentist. In the present case, the patient is fearful and anxious, but fear and anxiety are often reasonable responses to a situation, not signs of incapacity. For the time being, we are assuming that this is the case with Mr. Vianni in order to ask if, even though we assume Mr. Vianni is capable of autonomous decision-making, there are still values at stake in this case that are important enough that a dentist may ethically choose to prioritize them for the patient rather than respecting his autonomy. In terms of the discussions earlier in this chapter, the question here is whether this is a situation in which paternalism—interfering with a capable person's exercise of his or her autonomy precisely because this would be better for that person—is ethically justifiable.

With this focus, one additional feature of the case, not yet stressed in this commentary, needs attention. Mr. Vianni's fear and anxiety are not news to Dr. Clarke. Nor is it news that there is little sound enamel left on the first molar or that it contains a large restoration that is getting very old. It would have been prudent of Dr. Clarke to warn Mr. Vianni gently but regularly, as she got to know him, that this tooth would probably not hold up forever and that endodontic therapy, performed in a pain-free manner, would be the best therapy for it. More importantly, Dr. Clarke should not have waited until now to wonder what to do about Mr. Vianni's fears and anxieties. She should have established a plan with him some time before to begin addressing these concerns of his so that he could be better prepared for the major restorative, endodontic, or periodontal work that he would likely need as he grew older. Dr. Clarke has been willing to leave the relationship very one-sided, with Mr. Vianni acting very much like the passive patient of the Guild Model, instead of working to address the factors in Mr. Vianni's case that were making the relationship so. Dr. Clarke does not seem to have worked as hard at producing an Interactive Relationship as Mr. Vianni's limitations required.

Of course, Dr. Clarke might well be able to say she did try to bring their relationship around to being more interactive and that Mr. Vianni was unwilling or unable to let that happen. She might also be able to say there is only so much time and effort that she owes this particular patient. It might be that she has already met or even gone beyond the basic commitments of time and effort that she owes to each of her patients within the ordinary dentist-patient relationship, so much so that further time and effort spent trying to bring about more of an Interactive Relationship with Mr. Vianni would either take time away from other patients in need or from other commitments and aspects of Dr. Clarke's life that legitimately compete with this patient's needs.

These two issues, how much time and effort a dentist owes to each patient in comparison with other patients in need and how much personal sacrifice of other commitments and concerns a dentist owes to his or her patients are very important questions that do not lend themselves to easy answers—nor can they be addressed simply within strict business time and resource management principles and practices. They clearly play an important role in the ethics of this case, and they will be discussed more fully in chapter 6.

But the importance of these issues does not eliminate or provide an answer to the question that is the central focus of this chapter: What is the Ideal Relationship between dentist and patient? If the Interactive Model is the ideal, as has been proposed here, then it is the relationship that a dentist ought to try to achieve with whatever resources of expertise, time, effort, hard work, and common sense he or she has available. It will often be impossible to achieve this ideal fully, given the patient's situation and the resources reasonably available to the dentist. That does not lessen its claim, however, to being the kind of relationship that dentists should strive to achieve. For with whatever resources the dentist has available, and to the extent possible given the patient's actual situation, it is an Interactive Relationship that the dentist should be working to bring about.

So what should Dr. Clarke do in the case as it has been described, given the current assumption that Mr. Vianni is capable of autonomous decision-making about endodontic therapy? One option might be to work for additional time in order to persuade Mr. Vianni to choose the best treatment. She might, for example, provide temporary pain relief and antibiotic therapy (to prevent further infection) in order to have several days' time to actively address Mr. Vianni's unreasonable fears of endodontic therapy. The risks of this option include the delayed relief of Mr. Vianni's pain, the chance of not prescribing an effective antibiotic and increased medical complications, and the risk that the task of refocusing Mr. Vianni's attention on his commitment to dental health (and then explaining the benefits of endodontic therapy in the present situation) may well take more time than Dr. Clarke's temporizing efforts can provide. She will also have lost the option of beginning endodontic therapy here and now, and she may not be able to persuade him to choose endodontic therapy anyway.

But it is worth asking if Dr. Clarke would really be working effectively for a more Interactive Relationship if she opted for this path. Much would depend on how she used the time that temporizing would provide. If it were devoted to an aggressive effort to persuade him to choose endodontic therapy, it is doubtful that the fundamental equality of the two parties and the mutual respect of each other's values, on which an Interactive Relationship rests, would be effectively honored. On the other hand, it might be possible, if time for thoughtful conversation were available (although it might be the case that neither party would have time for this anyway), that the value of Mr. Vianni's oral health, which both parties wish to honor, could bring them to a shared decision about his treatment.

This brings us to the further question of what, if shared deliberation did result in a decision by Mr. Vianni, Dr. Clarke ought to do if Mr. Vianni chose not to have endodontic therapy. Still assuming that Mr. Vianni's refusal of endodontic therapy would be an autonomous one, Dr. Clarke might take the position that the moral and professional importance of respecting Mr. Vianni's autonomy requires that she abide by that choice. How she should proceed after that would depend on her judgment about the suitability of alternative therapies—for example, simple extraction or extraction with some replacement option to fill the space and to maintain the occlusion and integrity of the dentition.

If Mr. Vianni chooses not to have endodontic therapy after careful interactive deliberation, Dr. Clarke would have reason to view the choice as one she and Mr. Vianni have made together. But notice that, without conversation between them of the sort mentioned in the previous paragraph, it seems more likely that she will view herself as unwillingly supporting a mistaken choice by Mr. Vianni. In other words, the mere fact that a patient's autonomous choice has been carried out by the dentist does not automatically mean that the ideal of an Interactive Relationship has been achieved. The proposal that the Ideal Relationship between dentist and patient is an Interactive Relationship will often require far more communication and collaboration from both parties than is needed to reach the lower ethical norm and minimal legal standard of Informed Consent.

Finally, however, even on the assumption that Mr. Vianni's imagined refusal would be an autonomous one, Dr. Clarke might still take the position that she ought to initiate endodontic therapy here and now, without the interactive conversation just referred to and without fully informing Mr. Vianni about what is happening until the worst is past. She might judge, in other words, that this is a situation of *justifiable paternalism*—that is, that violating Mr. Vianni's autonomy for his own greater good would be ethically justified. Suppose Dr. Clarke reasoned that since there are values she is committed to as a dentist—which are called dentistry's Central Practice Values in this book—that are an accepted part of the dentist-patient relationship (which is the relationship that Mr. Vianni has chosen to enter into), then if some of these are more important than respecting a patient's autonomous choice, she should choose to produce them for Mr. Vianni rather than respect his autonomy in this particular matter.

In order to justify reasoning in this way, Dr. Clarke would have to think carefully about two things. One is to ask herself whether a dentist's obligation to strive for an Interactive Relationship can ever be outweighed by other components of dentistry's ethical commitments. This topic, about situations in which one's professional obligations conflict with one another, is examined in chapter 6. The second is to identify the Central Practice Values of professional dental practice and determine if they are ranked in importance and then ask if any of them outrank the patient's autonomy. This is the topic of the next chapter.

5

⋙⋙

The Central Practice Values
of Dental Practice

CASE: THE CHEAPEST WILL HAVE TO DO

Ina Kirchland, a sixty-eight-year-old widow in good general health, is in severe pain. She is squeezed in at 9:40 a.m., before another patient's 10:00 a.m. appointment. Although her teeth are generally in good shape, her upper-left first premolar has been a problem for some time. Dr. Luban and Mrs. Kirchland have discussed it being only a matter of time before it will need a root canal or removal and replacement. After a quick examination, Dr. Luban says that time has now come; the lingual cusp has fractured and exposed the pulp.

Mrs. Kirchland does not have much money and is without dental insurance. She lives on her deceased husband's social security benefits, which she supplements to some extent by providing day care in her home several afternoons a week. Her resources for dental care, as for everything, are very limited. Her constant anxiety about how to make ends meet is voiced at the outset of every dental appointment.

Dr. Luban prefers for Mrs. Kirchland to choose a root canal, post, and crown because of the importance of filling the space if the tooth ever has to come out, which they have discussed previously. But the root canal, even without an immediate post and crown placement, will certainly cost more than a simple extraction. Mrs. Kirchland can still elect to have an extraction with one of several kinds of fixed prostheses, but any one of those, considering the condition of the abutment teeth, will be even more expensive than the root canal, post, and crown, and an implant will be more than that. So Dr. Luban judges that the alternatives to the root canal, post, and crown are not useful options. Another possibility would be an extraction with one of several kinds of removable partial prostheses; this would cost Mrs. Kirchland less than the root canal, post, and crown, but the removable prosthesis might need replacement later on in the event of accidental breakage, carious abutment teeth, and so on, although such events could affect the other options as well.

Before going into all this, Dr. Luban thought he ought to mention the option of an extraction with nothing to fill the space; some of his older patients viewed this as the obvious thing to do. But Mrs. Kirchland immediately cut him off, saying, "Heaven forbid, not after all these years."

Now, if Dr. Luban simply presents Mrs. Kirchland with just the facts about only three of these options—root canal with post and crown, extraction with some kind of prosthesis, and simple extraction and no replacement—he is quite certain that she will simply choose the cheapest therapy, even if she has talked in the past about filling the space if the tooth were ever lost and even if she is made aware of the minor risks of shifting teeth and altered occlusal function. "I am getting old," she has said many times, "the cheapest and simplest will have to last me."

Endodontic therapy can also be tricky; unusual canal anatomy or an as-yet-undetected fractured root might later mean removal of the tooth anyway. Dr. Luban certainly has to mention these possibilities in some way, but too much talking about what could possibly happen may cause the simple extraction to now look better to Mrs. Kirchland.

On the other hand, he can definitely control how much to stress this aspect of root canal therapy in his explanation. In fact, he can probably make his explanation of the alternatives persuasive in any direction he chooses. Dr. Luban can probably lead Mrs. Kirchland to choose the root canal by strongly emphasizing the benefits of endodontic therapy, post, and crown followed by the risks of an extraction and no replacement and the inconvenience of caring for a prosthesis—and its possibly needing to be replaced later on. He has serious reservations about doing this, though, because under such circumstances Mrs. Kirchland's choice might not be very autonomous.

He could refrain from returning to the option of a simple extraction. But wouldn't that leave Mrs. Kirchland even less free to choose? Doing so will keep her from knowing about a possible treatment that is still within the range of clinically acceptable therapy, even though it is not the preferred treatment for her clinical situation.

Yet Dr. Luban is certain that the root canal with post and crown is really worth her money. He also has doubts that a choice of either cheaper therapy would be any more of a free choice on her part—given her view of her financial situation and her evident anxiety about it.

What should Dr. Luban do and why?

A PROFESSION'S CENTRAL PRACTICE VALUES

The practice of each profession—that is, the application of its expertise for the benefit of its clients—is necessarily focused only on certain aspects of the well-being of those clients. No professional group is expected by the larger community to be expert in their clients' *entire* well-being. Consequently, no profession is committed to securing for its clients everything that is of value for them. Of course, the achievement of any values for a profession's clients will depend on an understanding of the relation of these values to each client's whole person. It is precisely in this way that the expressed concern of many professions about being attentive to the "whole" client can contain an important element of truth. But there is always necessarily a certain limited set of values that are the specific focus of each profession's expertise, and it is therefore the principal job and obligation of that profession to secure these for its clients. In this book these values are called the Central Practice Values of a profession's practice.

The aim of this chapter is to propose an answer to the obvious question: What are the Central Practice Values of dental practice and of the dental profession? What specific aspects of human well-being is each member of the dental profession tasked to secure— as much as is possible under the circumstances—for each of its patients? In addition, if there are a number of Central Practice Values, it is important to ask if these are of equal importance or if some of them take precedence over others when all of them cannot be achieved simultaneously. That is, do they form some sort of ranked hierarchy?

Before considering these questions, however, two other questions must be addressed. First, who determines a profession's Central Practice Values? Second, how can we identify the values currently accepted as the Central Practice Values for a particular profession's practice in a particular society? Clearly, it is not the individual practitioner who determines what values are Central Practice Values for the dental profession and dental practice in a given society. Of course, each individual dentist does make a personal choice to accept the obligations of professional practice as a dentist, and in this respect each dentist's commitment to the Central Practice Values of dental practice is his or her own doing. But the contents of this commitment, as chapter 2 explained, are the product of an ongoing dialogue between the dental community and the community at large. So when a person chooses to become a dentist, he or she accepts and commits to the values identified in that ongoing dialogue— that is, the Central Practice Values of dentistry as a recognized profession in this society, not to some set of values of the individual practitioner's own devising.

The person who becomes a dentist may even consider the values currently accepted as Central Practice Values for dental practice in a given society to be in need of revision or significant adjustment. Such a person may therefore choose to work, as a member of the dental community, to change or adjust the values that both the dental community and the community at large accept as central for dental practice. Some subtle ethical questions can arise for such a dentist about the extent to which a member of a profession may, and sometimes even ought to, engage in conscientious refusal to serve values that he or she judges incorrect for that profession's practice. But the starting point of all such reflections and choices must be the fact that the content of professional norms for a given profession in a given society is first of all the product of an ongoing dialogue between that professional group and the larger community. It is not the product of unilateral choices on the part of an individual practitioner or even on the part of the professional group alone.

VALUES FOR PATIENTS FIRST OF ALL

The expression "dentistry's Central Practice Values" may seem to refer most importantly to the *dentist's* values. But the intention of this expression is that it refers first of all to values *for dentists' patients*. That is, dentistry's Central Practice Values, as this concept is being offered here, refers first of all to the kinds of benefits *that patients receive* from dentists engaged in the practice of their profession (and that can directly or indirectly impact persons in general that may not yet be, or may never be, patients of a particular dental practice). It was stressed above that every aspect of dental practice is value laden, and this is the case in part because everything a dentist does in relation to a patient should be directed first and foremost to the achievement of a certain set of values for the patient. These values are called "central" to the practice of dentistry because it is they that should principally shape every aspect of a dentist's professional practice. They are called "practice values" because what they should shape is whatever the dentist does in caring for the patient; they are the values that the dentist is striving to bring about for the patient and that the dental profession is striving to bring about for the whole society.

Of course, it would not only be very strange but probably psychologically impossible for someone to become a dentist who does not personally value the kind of benefits that dental expertise enables a dentist to bring about for his or her patients. So we can expect dentistry's Central Practice Values to be aspects of human life that a dentist personally values as well. But throughout this chapter and in their use as guidelines for ethical dental practice, it should be remembered that the first reason the Central Practice Values of dentistry should be pursued is because they are precisely the values that dentistry has committed to the larger society to strive to bring about *for those they serve*—that is, first and foremost, dentistry's patients.

IDENTIFYING A PROFESSION'S CENTRAL PRACTICE VALUES

How, then, can we identify the values that are currently accepted as central for the dental profession and dental practice in our society? The short answer is that we must carefully examine the *conduct* and the *discourse* of the members of the society and the members of the profession, as well as their interactions with one another. That is, we can identify the Central Practice Values by carefully examining the conduct and discourse of members of the dental profession and their patients as these parties discuss and then make decisions about dental treatment. These values can be identified, in part, by examining the kinds of reasons that dentists and those they serve offer for their recommendations, choices, and actions and the reasons that they accept from one another as reasonable, along with the kinds of reasons that are given and accepted in the society at large for justifying dentists' and patients' decisions in practice and in their relationships with each other.

In spite of its length, this is the "short" answer because the long answer involves the actual work of sifting through and sorting out all the data about conduct and discourse that pertains to the practice of dentistry in the society. In fact, without noticing it, all of us who deal with the dental profession in our society, and certainly both the established and the aspiring members of the dental profession itself, constantly absorb and contemplate this data to form an understanding of what is taken for granted about the Central Practice Values of dental practice in our society.

Ideally, those who are most concerned about the dental profession and dental practice perform this work of sifting and sorting much more explicitly and self-consciously. They then try to articulate what they observe in accepted patterns of conduct and discourse so that other concerned parties can evaluate their proposals and offer the evidence of their own observations and experiences until a genuine consensus about the contents of accepted professional norms can be formed. The accounts of the accepted norms of dental practice that appear in the codes of ethics of professional organizations and the sets of advisory opinions about such codes are examples of such efforts. The historical strength of each organization's contributions to these deliberations, of course, varies. The account of the accepted norms of dental practice offered in this book (and the discussions in articles and books by other scholars of dental professional ethics) is thus another part of this process.

The codes of ethics proposed by organized dentistry have a special importance in this effort because they are commissioned and supported by large and longstanding historical groups of dentists. Thus, their authors have far more claim to be representative of the dental community than the three authors of this book have or the authors of other scholarly articles and books have. At the same time, the details of their deliberations in determining the content of such codes are rarely made known to the larger society, and it is extremely rare that members of the nondental community are represented at all in the creation of such codes. Consequently, the codes are often representative of only one side of the dialogue. On the other hand, a book like this or a scholarly article on a particular topic in dental professional ethics can examine the accepted norms of dental practice, raise questions about the reasons supporting them, and propose possible alternatives to them and other considerations—in far more detail than any published code or set of advisory opinions can do. Thus, both efforts are needed to help make the contents of the ongoing dialogue more articulate.

From what has been said, it follows that the many statements about professional norms and obligations made in this book should be read as hypotheses about the contents of the current dialogue between the dental community and the community at large. These statements aim to focus on and help clarify the norms and values that the two groups accept as shaping the dental profession and dental practice in our society. Yet, while these are "only" hypotheses, the accounts of professional norms and obligations offered here are not mere constructions of the authors' imaginations. They are based on extensive and careful analysis of our society and its dental community using the most sophisticated concepts about the nature, basis, and implications of professional obligation available, many of which are also summarized in this book so that they, too, can be thoughtfully evaluated by the reader.

The authors believe that the claims made in these pages about the contents of dentistry's professional norms are in fact well supported by the data; that is, they are supported in the conduct and discourse—in the actions undertaken and in the reasons given—of dental professionals, their patients, and other members of the larger community.

DENTISTRY'S CENTRAL PRACTICE VALUES

As dentists care for patients, they make numerous decisions that are inherently value laden. Most of these do not involve conscious examination of competing values by the dentist, because the values the dentist is guided by are the fruit of well-established habits of professional practice. But whether the value content of a particular judgment is explicit or implicit, a dentist cannot practice without making numerous decisions in which values play an important role. The practice of dentistry, in other words, is not only a matter of technical judgment and skill; it is also an activity in which the dentist strives to bring about certain values, either directly for the patient or as part of his or her relationship with the patient.

To make the same point in another way, consider a dentist who focuses his or her efforts principally on entertaining the patient and receiving the patient's plaudits as a result, even if this means forgoing procedures needed for the patient's oral health. Or consider a dentist who works chiefly to give patients the excitement and exhilaration that some people experience when facing a serious risk head-on, so the dentist therefore makes little or no effort to control or minimize the risk to the patient in advance. Such dentists would have a limited clientele, of course. The risk-adverse would not be interested in the latter dentist, and patients who go to dentists for more familiar reasons would probably avoid both of them. But many people enjoy being entertained, and there seem to be people who enjoy risk-taking enough that each kind of dentist might still have regular patients. Would either of these practitioners be practicing in a professionally acceptable way, even if they had patients? The answer to this question is clear. Neither of these ways of employing dental expertise is professionally appropriate under the accepted standards of dental practice in our society. Regardless of whether a person could actually earn a living doing such things, these ways of acting are not proper ways for a person who claims to be a dentist to act. They are misdirected; in fact, precisely what is wrong with them is that they are directed at the wrong values.

As in every profession, there are certain values that are central to the proper practice of professional dentistry, and every dentist is committed, as a professional, to working to achieve these values above all for his or her patients. What are dentistry's Central Practice Values? There are six values that appear to be the accepted Central Practice Values for dental practice in our society:

1. The Patient's Life and General Health
2. The Patient's Oral Health
3. The Patient's Autonomy
4. The Dentist's Preferred Patterns of Practice
5. Aesthetic Values
6. Efficiency in the Use of Professional Resources

The question of whether these six values are hierarchically ranked will be discussed later in this chapter. But before that, each of the six must be explained in its own right.

The Patient's Life and General Health

One value that certainly plays an important role in dentists' judgments in practice is the value of the patient's Life and General Health. Although this value is not discussed as much as that of the patient's Oral Health, nevertheless every patient that a dentist examines and every treatment that a dentist recommends or performs must be evaluated on the basis of this value. A dentist who recommends a treatment or ignores or denies a condition that places a patient's life at risk without any consideration for this fact would certainly be acting unprofessionally. Moreover, a dentist who pays no attention to the connections between a patient's oral condition and other aspects of the patient's health would be similarly guilty of a serious professional failure.

It will be important to reflect on the relative importance of this value—the patient's Life and General Health—in comparison with other values in dental practice. Is it correct to say that the patient's Life and General Health should take priority over all other values that a dentist strives to achieve, or are other values more important than this in the practice of dentistry? This question will be examined in detail in the next section. But first, a description is needed of the other five Central Practice Values for dental practice.

The Patient's Oral Health

The patient's Oral Health is the most obvious value that dentists aim to achieve for their patients. Although it may appear to be a fairly simple idea, *oral health* is actually quite a complex notion. There are general standards of appropriate oral function, of course, but the specific character of appropriate functioning for a particular patient will depend on many variables, including the patient's age, the pattern of development of the patient's dentition, other health conditions, the patient's physiological and functional needs, the patient's underlying anatomy, and so on. Oral health also includes the notion that oral functioning is pain free. But pain and discomfort are also relative terms, and the specific standard that a dentist should apply to a given patient will also depend, at least in part, on variables like those already mentioned. Nevertheless, in spite of the complexity of its content, oral health plays a very important role in the judgments dentists make every day in practice. For present purposes, the Central Practice Value of "Oral Health" will be defined as appropriate and pain-free oral functioning.

The complexity of the notion of oral health is in fact just an extension of the complexity of the idea of health itself. Health is not merely a factual concept. It is an evaluative concept as well because it is used to identify certain characteristics and conditions as being preferable for humans, as the ones humans are better off having. It is beyond the scope of this book to study the larger concept of health in any detail, but all who are health care providers, including members of the dental profession, would do well to think carefully about the meaning of this concept and its implications for their professional practice.

The Patient's Autonomy

"Autonomy" was discussed at some length in the preceding chapter. The brief definition adopted there, "choosing and acting on the basis of one's own values, goals, purposes, and principles of conduct," will continue to be operative in this discussion of Autonomy as one of dentistry's Central Practice Values.

The prominence of the professional-legal principle of Informed Consent and the reasons given in chapter 4 for considering the Interactive Model to be the ideal model for the dentist-patient relationship should be reasons enough for this list of dentistry's Central Practice Values to include the patient's Autonomy. However, later in this chapter, when the relative importance of dentistry's Central Practice Values becomes the focus of discussion and they are ranked, the question of the relative priority of the patient's Autonomy will be shown to be more complex.

The Dentist's Preferred Patterns of Practice

The dentist who practices in a technically competent manner still has many choices to make. Among these choices are some that might be noticed by a thoughtful layperson. For example, the dentist must choose among various kinds of dental chairs and various ways of laying out an operatory. But dentists make many more choices that laypeople are rarely aware of, and many of these choices are much more important. There are, for example, choices among various styles and brands of hand instruments, various kinds and brands of medicaments, various dental materials, and so on. There is a wide range of choices to be made regarding the worth and maintenance costs of major dental equipment because the available technology changes and advances so rapidly. Still more complex than these are the dentist's choices among various acceptable approaches to most of the diagnostic, operative, and other procedures in dental practice. A dentist must make choices in all these areas, weighing the options in terms of patient outcome and patient comfort, of course, and also in terms of the dentist's own output of time, effort, and money, and the dentist's degree of comfort with and trust in each alternative as well as the dentist's ability—determined in practice through repeated use of the procedure or technique—to become able to habituate its use rather than continuing to have to focus on every step or detail of its use, as at the start.

It might seem that no special values are involved in these choices other than those mentioned under the other headings in this section—that is, dentistry's other Central Practice Values. It might seem, in other words, that once those other values have been fulfilled, nothing else is at stake but the dentist's own preferences, which will vary from dentist to dentist. But in fact, there is a subtle professional value at stake in these choices that needs careful articulation because it is so easily overlooked.

No one can effectively apply complex expertise to concrete situations, such as the specific clinical needs of a particular patient, if every detail of that application must be self-consciously judged and chosen each time it arises. For this reason, becoming a competent and effective professional is, in significant measure, a process of becoming capable of applying many aspects of one's expertise *habitually*, without self-conscious attention. The initial development of such habits—habits of dental perception, valuation, judgment, and action—is the principal goal of dental school training. Further development of a young dentist in the early years of practice requires deliberate attention to the many more details of competent practice and the pursuit of continuing education where needed. It is only when most of the ordinary details of a particular procedure—whether diagnostic or operative or something else—can be addressed without self-conscious reflection and judgment that a dentist is able to then attend effectively to the unusual, the unique, and the problematic in this particular patient or respond effectively when an apparently ordinary situation for some reason goes awry.

Consequently, a dentist's comfort with, trust in, and preference for a particular pattern of practice—in any area in which, within the range of technically competent practice, important choices remain—is not something merely subjective and professionally value neutral. Instead, the dentist must learn from experience whether a particular pattern of practice is one that he or she is able to effectively habituate and is therefore one that the dentist wants to have as part of his or her habitual way of practicing. Such judgments are not only objectively significant for professionally adequate dental practice from the dentist's point of view. They are clearly of real value to patients as well and are, in fact, of far greater value to patients than patients themselves are likely to realize. Therefore, our account of dentistry's Central Practice Values must include these patterns of practice because of the subtle but significant benefits they bring about for patients. To take one example, many dentists recommend an implant to replace a missing tooth instead of a bridge, especially in those cases where the teeth adjoining the space where the missing tooth was are unrestored and have adequate bone support. Such dentists believe that this is the more conservative approach to the situation because, in addition to other benefits, there is then no need to remove healthy enamel on the adjoining teeth that would be used as abutments for the bridge. But there are disadvantages to utilizing a tooth implant: perhaps a greater overall cost to the patient, the need for the patient to undergo a surgical intervention, and a wait—sometimes more than six months—for the first stage to heal. Either approach and a few others fall within the standard of care. In practice, though, a dentist will ordinarily make a recommendation—one way or the other—according to his or her best judgment of the relative weight of these benefits and disadvantages and how experienced he or she is in doing implants—that is, the extent to which the dentist has mastered and thus habituated the details of this procedure. This experience-based preference is an example of a Preferred Pattern of Practice.

The same is true, at a different level of generality, of what is sometimes called a dentist's philosophy of practice. Dentists who practice in a technically competent manner differ not only in their choices regarding particular elements of dental practice, such as choice of hand instruments or disinfectants or how to approach a three-unit bridge, but dentists can also choose different "philosophies" of dental treatment within the range of technically competent practice.

For example, one dentist may do everything possible to save and work with natural teeth, refusing to extract a natural tooth unless there is no other clinically acceptable option and, in all other cases, referring any patient who is unhappy with so narrow a range of clinical options to other dentists. Another dentist may be less restrictive in this regard, urging the patient to preserve natural teeth but being willing to provide any technically acceptable form of treatment that the patient might choose. Yet another may routinely present the technically acceptable treatment options for a given oral condition as being equally commendable. So long as all three of these dentists are functioning within the range of technically acceptable practice, none of them is in violation of the Central Practice Values of Life and General Health and of Oral Health. (It is also true, however, that different dentists may have different opinions about what constitutes "technically acceptable practice." In general, if it is determinable, the proper criterion here will be the judgment of the dental community as a whole.)

A dentist's philosophy of practice is a drawing together of many narrower choices within the range of what is considered technically competent, and it focuses and determines those choices in a number of ways in practice. Like the more technical choices already discussed, a dentist's philosophy of practice affects dental practice through becoming habituated so that fundamental questions about the proper goals of dentistry—within the range of what is technically competent—do not have to be debated by the dentist in regard to every patient. For the same reasons already given, then, respect for a dentist's choice of philosophy of practice is also part of the Central Practice Value under discussion here.

In a similar way, each dentist must determine the type of setting he or she is able to practice in most effectively and, having identified it, proceed to habituate his or her interactions with the elements of that setting. The preferred setting for many dentists is the typical dental office, but there are many different kinds of these: solo practices where the dentist does all of the oral health work personally; solo practices where the dentist is assisted at chairside by a dental assistant; practices that include the services of a dental hygienist; practices that include a number of dentists, which in turn come in a variety of organizational arrangements; public health and military dental practices; and so on. A dentist's goal in choosing from among these options—even when the most desirable of these for a given individual may not be available to a young dentist starting out—is the practice setting in which he or she is most "comfortable," meaning in which he or she is most able to habituate his or her most effective modes of dental care for patients.

All of these kinds of choices of habitual patterns of practice, provided they are within the range of what is judged technically competent by the dental profession as a whole, will here be called Preferred Patterns of Practice. The relative importance of this Central Practice Value in comparison with the other five values will be discussed below.

Aesthetic Values

A dentist who paid no attention to the oral and facial appearance of patients or to their judgments about their oral and facial appearance would surely be failing professionally because one's oral and facial appearance ordinarily has important connections to the psychological components of General Health. But there are also accepted standards of form within dentistry (regarding the size of teeth, their shape, color, placement, and so on) over and above considerations that are directly related to General and Oral Health. These are standards that the dental profession subscribes to and that a dentist learns initially in dental school and more fully through practice and contact with other dentists. Therefore, a dentist who paid no attention to these standards in his or her practice would also be failing professionally. Clearly, then, dentistry's Central Practice Values include Aesthetic Values.

It is important to note, however, the differences between these Aesthetic Values and patients' personal judgments of oral and facial appearance. For there is no single standard of appropriate appearance to which all patients or even the majority of patients adhere, even though a preference for teeth that are whiter than their natural color has become fairly widespread in recent years. In relation to patients' own aesthetic judgments, then, the dentist honors this Central Practice Value principally by guiding each patient to judge oral and facial appearance according to the patient's own aesthetic standards.

However, the dentist's interpretation of the larger community's standards of appearance should also play a role in determining what services to offer, for serious violation of the community's standards might have an impact on the patient's psychological well-being, which, as noted above, the dentist must consider as one element of the patient's General Health. Even more importantly, acting on the patient's judgments of good appearance never justifies doing serious damage to healthy teeth because Oral Health is more important professionally than Aesthetic Values. This conflict will sometimes create difficult judgment calls: for example, the determination of whether to remove part of a tooth to make it whiter or to apply gold or a gem to a tooth solely because the patient has a positive aesthetic or cosmetic judgment about increasing its whiteness or adding gold or a gem. There is no standard set by the profession that is currently operative in matters of a patient's own cosmetic judgments except that of honoring the patient's choice unless bringing it about would be harmful to the patient.

But there is still an accepted standard, or set of standards, within the dental profession regarding the proper and natural shaping of a restoration and numerous other matters of form, color, and function in restorative work, prosthetic work, and many other aspects of dentistry. Some of these standards may be relevant to Oral Health, but many of these aesthetic standards pertain specifically to form or color and function independently from the context of Oral and General Health. Nevertheless, these accepted standards constitute an objective criterion for judging practice—*objective* because these are the actually accepted criteria for practice within the dental community in our society.

A number of other ethical concerns relating both to the relative priority of aesthetic values, especially when they compete with dentistry's other Central Practice Values, and to other aspects of dentistry's professional ethics will be examined in chapter 13.

Efficiency in the Use of Professional Resources

Efficiency is a common value, so it might not seem to have any more importance for the professional practice of dentistry than it has for any other occupation. But it does in fact have a special place in dental practice. The larger society has expended a lot of resources over time to support the development of the dental profession's expertise and the specialized physical resources used by dentists to care for patients. The larger society has also made subtle investments of other sorts in establishing dentistry's special social authority in matters of oral health and in according dentistry and its members the social power that accompanies such authority. These investments have been made within society's many educational, research, political, and civic groups in order to respond to a certain set of important human needs. The social importance of these needs and of the resources the larger society has expended to meet them, plus the fact that the professional resources of dental expertise, time, energy, and the physical resources of dental practice are not in unlimited supply and the fact that special effort has been necessary to make them available at all, indicate that a dentist who used these resources to no particular good or who squandered them thoughtlessly, even when pursuing an appropriate benefit for a patient, would be acting unprofessionally. And the same is true, for parallel reasons, of every other profession.

Of course, few dentists would seriously consider wasting professional resources in this way because a dentist's living—like that of the members of other professions—depends on him or her doing professional work efficiently. But one reason for including Efficiency in the Use of Professional Resources among a profession's Central Practice Values is that, for the reasons just mentioned, such efficiency is not only a matter of self-interest for the dentist but also an obligation to the larger society. This value, furthermore, is owed to the dentist's own patients, both in terms of how they are cared for by the dentist and in their capacity as members of the larger society who are dependent on the effective utilization of the profession's resources in order to receive oral health care at all. But this leaves us with the question of how important Efficiency in the Use of Professional Resources is in comparison with dentistry's five other Central Practice Values and how important they are in comparison with one another. That is the topic of the next section.

RANKING DENTISTRY'S CENTRAL PRACTICE VALUES

What is the proper ranking of these six Central Practice Values? Does one or another of them consistently take precedence over some or all of the others?

In some dental practice judgments, the ranking of these values will not be very important because all Central Practice Values that are achievable in the situation can be achieved simultaneously without diminishing any one of them in the process. But when two or more of these values are simultaneously at stake and the alternative interventions available to the dentist are such that these several values cannot all be maximized at once—that is, when the Central Practice Values of dentistry conflict with one another by pointing to mutually exclusive courses of action—then the question of whether they are ranked in priority and therefore form a hierarchy of importance becomes crucial to acting in accord with a dentist's professional commitments.

To stimulate careful discussion of these issues, the following ranking of the six Central Practice Values is proposed, beginning with the most important:

1. The Patient's Life and General Health

2. The Patient's Oral Health

3. The Patient's Autonomy

4. The Dentist's Preferred Patterns of Practice

5. Aesthetic Values

6. Efficiency in the Use of Professional Resources

The following discussion identifies our reasons for proposing this particular ranking of these values as normative for dental practice.

Let's begin with the first value. A dentist who recommended a treatment that involved significant risk to a patient's life or severely compromised a patient's general health—or who ignored or denied such a risk for the sake of any of the other values among dentistry's Central Practice Values—would be acting unprofessionally. In fact, the only circumstances in which a dentist might ethically recommend a treatment posing serious risk to the life or health of a patient are those in which the oral condition to be treated itself poses significant risks to life or health of that patient and the proposed dental treatment would diminish those risks. That is, risk to Life or General Health via dental interventions is justifiable only for the sake of Life or General Health itself. Consequently, it is clear that the patient's Life and General Health is the highest ranking of the Central Practice Values of dentistry.

The patient's Oral Health—that is, appropriate and pain-free oral functioning—is the dental value appealed to most frequently in dental practice; it is the second or next-most important value that dentists are committed to achieving for their patients. Relatively minor trade-offs of oral function may be acceptable for the sake of the patient's Autonomy or Aesthetic Values and possibly for Efficiency in the Use of Resources. But a dentist who accepted a trade-off that would leave a patient with significantly impaired or painful oral function, even for the sake of values lower on the list, would be practicing unethically. Therefore, the patient's Oral Health ranks second on the hierarchy of Central Practice Values.

The relative importance of the patient's Autonomy in the hierarchy of Central Practice Values for dental practice is, in one respect, easy to state, but in several other respects it is a complex matter. If a patient asked a dentist to perform a procedure that, in the dentist's professional judgment, would significantly harm the patient's Oral Health or the patient's Life or General Health, and if the dentist acted on the patient's request out of respect for the patient's Autonomy and performed the procedure, the dentist would be acting unprofessionally. Instead, the dentist ought to refuse to act on the basis of the patient's autonomous choice if the action chosen would be contrary to the patient's Oral or General Health. It seems obvious, then, that the patient's Autonomy ranks lower in the hierarchy of Central Practice Values than both the patient's Oral Health and the patient's Life and General Health.

In addition, if there are alternative treatments for a patient that support the patient's Oral and General Health and the patient chooses one of these and then the dentist fails to respect the patient's autonomous choice among these alternatives in order to prioritize Aesthetic Values or Efficiency in the Use of Resources, it seems clear that the dentist would be acting unprofessionally. The latter values, though among dentistry's Central Practice Values, are nevertheless below the patient's Autonomy in the hierarchy.

The issue grows more complex, however, when the value of the patient's Autonomy is compared with value of the dentist's Preferred Patterns of Practice. In fact, some dentists hold that the dentist's Preferred Patterns of Practice has a higher position in the hierarchy of Central Practice Values than the patient's Autonomy, in spite of all the arguments (summarized in the previous chapter) about the great moral importance of respecting patient's Autonomy.

In examining this issue, however, it is important to remember that dentistry's Central Practice Values are the values that the profession is first of all committed to bringing about for patients, not for dentists themselves. That is, the value of the dentist's Preferred Patterns of Practice is not to be measured by how attached a dentist might be to his or her practice patterns but rather by the benefits it secures for patients. The previous section explained why a dentist's development of habituated patterns of practice that are referred to by the expression "preferred patterns of practice" is important to effective dental treatment. The relevant question here, then, is whether the fact that the dentist has a habit of practicing a certain way (i.e., a Preferred Pattern of Practice) is reason enough for the dentist to refuse to act on the basis of a patient's autonomous choice, provided that Oral and General Health are not put at risk by doing so.

Of course, there are situations in which the patient's Oral or General Health depends on the dentist's following a Preferred Pattern of Practice. That is, there are situations in which the value to the patient of a dentist's Preferred Pattern of Practice lies in its being necessary under the circumstances for the Oral or General Health of the patient rather than primarily in the value of the dentist's habituated, and therefore preferred, Patterns of Practice. But if the matter hinged solely on the relative importance to the patient of his or her Autonomy being respected compared with the value to the patient of the dentist following a Preferred Pattern of Practice, can a reasonable case be made for saying that the patient's Autonomy ranks higher in dentistry's Central Practice Values than the dentist's Preferred Patterns of Practice?

Suppose, for example, that it is part of Dr. Jones's philosophy of dental practice that she does not believe in amalgam buildups, even in situations in which this sort of restoration would be within the range of minimally acceptable treatments. In such cases, Dr. Jones prefers to place a gold or porcelain-fused-to-gold crown. Consequently, when clinical circumstances arise in which she needs to mention an amalgam buildup as a treatment option, she invariably mentions that she does not recommend or perform them and would therefore need to refer the patient to another dentist if the patient were to choose that option.

But consider Mr. Smith, whose regular dentist of many years has recently died. He is now in Dr. Jones's chair and is asking for an amalgam buildup rather than a more expensive crown because his previous dentist was willing to provide them. In this particular case, however, Dr. Jones is certain that the amalgam buildup would be unstable and would fracture in a short time. She therefore declines to provide it, not because she prefers alternative therapies but because, in this instance, it is the wrong therapy under the circumstances. That is, she believes it would be a violation of the Central Practice Value of Oral Health to provide Mr. Smith this treatment under these clinical circumstances, regardless of Mr. Smith's wishing it otherwise. In such a case, the Pattern of Practice may seem more important than the patient's Autonomy, but the amalgam buildup is primarily rejected not because it is not Dr. Jones's Preferred Pattern of Practice but because it jeopardizes Mr. Smith's Oral Health. Consequently, such situations do not resolve the question of whether the patient's Autonomy ranks higher on the hierarchy of dentistry's Central Practice Values than the dentist's Preferred Patterns of Practice.

But suppose Dr. Jones's preference for crowns in a case like this was the only reason she refused the buildup. Suppose, for example, that she knows she is very skilled at placing crowns and considers the lack of long-term endurance of amalgam buildups to be a less excellent form of dentistry, even though that would be an acceptable treatment under the circumstances. In other words, what if the matter hinged solely on the relative importance of the patient's Autonomy being respected compared with the value to the patient of the dentist following his or her Preferred Pattern of Practice? Can this be a reasonable case for arguing that the patient's Autonomy ranks higher in dentistry's Central Practice Values than the dentist's Preferred Patterns of Practice when the values of the patient's Oral and General Health are not significantly at risk?

The answer to this question seems to come from a point that has already been discussed, both in chapter 4 and again in the previous section. For the dentist may not ethically treat a patient capable of autonomous choice without the patient's participation in the choice, both because of the high value associated with respect for others' autonomy and because of the primacy of relating to the patient as interactively as possible. For these reasons, the patient's Autonomy ranks higher among dentistry's Central Practice Values than the dentist's Preferred Patterns of Practice.

This ranking does not prohibit the dentist from explaining his or her reasons for preferring one course of action to another, and the patient may need to be told that the treatment he or she is choosing will have to be provided by another dentist. Such explanations may, when taken into account by the patient, lead the patient to make a different choice. But what the dentist may not do in such circumstances is say—or even hint or suggest—that doing what the dentist prefers is necessary from the point of view of the patient's Oral or General Health, since that is not true.

Regarding Aesthetic Values, it is not clear—though it may be a close call—that the Aesthetic Values of the dental profession regarding the size of teeth, their shape, color, placement, and so on are of greater benefit to patients than the *value to the patient* of the dentist's Preferred Patterns of Practice. There may well be situations in which, for example, the proper shaping of a restoration will be of such sufficient importance that the dentist is required to make an exception to his or her Preferred Patterns of Practice. But the reason for the exception in such cases will almost always be based on the value of the patient's Oral Health rather than on the value to the patient of dentistry's standards for specifically Aesthetic Values.

Moreover, it seems reasonable to propose that the intrinsic value of the *patient's* judgments of oral and facial appearance, for which there is no objective standard, makes them less significant in the dentist's efforts to benefit the patient than the continued capacity of the dental professional to apply his or her expertise for the patient's benefit through Preferred Patterns of Practice. The latter benefits are of objective value to the patient and therefore they seem more important than the patient's more subjective judgments of Aesthetic Value. For this reason, Aesthetic Values, both those of the dental profession and those of dentistry's patients, rank below the dentist's Preferred Patterns of Practice in the hierarchy of dentistry's Central Practice Values.

However, when a patient is seeking a dentist's assistance specifically to achieve the patient's aesthetic goals for his or her teeth, it is most often the case that a refusal by the dentist to work for a particular outcome on aesthetic grounds will conflict not only with the patient's aesthetic judgment but also with the patient's Autonomy. In such situations, it is the value of the patient's Autonomy that is being compared with Aesthetic Values, and, for the reasons stated above, the patient's Autonomy is the more important of the Central Practice Values at stake in the situation. A dentist is, however, not only professionally justified but required to decline to carry out a patient's choice of aesthetic interventions if the dentist judges that doing so would violate the value of the patient's Oral Health or the patient's Life and General Health, for these Central Practice Values clearly outrank both the patient's Autonomy and Aesthetic Values.

The remaining question about the hierarchy of Central Practice Values concerns the relative ranking of Aesthetic Values and the value of Efficiency in the Use of Professional Resources. Here at the bottom end of the hierarchy, it may be that the ranking of these last two values is again a close call. But the conduct of a dentist who would pay no attention to the profession's accepted Aesthetic Values or who would not attend to a patient's valuation of a particular aspect of facial appearance solely to avoid expending the resources of the profession that would be involved seems inappropriate. That is, if none of the higher-ranking Central Practice Values were at stake in a given practice situation, then the proposal being made here is that Aesthetic Values take priority over a general commitment not to waste professional resources. The reason for this is that Aesthetic Values are among the Central Practice Values that dentistry is committed to furthering for patients; it follows that employing resources to accomplish Aesthetic Values is not a waste.

Of course, it is possible to imagine a situation in which an unusual amount of professional resources will be necessary to achieve dentistry's aesthetic standards or to accomplish a patient's aesthetic goals but in which accomplishing this would not violate the four higher-ranking Central Practice Values for the patient. The relevant question about such a case is whether dentistry's professional commitment to Aesthetic Values means that the dentist is professionally required (assuming also that the dentist is competent in the matter and that the aesthetic improvement is justifiable) to undertake whatever expenditure of professional resources is necessary to achieve this aesthetic improvement. It is hard to imagine such a case in which none of the other four Central Values of Dental Practice are at stake. But if such a case arose, would it be professionally acceptable for the dentist to refuse to work for the relevant aesthetic improvement for the patient solely on the grounds that too many professional resources would be required?

The best answer to this question, provided it is understood this narrowly to focus on the ranking of dentistry's Central Practice Values, seems to be yes. That is, using professional resources to accomplish a genuine aesthetic improvement for a patient is not a waste of professional resources, and therefore Aesthetic Values rank above Efficiency in the Use of Professional Resources in the hierarchy of Central Practice Values. Even if there were a case in which the other four Central Practice Values were not at stake, however, it is extremely difficult to imagine that other norms of dental practice would not be relevant, especially the Relative Priority of the Patient's Well-being. Chapter 6 will discuss such matters in detail, including how much sacrifice of personal effort and other personal resources a dentist is required to commit to the well-being of his or her patients which will affect the degree of sacrifice required by the primacy of patients' well-being when only lower-ranking values in the hierarchy of Central Practice Values are affected. But answering these questions correctly will not challenge the claim being made here— namely, that Efficiency in the Use of Professional Resources should be considered the sixth ranking value in the hierarchy of dentistry's Central Practice Values.

Anyone who is concerned about professional ethics in dental practice should carefully consider the theme of the Central Practice Values of dental practice. They should examine proposed accounts of the content of the values identified here as dentistry's Central Practice Values as well as the ranking of the six offered here. They should ask, first, whether any of dentistry's Central Practice Values have been omitted from the list and, second, whether the proposed ranking of these values for dental practice is incorrect or admits of important exceptions.

THINKING ABOUT THE CASE

Now we can apply this proposal about the hierarchy of Central Practice Values of dental practice to the case presented at the beginning of the chapter.

First of all, Dr. Luban's question about Mrs. Kirchland's current capacity for autonomous choice, given her anxieties about money, is an appropriate question to ask. For, as has been explained, the dental professional's proper relationship to a capable person differs significantly from his or her proper relationship to a patient with diminished capacity to participate in decision-making, and, as chapter 7 will explain, profound fear can diminish a person's capacity for autonomous choice. So Dr. Luban's question about Mrs. Kirchland's current capacity is ethically appropriate. This question is not one that can be directly resolved by referring to the hierarchy of dentistry's Central Practice Values. But it is, nevertheless, related to at least one of these values.

It is important to note, then, that Dr. Luban has known Mrs. Kirkland for many years. He has heard Mrs. Kirkland's continuing concerns on many occasions about finances and her need, in her judgment, to be satisfied with "the cheapest and simplest." If Mrs. Kirkland's fears in this regard should be examined from the point of view of her capacity for autonomous decision-making, then Dr. Luban should already have been addressing them out of a concern for her autonomy. But if, from his previous experience with her, he judges that these fears have not been signs of diminished capacity for decision-making in the past, then—unless he sees some dramatic change in Mrs. Kirkland in this regard—these fears cannot be consistently viewed as marks of diminished capacity in the present situation. Nor, obviously, can the mere fact that a patient chooses less-than-optimal therapy or therapy different from that recommended by the health professional be taken as conclusive evidence of the patient's incapacity for autonomous choice. Therefore, in the absence of additional evidence of the patient's lack of capacity for decision-making, which the case does not provide, Dr. Luban must judge Mrs. Kirchland to be as capable of autonomous choice as she has ever been.

To focus now on the contribution of dentistry's Central Practice Values to Dr. Luban's ethical thinking about the case, consider that Mrs. Kirchland is presently in "severe pain," pain serious enough that she has asked for an emergency appointment (and did so in spite of her limited financial resources). In fact, Mrs. Kirchland is very likely to be far more interested, at this moment, in relief of her pain than in any other benefit that Dr. Luban could offer, including the long-term treatment of this tooth.

Thus, the value of the patient's Life and General Health (which also includes pain-free functioning), the value of the patient's Oral Health, and the third-ranking value of the patient's Autonomy all require Dr. Luban to first of all address Mrs. Kirchland's emergent pain. In addition, it is likely that she will be able to make a thoughtful choice among the available long-term therapies only when she is out of serious pain.

Dr. Luban may have a strong preference that Mrs. Kirchland settle on a treatment plan during this visit rather than rescheduling her for a visit that might well be only a consultation to resolve the question of treatment. However, even if Dr. Luban is able to provide quick relief of her pain, Mrs. Kirchland's state of mind may not be well suited to moving directly into conversation about expensive long-term treatments. Thus, Dr. Luban's Preferred Patterns of Practice may have to give way to his efforts to support Mrs. Kirchland's Autonomy—to help her make as autonomous a choice in this matter as she can. That may require scheduling an appointment on another day.

On the other hand, since Mrs. Kirchland has been squeezed into a full day of patients, Dr. Luban may prefer to reschedule her before determining the long-term treatment for this tooth. What if, in that case, she wanted to hear about the pros and cons of the different therapies right away and make a decision while still in the chair? In such a scenario, it is not only Mrs. Kirchland's autonomy that is at stake but also her oral health and possibly her general health, as well as the autonomy of a number of other patients. Dr. Luban has obligations to the patients in the other operatories and to those in the waiting room, not just to the patient before him in the chair. There is no clear guideline for dentists to use in ranking the competing needs of different patients. The priorities of General and Oral Health do require that emergencies be addressed. However, among nonemergency patients, including Mrs. Kirchland after pain relief has been administered, rules of thumb like "patients with appointments get priority" and "first come first served" are reasonable but do not completely resolve the question of how a dentist should distribute his or her time and energy among them. Arguably, as long as each patient's General and Oral

Health and Autonomy are being adequately served, a dentist may distribute time and energy as he or she chooses. But it is worth asking if this is the proper way to understand this matter.

To change the scenario somewhat, suppose that Dr. Luban is able to provide Mrs. Kirchland with quick relief of her pain by perhaps a pulpectomy and medication, but she proves able to return later the same day during the time of a canceled appointment. Now unburdened by pain, she is ready to work out a long-term treatment plan. But her financial situation has not improved (and in fact is now worse, since she owes something for the emergency appointment and pain relief). What guidance could Dr. Luban receive from the proposed hierarchy of Central Practice Values for the conversation with Mrs. Kirchland?

First, given the hierarchy of dentistry's Central Practice Values, Dr. Luban may not recommend or do anything he believes would violate Mrs. Kirchland's General or Oral Health. (The norm of Competence requires, of course, that his judgment be well informed and that he not undertake anything that is beyond his level of competence.) Second, the value of the patient's Autonomy requires that Dr. Luban explain to Mrs. Kirchland all of the treatments, including the option of no treatment, if appropriate, that are at least minimally adequate responses to Mrs. Kirchland's needs, where adequacy is judged by the standards of dental professionals in our society generally. He must explain these alternatives in language she can understand, both in terms of the treatment and likely outcome and in terms of the likelihood of possible complications, accompanying pain or discomfort, and costs. All of this is well known.

But the value of the patient's Autonomy, like the ideal of an Interactive Relationship, requires more than just informing the patient of these matters. As explained in the previous chapter, it also requires that, to the extent possible given the time, human, and other resources available, Dr. Luban not only must not violate Mrs. Kirchland's Autonomy but also must work to *enhance* it. In the case at hand, one of the chief hindrances to maximizing Mrs. Kirchland's Autonomy is her financial situation. Whether he has addressed this issue previously or not, Dr. Luban needs to determine if there is anything he can do to address this difficulty so she can choose more autonomously.

One possibility Dr. Luban could offer Mrs. Kirchland is a payment plan to reduce the financial impact of her choice. Perhaps he could make adjustments to the cost of the more expensive options, especially for the treatment of choice. Perhaps he could make even greater sacrifices, providing treatment at cost or less than that, accepting day care services in partial or complete payment for the needed dental care, or other options. The hierarchy of Central Practice Values does not provide definitive guidance to Dr. Luban about which of these alternatives he ought to undertake, partly because the questions at issue include the question of how much sacrifice of other considerations a dentist is professionally committed to undertake in order for his or her patients to receive the best possible treatment. This question, the question of the Relative Priority of Patients' Well-being, will be addressed in the next chapter. But, in any case, simply offering her the needed information and waiting for her to consent will not be enough. The value of Mrs. Kirchland's Autonomy within the hierarchy of dentistry's Central Practice Values most assuredly requires Dr. Luban to at least *ask himself* these questions to see what options are available to him to *enhance*, not merely refrain from violating, her capacity for autonomous choice.

Third, a patient's Oral Health depends significantly on correctly understanding relevant facts. Mrs. Kirchland apparently views herself as quite elderly, and her comment that the cheapest and simplest will have to do suggests that she does not recognize that, at sixty-eight, she could easily need her teeth to be functional for another fifteen to twenty years. Consequently, the Central Practice Value of the patient's Oral Health requires Dr. Luban to try educate her—probably gently, but the manner depends on the particular patient, dentist, and their relationship—about these facts. In addition, he should try to do this independently of the particular treatment decision at hand. He should try to guide her to rethink her whole view of herself as being at the end of her life and challenge her view that care of her teeth, and perhaps other aspects of her health (since the Central Practice Value of the patient's Life and General Health is also at stake in her views about herself), is not as important as it used to be.

Finally, to take up the hardest aspect of this case, suppose that Dr. Luban and Mrs. Kirchland have a long and careful conversation about all these matters, and suppose that at its conclusion Mrs. Kirchland chooses a treatment that is inconsistent with Dr. Luban's philosophy of dental practice. Suppose, for example, that she chooses the extraction and partial denture rather than endodontic therapy, and suppose that Dr. Luban, in a way that the original case did not indicate, is strongly committed to preserving natural teeth. Suppose, for example, that he strongly prefers that patients who are candidates for endodontic therapy but who do not choose it be referred to other dentists who provide a form of treatment that is within the standard of care but contrary to his philosophy of practice. Does the hierarchy of Central Practice Values provide any guidance to Dr. Luban in this sort of situation?

If respect for Dr. Luban's Preferred Patterns of Practice, including his philosophy of practice, ranks below Mrs. Kirchland's Autonomy on the hierarchy of Central Practice Values, as the account of Central Practice Values given in this chapter proposes, this might seem to require that Dr. Luban provide a treatment that violates his philosophy of practice. But it is important to remember the setting in which Mrs. Kirchland seeks treatment for her tooth. In most urban areas of North America, the majority of people have fairly ready access to a large number of general dentists. In such a setting, Mrs. Kirchland could receive treatment consistent with her own choice from a dentist who does not share the philosophy of practice now attributed to Dr. Luban. In fact, there are probably specific dentists to whom Dr. Luban refers patients under just these circumstances, dentists whom Dr. Luban trusts and who also understand Dr. Luban's reasons for the referral. Because of the ready availability of dentists with different philosophies of practice, it may be the case that neither Mrs. Kirchland's Autonomy nor Dr. Luban's Preferred Patterns of Practice need to be compromised.

But suppose other dentists were not conveniently available, or suppose the treatment at issue was an emergency treatment so that there was not time to refer the patient to a dentist with a different philosophy of practice or that Dr. Luban could only recommend dentists who would not offer her a payment plan that she could afford. In any case, the setting would not eliminate the conflict between Dr. Luban's Preferred Patterns of Practice and Mrs. Kirchland's Autonomy. What ought Dr. Luban do then?

If the account of the hierarchy of Central Practice Values offered in the previous section correctly represents the content of the dental profession's norms in our society at this time, then in a situation of this sort, Dr. Luban would be professionally required to act according to it. First, if the situation were an emergency or other practitioners were not available, then dentistry's Central Practice Values of the patient's Life and General Health and the patient's Oral Health would require Dr. Luban to personally address Mrs. Kirchland's needs rather than delaying her care by trying to refer her to another dentist. Second, if several treatments were within the range of technically acceptable treatments for Mrs. Kirchland's condition, then the value of the patient's Autonomy requires that all of them be presented to her for choice. Dr. Luban may appropriately explain his reasons for strongly preferring one of these modes of treatment over the others, but if all are within the range of what is acceptable to the dental profession at large, then Dr. Luban is required to explain that fact to Mrs. Kirchland as well so she has a clear understanding of all the alternatives available to her.

But if, under these constrained circumstances where another dentist is not reasonably available to assist Mrs. Kirchland, she chooses a mode of therapy inconsistent with Dr. Luban's philosophy of practice, the priority ranking of the patient's Autonomy over the dentist's Preferred Patterns of Practice requires him to provide the treatment she chooses if it is within his competence. (If it were not within his minimum level of competence, of course, he should not indicate that it is available in his practice in the first place, although his own minimum level of competence and the availability under other, nonemergency circumstances from other dentists probably should be mentioned.) Because Mrs. Kirkland needs treatment that, on these assumptions, cannot be delayed or sent elsewhere, Dr. Luban cannot ethically refuse to provide this treatment (because of the highest ranking Central Practice Values of the patient's Life and General Health and the patient's Oral Health), and he cannot ethically require Mrs. Kirchland to accept the treatment he prefers if he is competent to perform other modes of treatment that are within the standard of care and she chooses one of them (because the value of the patient's Autonomy, as it is proposed here, ranks higher than the value of the dentist's Preferred Patterns of Practice).

In this way, the hierarchy of Central Practice Values does put constraints on the choices that a dentist can professionally make, although the circumstances in which these constraints will be felt may vary for dentists in different parts of our society. Of course, this discussion has not resolved the question of what counts as convenient accessibility of another dentist with a different philosophy of practice. If, for example, this scenario were carried out in a rural setting where the next dentist might be very far away, Dr. Luban's professional ethical deliberations would have to include a fair resolution of this accessibility question before he could determine whether or not professional ethics require him to perform a treatment contrary to his philosophy of practice.

It also needs to be pointed out that conflicts can arise *within* the scope of each of these Central Practice Values. All health professionals encounter situations in which different aspects of a person's General Health are in conflict, and both cannot be satisfied at the same time or to the same degree. Conflicts of this sort commonly arise for dentists regarding patients' Oral Health as well. A partial or complete denture may well involve some loss of comfort and function, even compared with the natural teeth that need to be extracted because they are compromised in some other way, but this loss is necessary to maintain the most important aspects of function that the natural teeth can no longer provide or could provide only at the risk of systemic infection.

Thus, it should not be surprising that conflicts will arise between different elements of other values in the hierarchy. For some patients, for example, a dentist may be able to preserve his or her range of clinical alternatives only by applying strong psychological pressure to get a patient to practice appropriate oral hygiene. One aspect of a patient's Autonomy, being free of psychological pressure about hygiene, is in conflict with another aspect of his or her Autonomy—that is, the opportunity to choose to keep his or her natural teeth functional.

The same could be true in regard to a dentist's philosophy of dental practice. Suppose Mrs. Kirchland was not a long-time patient of Dr. Luban's but a patient he has never seen before who came to his office because of her emergency. After he has relieved her pain, Dr. Luban's philosophy of practice may direct him to offer only endodontic therapy with a post and crown, with the indication that he will refer Mrs. Kirchland to another dentist if she chooses a treatment option that does not preserve her natural teeth. But his philosophy of practice may also include a strong preference for educating patients to practice effective self-care and to establish a continuing relationship with one dentist over years; this would be specifically for the sake of both continuity of care and the value of educating patients to promote better oral self-care over time. Suppose Mrs. Kirchland indicates very quickly, while Dr. Luban is still addressing her pain and explaining her situation, that she would value a stable relationship with a dentist and that she, in fact, trusts Dr. Luban and hopes he will accept her as his regular patient. But suppose she also resists his recommendation of endodontic therapy.

In this situation, two elements of Dr. Luban's philosophy of practice are in conflict. This is due to the particular facts of Mrs. Kirchland's situation and the particular stance that she, in the exercise of her autonomy, is taking. Dr. Luban can act on his commitment to preserve natural teeth and refer a different treatment to her with the hope that she will establish a stable relationship with the recommended dentist, but in doing so he would need to recognize that he, himself, is not establishing a stable relationship with a patient willing to do so. Or, he can choose to work toward a continuing relationship with this patient and, in doing so, perform a treatment that he prefers not to perform. Although neither of these choices is ideal, either of them is still professionally justifiable. As long as a higher-ranking Central Practice Value of dental practice is not violated in such choices, either element of the dentist's philosophy of practice may be chosen over the other.

There is no simple algorithm that can guide judgments in such matters. What is admirable about the dental profession is that it is committed to conduct in accord with certain norms and, among them, to a certain set of Central Practice Values. The account of these values offered here is certainly not the last word about them. It is hoped that this account will stimulate careful reflection and discussion, within the dental profession and in the larger community, and that such reflection and discussion will lead to an increasingly clearer understanding of dentistry's Central Practice Values. Even the clearest account of dentistry's Central Practice Values and the other norms of dental practice, however, will not eliminate the need for careful thinking and conscientious judgment in the face of each unique set of circumstances that daily practice produces.

6

❈❈❈❈❈❈

Ethical Decision-Making and Conflicting Obligations

CASE: HOW MUCH SACRIFICE?

When Dr. Sharon Sullivan returns from lunch around one o'clock, she notices a new patient in Operatory 2. "Who's in Op. 2?" she asks her hygienist, Elizabeth Minowski. "The day list says she's Edith Blake, but I don't recognize her."

"She's an emergency," Elizabeth explains, "says she's been in pain for three or four days, but it's obvious she hasn't seen a dentist in a long time. Every quadrant has caries and perio involvement. She lives at the Transition Home. Someone there sent her over."

"Where's the pain?" asks Dr. Sullivan.

"Upper left. I saw a large lesion in #13, but the gums are also swollen and red. She was squeezed in as an emergency patient before Mrs. Livingston at 1:15. I just glanced over her history form, introduced myself, and got her in the chair. I had a quick look when she was pointing out her problem, then I heard you come in. Do you want me to take radiographs and do the charting before you look at her?" asks the hygienist.

"No, Liz," says Dr. Sullivan. "Mrs. Livingston isn't here yet, so I might as well see her myself. But what do you mean they sent her over from the Transition Home? What's that?"

"The Salvation Army runs a home over on Third Street for women trying to get out of prostitution. I thought you knew about it. Carolyn Elward was a patient of ours before Dr. Bingley retired, and she used to be one of the supervisors there. Anyway, Ms. Blake is a resident at the Transition Home. She says her hall leader told her she should see a dentist when aspirin wasn't controlling her pain. She was sent here because she could walk here from there."

"Okay. When Mrs. Livingston gets here, have Jane explain to her that she may have a little wait because of a patient with an emergency," says Dr. Sullivan. "She's better in the waiting room than in a chair because she gets so anxious once she's back here in the operatory."

99

"Hello, I'm Dr. Sharon Sullivan," Dr. Sullivan says to Ms. Blake. "Ms. Minowski says you've been having quite a bit of pain in the top-left part of your mouth. What do you want us to do?"

"Yes, it's been hurting for three or four days, but this morning it got so bad that even aspirin wouldn't help it."

"Do you mind if we chat while I take a look around your mouth?"

"Oh no, go ahead, I already like you guys and I love to talk."

"How long is it since you've seen a dentist?"

"It's been a long time," says Ms. Blake. "Since I was in high school."

"How old are you now?" asks Dr. Sullivan.

"I'm twenty-six, so almost ten years, I guess."

"Well, I'm sorry to say, your teeth do have some problems."

"I'm not surprised," says Ms. Blake. "I really didn't take good care of myself for quite a long time. I was on the street, if you know what I mean, and I didn't care very much about things like that. Actually, I didn't care much at all what happened to me then, to be honest."

"I think I understand," answers Dr. Sullivan. "Ms. Minowski mentioned that you're staying at the Transition Home now. Is that helping you get a better hold of things?"

"Oh, yes," says Ms. Blake. "I feel safe there. I'm even starting to think it's worth it to take care of myself. The counseling, the other girls who live there, and the girls who finished the program and come back to talk with us all help a lot. They really know what it's like to be on the street and what it does to you and how you think about yourself. The Little Handbook they give out says the first goal for every girl is to restore her self-esteem, and I certainly need that."

"How long have you been living there?"

"I found out about it about three months ago and talked to them on the phone. But it's not easy to get off the street. You can't just walk away. But something told me I had to try it, and I went there five weeks ago and they accepted me into their program."

Meanwhile, Dr. Sullivan completes her examination. Besides the deep cavity in the upper-left second bicuspid that is very tender to touch and the likely cause of Ms. Blake's pain, there are other carious lesions in half a dozen other teeth and generalized periodontal involvement with deep pockets in several sites as well, plus several other areas that need a closer look once all the X-rays are taken. At first glance, though, it seems that all of the teeth are probably salvageable, but Ms. Blake clearly needs a lot of dental work. Dr. Sullivan excuses herself to see if Mrs. Livingston has arrived and to ask Ms. Minowski to take the needed X-rays.

"Excuse me for asking, Dr. Sullivan," says Ms. Minowski, "but have you talked to her about paying for this?"

"Actually, no, Liz," says Dr. Sullivan. "I was focused on getting the exam done before Mrs. Livingston got here, so I haven't even considered money yet. Since she is already in the chair, let's see what it will take to get her out of pain and then we can figure out the money part."

"That's why I mentioned she was from the Transition Home. I doubt she has money to pay for a lot of dental care," says the hygienist, "and she doesn't have a medical card or any insurance."

"And you were trying to clue me in by mentioning the Home?"

"Yes."

"Well, I appreciate the effort, but I didn't get the hint," says Dr. Sullivan. "Let's do the X-rays first so we know what we are talking about and I will get started with Mrs. Livingston."

Mrs. Livingston's checkup goes quickly, and Dr. Sullivan returns to the operatory to talk with Ms. Blake about what she has found during her examination. "I haven't had time to look at your X-rays to make sure there aren't any other problems that I can't see, but even if there aren't, it would take at least three or four visits to do a proper cleaning of all your teeth and then deal with the other large cavities that I can see just by looking. Then we would have to decide how much additional treatment you will probably need for the gum problems."

"I don't have that kind of money," says Ms. Blake. "I told the woman at the front desk that I didn't know if I could pay for this, but she said you wouldn't send me away in pain. Then you were so nice and talking with me that I forgot to say anything. I'm sorry."

"Well, I enjoy talking with you, too," says Dr. Sullivan, "and that's probably why I forgot to mention it myself. But you really do need to get your teeth fixed or you will have more bouts of pain and maybe something worse. We could arrange a long-term payment plan so you wouldn't have to pay a lot of money right away. We do that with many of our patients."

"The work I do at the Home helps pay my room and board. I only get $30 a week for spending money from that. That's what I brought to pay for this appointment. I just got paid this morning. I hope it's enough. If I do well in the program, the Home will help me find a real job after three months. All the girls who have left the Home have left with real jobs, and the Home helps them find an apartment and then they come back for counseling and to help the girls who are still there. But I won't be able to do that for at least two more months or maybe more."

"I don't want to take your $30, Ms. Blake," Dr. Sullivan says. "If you can stay for a while this afternoon, I will work around the other patients in my schedule and take care of the big cavity in your upper-second bicuspid because that's probably what's causing your pain. I won't need to charge you for that if you can stay here and I can fit it in between my other patients."

"That's very kind of you, doctor. You really should take some payment for that, even if it isn't close to enough. I really appreciate it," says Ms. Blake.

"My real concerns," says Dr. Sullivan, "are your other teeth. You will be in here again in no time if they aren't attended to, and your teeth need a good cleaning so you can start taking proper care of them again. They're worth it and so are you."

"Well, I will start brushing them like I am supposed to, but they hurt and bleed when I do. Anyway, I really couldn't pay for a lot of appointments, and it isn't fair for you to have to do all that work for nothing. I think it will just have to wait until I get on my feet."

"I really don't think that would be the best thing for you," says Dr. Sullivan. "Let me think about it. My next patient is here now. I will be back to work on that cavity as soon as I can. Do you mind hanging around? In the meantime, I will ask Ms. Minowski to do a basic cleaning, just to get you started."

"Will you at least take my $30?" asks Ms. Blake. "I'm sure it's nowhere near enough, but I want to be fair to you, and you have already been too kind to me."

"Let me think about that," says Dr. Sullivan. "I'll be back in a little while. I'll get Ms. Minowski in here shortly."

Dr. Sullivan actually has a lot to think about. First, there is the financial question, not just about the $30 but also about Ms. Blake's need for considerable dental work. For now, let's set aside the possibility of Medicaid benefits, which vary from state to state and from one time to another. One obvious possibility would be for Dr. Sullivan to accept a major financial loss and address all of this patient's dental needs in the best way possible for no payment or a little symbolic payment for each visit. Or she could find a way to help her some but not provide the best possible care—for example, by using composite buildups instead of crowns so that it would be less of a loss for her. Or maybe she should let Ms. Blake postpone the rest of the care she needs until she has a job and then work out a payment plan for at least some of it while taking the rest as a loss. Or she could just tell Ms. Blake what she needs and leave the decision up to her, regardless of whether the patient can afford it or not.

Besides that, Dr. Sullivan has seen some marks on Ms. Blake's arms that suggest she might have been an IV-drug user at some time, probably during her days on the streets, and bruises that might indicate previous instances of abuse. Dr. Sullivan wasn't comfortable raising these questions with Ms. Blake in this first visit. But a dentist's observations can raise potential questions about other risks to the patient that may or may not be appropriate to raise once a more lasting relationship between patient and dentist has been established. The possibility of Ms. Blake having become HIV positive also raises a question about whether this could involve risks for Dr. Sullivan and her staff if they were to treat her.

All in all, Dr. Sullivan has a lot of thinking to do. What level of charity care is she professionally obligated to provide for Ms. Blake? Are there limits to her professional obligations in a case like this? Are there things she could do that would be above and beyond the call of her professional obligations, and should she do them even though it is beyond what is required of her? And, for each of these options, are there other factors besides being an ethical professional that should impact how she weighs the pros and cons?

DIFFICULT PROFESSIONAL-ETHICAL JUDGMENTS

Many professional-ethical judgments are easy and straightforward and, like most actions in other areas of our lives, they are mostly the result of good habits; rarely do they need to be carefully thought out and self-consciously chosen each time they arise.

Of course, thoughtful people carefully examine their professional habits from time to time, as well as their other moral habits. As chapter 1 indicated, it is precisely reflection of this sort that legitimates the claim that actions done from habit are still rationally chosen actions, even though they are not the product of explicit deliberation in the situation. The examples used in this book, however, all focus on what a dental professional, thinking carefully about a particular case, might consider when determining how to act in the case. But this book also hopes to stimulate careful reflection on the reader's *habits* of professional conduct and ethical reflection. It is always good to ask, after thinking carefully about a particular case, whether what was learned in the case tells us anything valuable about habits that we have (or don't have) that impact our professional-ethical lives.

For all the centrality of habits in our moral and professional lives, though, there are three kinds of circumstances that can arise where determining *what one professionally ought to do* definitely requires explicit and careful deliberation on the alternatives at hand; these are (1) when a situation requires a professional to think about the limits of his or her professional obligations and, then, the extent to which he or she is committed to sacrificing other things for the sake of a patient, (2) when one's professional obligations are themselves in conflict, and (3) when a person's professional obligations conflict with other commitments or his or her obligations to other people.

The most difficult ethical dilemmas professionals ordinarily face involve one or more of these circumstances. Yet none of them has been discussed very carefully in the dental ethics literature or the literature on professional ethics generally. Discussing them here will not yield some tidy algorithm that readers can apply to resolve difficult ethical questions. This chapter aims, instead, to shed useful light on dentists' most difficult ethical decisions by first reflecting on the general structure of ethical thinking and then on the characteristics of each of these three sets of circumstances.

A MODEL OF PROFESSIONAL-ETHICAL DECISION-MAKING

When a dentist is faced with making an ethical decision in an unusual or ethically complicated situation, it can help a lot if the dentist has already reflected on the components of a carefully thought-out ethical decision. What will be proposed here, then, is a *model* of the steps of professional-ethical decision-making. Any model of decision-making is necessarily an oversimplification because it focuses on specific aspects of ethical thinking and treats them as separate "steps" of the decision-making process. In actual ethical reflection, these "steps" are highly interdependent and we do not completely finish Step Two, for example, before beginning Step Three. Instead, we move back and forth between the different steps, learning from one of them that we haven't adequately answered another and gathering data from one of them that proves informative for another, and so on. It is still worthwhile, though, to carefully separate and describe the several distinct kinds of thinking involved in ethical decision-making. This is because, when an ethical decision is particularly complex, having a kind of "road map" of the steps involved can often be very useful.

Step Zero: Getting the Facts

This model presumes that the person using it has already carefully identified all the relevant facts—that is, about the situation, the people involved, the possible actions that might be chosen, the probability and possible outcomes of these actions, and so forth. It would obviously be a mistake to learn the steps of this model and then use it without always stopping to ask, "Do I have all the facts I need, and have I understood them all correctly?" As with the other steps in this model, however, there is no assumption here that we always finish Step Zero completely and only then begin the rest of the process. Often our need to address the issues in a later step in the process requires us to "go back" and get some more facts or to check our facts again. This is because of factors we did not notice at first. This model will not, however, attempt to describe the methods that careful thinkers use to "get the facts" they need. Therefore, "Getting the Facts" will be considered "Step Zero" in this model of Professional-Ethical Decision-Making.

Step One: Identifying the Alternatives

Step One consists of determining what courses of action are available to choose between and then identifying their most important aspects. Sometimes options are obvious from the facts of the situation and do not require one to stop and think carefully about it. But at other times it can be difficult to see what the alternatives are. Certain circumstances about the situation, or our own habitual ways of perceiving and acting, can cloud our vision of what actions would be possible for us. So it is always useful to make a point of explicitly asking what courses of action are available to us and what would be the likely outcomes of each of these alternatives. In addition, we will often need to ask about each of our alternatives, what other choices, for ourselves and for others, are they likely to lead to. It is also important to ask, in most situations, how likely it is that the various possible outcomes and future choices that we can envision will actually occur.

Dentists are typically well trained to identify the clinical alternatives for a given patient's presenting condition. Professional-ethical decision-making requires that dentists also carefully identify the alternative ways in which the dentist might act in relating to the patient or other persons involved and in responding to other nonclinical aspects of the situation.

Step Two: Determining What Is Professionally Important

Once the alternative ways in which a dentist might respond to a situation have been carefully identified, the dentist needs to examine them from the point of view of what ought and ought not be done *professionally*. Each of the identified alternatives must be examined from this point of view. The criteria to be used in this step of the decision-making process are the ethical standards of one's profession (i.e., the content associated with each of the nine categories of professional obligation that were identified in chapter 3). The principal purpose of this book is to help readers come to a more detailed and more sophisticated understanding of dentistry's ethical standards so that determining what is professionally important about each of the alternatives and their likely outcomes can then be done with greater precision and professional confidence.

Step Three: Determining What Else Is Ethically Important

Each alternative must be examined specifically from the point of view of the broader criteria of what ethically ought and ought not be done. This step goes over and above the specific ethical standards of the person's professional life, for one's professional obligations never constitute the entire moral content of a person's life. Moreover, the professional standards themselves have become dentistry's professional standards for *certain reasons*; that is, they have been accepted by the profession and the larger community in dialogue as dentistry's ethical standards so that the dental profession and its members will serve their patients and the larger community well. Therefore, if in a given situation specific professional-ethical standards conflict with one another, or if they fail to adequately direct which possible action would be professionally and ethically best in the situation, then the *reasons* behind the specific ethical standards should be considered—that is, the thinking that goes into determining what constitutes dentistry's serving its patients and the larger community well. Situations will also arise when a dentist's other commitments conflict with his or her professional commitments; in these situations, even more fundamental moral categories will need to be considered.

The details of the thought process in such situations will depend on the particular approach that a person takes to ethical reflection in its "largest" or "deepest" sense. Ordinarily, at the most general level, people do their moral reflection chiefly in terms of maximizing certain values for certain people or possibly for everyone affected, conforming to certain fundamental moral rules, respecting certain fundamental rights, or actualizing certain human virtues. So the details of this process will ordinarily have one or the other of these structures, or it may combine several of them together.

Many professional-ethical decisions will not require the kind of ethical thinking described here as Step Three. This is because the decision can be properly made solely on the basis of the ethical standards of the dental profession. The careful professional-ethical thinker will make a point, though, of at least asking whether anything about the situation is ethically important in some other way or for some other reason.

Step Four: Determining What Ought to Be Done (Ranking the Alternatives)

The process of determining what is professionally important and, if needed, what is ethically important for other reasons will sometimes lead, without further effort, to the conclusion that one of the alternative courses of action is what ought to be done. At other times, matters will be more complex because the relevant professional standards, on the one hand, and other ethically important values, rules, rights, virtues, or other kinds of ethical reasons that you judge to be relevant, on the other hand, favor different courses of action. Then one's determination about what ought to be done becomes a careful judgment about which of these competing sets of ethical norms is more suited to be the determining factor in one's decision about the situation.

Trying to determine what ought to be done sometimes leaves a person with a choice between several equally superior alternatives. For example, one's leading alternatives can be functionally equal because of the person's inability or lack of time to get all the information needed to judge more carefully between them. Or the leading alternatives may be equal precisely in that, with regard to competing professional and ethical standards, neither is more suited than the other to be the determining factor in one's decision. In such cases of equally superior alternatives, one may morally choose either of them because they are equal in professional or ethical merit and they are superior to every other alternative considered.

When a person does carefully judge that several alternatives—that are ethically superior to all the others—are either equally suited to the situation or functionally equal because of lack of time or information, then the person must resolve the situation by *choosing* between them; the faculty of judgment will then have done the best it can under the circumstances. It is a presupposition of this model of professional-ethical decision-making that *choosing* to act in a certain way is a specific kind of activity that is distinct from the activity of professionally or ethically *judging* about possible ways of acting.

ON THE PRIORITY OF PATIENTS' WELL-BEING AND THE LIMITS OF PROFESSIONAL SACRIFICE

Most sociologists who have studied the institution of profession mention "commitment to service" as one of the essential features of professions. Similarly, most health professions describe themselves, in their codes of ethics and elsewhere, as giving priority to patients' interests or being in the service primarily of the patient. To cite one example, the preamble to the American Dental Association's (ADA's) *Principles of Ethics and Code of Professional Conduct* (hereafter ADA Code) begins: "The American Dental Association calls upon dentists to follow high ethical standards which have the benefit of the patient as their primary goal."

But expressions like "service to the public" and "benefit of the patient" as one's "primary goal" admit of many different interpretations with significantly different implications for actual practice. Four different interpretations of such expressions will be examined in this section in order to provide a framework for discussing the extent of dentists' professional-ethical obligations and the amount of sacrifice of other interests that a dental professional ought to undertake.

A Minimalist Interpretation

The dentist's commitment to serve could mean only that dental professionals have an obligation to consider the well-being of their patients when deciding how to act in particular situations and when forming the habits that shape their daily work with patients.

This statement has to be considered a Minimalist Interpretation of the professional commitment to serve because the patient's well-being would not have any special importance in the dentist's professional life if the dentist gave the patient any less consideration than this. But obviously, in this interpretation, the well-being of dentistry's patients would not be given priority over any other of the dentist's concerns. In fact, in this Minimalist Interpretation, only two situations would clearly violate a commitment to the priority of the patient's well-being. First, a dentist's *failure to consider the patient's well-being* when the patient's well-being would certainly be affected by that dentist's choice, and, second, a dentist *knowingly choosing an action that was detrimental to the well-being of the patient* and doing so for the sake of something the dentist truly thought was not very important at all. However, given how health professionals in general, and dentists in particular, view themselves, and given what the larger community routinely believes and expects about health professionals' obligations, it is clear in our society that dentists are regularly understood to be committed to giving some kind of *priority* to the patient's well-being in the decisions they make. Therefore, the Minimalist Interpretation is clearly an incorrect understanding of dentists' professional obligations. The same conclusion is supported by sociologists' research into the health professions. We must, therefore, set aside the Minimalist Interpretation and consider others more carefully.

The Maximalist Interpretation

At the opposite extreme is the Maximalist Interpretation. This is what the common expression "putting patients first" (stated in just this way, i.e., without any qualification) seems to be saying about dentist's professional obligations. In this interpretation, the commitment to the priority of the patients' well-being would mean that dental professionals are obligated to place the well-being of their patients *ahead of every other consideration*—that is, not only ahead of all their own other interests and concerns but also ahead of *every* other concern and obligation they might have regarding any other person or group. This is a very extreme view of the professional's obligation to serve others. It deserves examination here because the rhetoric of the professions—especially the phrase "putting patients first"—so often seems to be giving the public and dentists just this message.

This Maximalist Interpretation, however, cannot reasonably be the correct view of the dentists' professional obligations to their patients. There would be very few health professionals if the Maximalist Interpretation were to be taken as accurate, and people would obviously suffer greatly if this was the case. Moreover, few health professionals, and very few members of the larger community, actually believe that dentists—or any other health professionals—really are obligated to place their patients' well-being ahead of literally everything else in their lives. So the question about how much priority dentists owe to patients' well-being needs to be carefully examined, precisely because we know the correct answer cannot be that dentists are obligated to make everything—absolutely everything—subordinate to the well-being of their patients. This Maximalist Interpretation must also be set aside. We must now examine interpretations of the priority of the patient's well-being that fall between these two extremes.

The Parity Interpretation

One intermediate interpretation can be called the Parity Interpretation, where the word "parity" refers to the *equal* importance of the patient's well-being and the dentist's other valued concerns. In this interpretation, the dentist is professionally obligated to hold the patient's well-being to be *at least equal in importance to his or her own well-being and any other important concerns or responsibilities the dentist might have*. The dentist would thus be obligated to choose the patient's well-being over any aspect of his or her own well-being or other concerns that the dentist judged to be of *lesser* significance than the effects of the dentist's actions on the patient's well-being.

With this interpretation, it is important to note, the dental professional is ethically permitted to choose his or her own well-being or other valued concerns over that of the patient in any situation in which the aspects of well-being at stake for the patient and dentist are of equal importance. That is, if the effects of the dentist's action are equal in their impact on the patient and on whatever the dentist holds highly valuable, then, in the Parity Interpretation, the dentist is not professionally obligated to accord greater significance to the patient's well-being than to his or her own important concerns. In such a case the dentist would be choosing between ethically equal alternatives and may therefore ethically choose either one.

Consider using the Parity Interpretation in a situation where all other things are equal (i.e., an appropriate relationship with the patient is established, the patient is a capable, chooser, and so on) and two courses of treatment that are equally beneficial to patient (e.g., they are equally effective and involve equal risks or the differences in effectiveness are balanced out by the differences in risk, etc.), then a dentist could ethically recommend the one that yields the greater profit for the dentist if the dentist judged his or her financial well-being and the patient's financial well-being to be equally important. By a similar reasoning, a dentist might ethically decline to care for a patient with a serious infectious disease in order to protect himself or herself from serious infection or decline to see an emergency patient in severe pain and even refuse to take time to advise the patient on where to receive emergency care if doing so would make the dentist late for an important lunch with a close friend.

The reasons for thinking this interpretation is not a correct interpretation of dentistry's commitment to service, as it is currently understood in American society, are definitely more subtle than the reasons for rejecting the two extreme interpretations. But the way most members of the larger community would react to dentists who are thought to be acting—or who actually do act—along the lines of the examples just given is indicative of their rejection of this interpretation, and many dentists would react similarly. That is, dentists who act in these ways would be widely judged—by patients and the larger society and by many dentists as well—to be violating their professional commitments. As will be explained below, for example, dentists and health care providers generally are widely understood in our society to have undertaken an obligation to accept more-than-ordinary risk of infection if the patient's well-being requires it and if sufficiently important aspects of the patient's well-being are at stake in the matter.

Similarly, a dentist would ordinarily be considered to be acting unprofessionally if he or she recommended one professionally acceptable treatment over another simply to increase earnings. (The issues associated with charges, profit, dentistry as a business, and patients' access to health care resources will be examined more fully in chapters 10, 11, and 12.) Similarly, dentists are widely understood to have an obligation to provide emergency care or at least to direct the patient to receive it elsewhere. The point here is that these examples, and many others that could be cited, strongly indicate that the Parity Interpretation is not an adequate account of how our society and the dental community in dialogue understand the dentist's professional commitment to give some kind of special priority to the patient's well-being.

The Greater-Than-One's-Own-But-Within-Limits Interpretation

This clumsy name for the fourth interpretation of dentists' professional obligation to give priority to their patients' well-being is an effort to say that the correct interpretation of this obligation places the degree of obligation on the dentist's part somewhere between that of the Parity Interpretation and the Maximalist Interpretation. The Parity Interpretation clearly requires too little of the dentist; the Maximalist Interpretation clearly requires too much. The Greater-Than-One's-Own-But-Within-Limits Interpretation clearly does not obligate the dentist to sacrifice *every* aspect of his or her own interest and other commitments for the sake of the patient. Yet the dentist *is* obligated to assign *greater* importance to *certain aspects* of the patient's well-being than to his or her own, and the dentist is also obligated to assign greater importance to the patient's well-being than to *some* of the dentist's other concerns and his or her commitments regarding other people.

Can this rather vague idea be made any more precise? Not in any simple way. There is no simple formula for determining how much sacrifice the dentist as a professional is obligated to bear for the sake of his or her patient. As in all matters touching the ethics of the professions, though, there are two complementary ways of making general ethical standards more useful. One is to observe—and if possible discuss—the ways most ethically admirable members of a profession act and how they explain their choices. This mode of ethical learning was mentioned in chapter 1 and will be discussed in chapter 15. The second way to make general professional-ethical standards more precise and more useful is by examining, comparing, and seeking out common threads in relevant examples, especially examples in which there is general agreement among dentists and within the larger community. Three such examples were just discussed. Several more will be offered here.

In the United States, patients' access to needed dental care ordinarily depends either on their own ability to pay or on some third-party payment arrangements. Some patients, consequently, have very little access to dental care. In such a society, a dentist who did not offer charity care and was unwilling to offer payment plans and other flexible financial arrangements for treatment would likely be judged by most dentists and by the larger community to be acting unprofessionally. Only very special obligations—for example, to one's family—would justify making no professional sacrifice for the sake of meeting patients' dental needs when there are so many patients who cannot get their dental needs met without such assistance.

The larger community does not presume, though, that a dentist must make extreme financial sacrifices to fulfill this obligation. A dentist in our society is not obligated, for example, to ask his or her family to live in poverty in order to meet more patients' unmet dental needs. A dentist's or other health professional's family might, of course, choose to make additional sacrifices in order to provide more needy people with treatment. Such actions would be above and beyond the dentist's professional duty, however, and the health professional could not justifiably claim that such sacrifices were required by his or her professional commitments. (See chapters 11 and 12 about patients having or not having access to needed dental services.)

As a second example, dentists are surely obligated to make their services reasonably available to their regular patients for routine care. There are surely circumstances, though, in which it is ethical for dentists to close their practices to new patients, and dentists are not obligated to be available at all times for routine care, even to their regular patients. They are also not obligated to never make exceptions in their schedules for personal and family reasons, nor must they simply make themselves subject to the convenience and schedules of their patients. At the same time, though, there might be exceptions to some of these statements if the frame of reference were a geographical area with very few other dentists or in the event of a natural disaster or if other conditions transformed adequate dental care into a scarce resource. Under such circumstances, the special ethical considerations that apply to the just distribution of scarce health care resources might supersede what is ordinarily permissible for health professionals.

Every profession's ethical commitments include giving some kind of priority to the well-being of those whom the profession and its members serve. However, few professions have made any attempt to articulate, even in general terms, the kinds of sacrifices this professional commitment might require of the profession's members—that is, sacrifices of the professional's other interests and obligations to other people for the sake of those whom the profession serves. One legitimate reason for this reticence is that these norms can rarely be expressed as precise rules for conduct. The most that can be offered, ordinarily, is the kind of careful examination of potential interpretations of this ethical standard that has been offered here in the hope of identifying at least some general guidelines. Even this brief discussion should have made it clear, however, that in regard to dentistry dentists have made a commitment to the larger society to ordinarily—and almost always—place their own well-being and other important commitments second to that of the patient's well-being. In practice this means the dentist accepts significant professional sacrifices for the sake of the patient. At the same time, however, the dentist's obligation to do this is not unlimited or unqualified.

CONFLICTING PROFESSIONAL OBLIGATIONS

Efforts to articulate the norms of a profession and offer explicit guidance for resolving difficult ethical judgments by establishing relevant priorities will never be inclusive enough to resolve all conflicts between obligations that arise in professional practice. One set of conflicting obligations these norms will rarely resolve precisely is conflicts between the different elements of the dentist's professional commitment itself. For a dentist's professional obligations, as chapter 3 has explained, can be differentiated into nine fairly distinct categories, and there is nothing to guarantee that conflicts will not arise *between* a dentist's obligations from different categories.

Suppose, for example, a pediatric patient old enough to comprehend the need for care and the value of cooperation nevertheless behaves uncooperatively in the chair, and the reactions of the patient's parents exacerbate rather than improve the situation. A dentist's efforts to establish a relationship with the patient and with the patient's parents that is as close to the ideal Interactive Relationship as possible may be in conflict with the dentist's efforts simply to practice within the norm of Competence. Or, consider a dentist's efforts to maintain appropriate relationships with other dentists, his or her own staff, or other health professionals (which will be discussed in detail in chapter 8). These nonpatient relationship obligations can conflict with the dentist's efforts to maintain an Interactive Relationship with a patient. Similarly, giving proper priority to the patient's Oral Health in the face of other pressing considerations can also raise complex questions about what ought to be done, and so on.

Similarly, there is no guarantee that there will not be conflicts between obligations within the same category of professional norms. One category, the category of dentistry's Central Practice Values, as it has been proposed here, includes a hierarchical ranking of the six central values. Conflicts between different values in the hierarchy can often be resolved simply by referencing the hierarchy—as examples in the previous chapter were used to demonstrate. Even so, there can be conflicts between different aspects of the same value in the hierarchy. Internal conflicts between different elements of the other eight categories of professional norms, moreover, have no clear hierarchy to assist in the resolution of conflicting norms.

One way to read the case in chapter 4, "The Dreaded Root Canal," for example, is as a conflict between two different elements of the patient's Autonomy within the hierarchy of Central Practice Values. Autonomy is actually a very complex feature of human experience, as the discussion in chapter 7 will make clearer, and it is not uncommon for the elements of autonomy to come into conflict such that they cannot all be achieved together. Dr. Clarke's choice in that case could easily be interpreted as a choice between respecting Mr. Vianni's consistent indication that he values having the highest degree of dental health over the years, which is one aspect of his autonomy, and respecting Mr. Vianni's likely choice not to have endodontic therapy, which is another aspect of his Autonomy. Sometimes a profession's norms will provide guidance in such cases. For example, an error-control rule can be offered that tells the professional to err, if erring is a serious risk, on the side of [something]. But often, conflicts that are internal to a category of professional norms, or even to a single norm like dentistry's Central Practice Value of Autonomy, will not be resolved by other norms of the profession. The focus of this section is to offer some insight into what a careful ethical thinker might do in such situations.

When there are conflicts between the elements of a set of norms that the norms in the set do not themselves provide a method for resolving, then one must ask a different kind of question about the profession's norms, a question about *why* the community has established this profession and *why* the community and the profession in dialogue have accepted these particular norms to govern its practice. For every profession, and for every norm of every profession, there are benefits to be gained and harms to be avoided that are the *reasons* why the profession and its particular norms for practice have been established. It is these benefits to be gained and harms to be avoided to which the thoughtful ethical thinker must turn when an internal conflict between elements of the profession's accepted norms is identified.

In the example of the disruptive pediatric patient, the dentist will have to consider a number of such factors—for example, the possible harm to the patient and its likelihood because of the dentist's inability to practice with ideal attention to the procedure; the possible harm to the patient and its likelihood if the diagnostic and treatment interventions that the patient needs are not performed at this time or by this dentist; the possible benefit or harm to the patient insofar as current actions impact the patient's ability to work cooperatively with dentists (and other health professionals) in the future; the relative value and likelihood of actually educating the patient to a different pattern of behavior and the impact of such education, or lack of it, on the patient's future health care; the relative value and likelihood of involving the parents in a more effective role regarding their child's dental care; and the impact of efforts to achieve these ends on the dentist's ability to serve other patients who are presently awaiting treatment, scheduled later in the day.

Certainly, preventing harm to the patient in the chair that is serious and otherwise unavoidable will always take precedence over other considerations. Yet as soon as the possible harm is avoidable or not so serious, many conflicting ethical considerations will need to be considered. So, when the profession's accepted norms do not provide clear guidance about the relative priorities of conflicting considerations, the dentist must return to the most fundamental values and principles behind his or her commitment to becoming a dentist and to the values and principles behind society's establishment of this profession in the first place.

CONFLICTS BETWEEN PROFESSIONAL AND OTHER OBLIGATIONS

Some people live psychologically sound and happy lives focusing almost exclusively on the values and norms of a single role and set of relationships. For most people, however, a broader range of values and norms of conduct is esteemed. This is because participation in a broader range of communities and relationships—and therefore in a broader range of roles—is needed for happiness and psychological health. Thus, most people make a commitment to another person as a spouse or committed life partner. Most establish lasting relationships of friendship with other adults. Many make the commitment of parenting children, accept obligations as adult children to care for their parents, make commitments to other family members or others for whom they become responsible, and so on.

All of these relationships and numerous other roles—with their values and norms—are part of the ordinary lives of most dentists.

Every dentist, and every professional in any field, has experienced conflict between his or her professional obligations and obligations based on other commitments that he or she has made. One category of the accepted norms of the dental profession—the relative prioritization of the well-being of a dentist's patients—is intended to guide dentists when care of the patient conflicts with other ethical considerations and commitments. But, as has been argued, just like the other categories of professional norms, this category cannot answer every question that might be posed. It cannot resolve every kind of conflict that can arise between professional and other obligations. In some cases, its guidance in the form of the Greater-Than-One's-Own-But-Within-Limits Interpretation proposed above does not so much provide answers as it suggests useful questions for the thoughtful dentist to pose in trying to determine what he or she ought to do. Just as in the case of an *internal* conflict between the aspects of one's professional norms, so, too, can professional obligations conflict with *other* obligations. One must look to the *reasons* behind the two sets of obligations, to the benefits they support and the harms they try to avoid, and to the most fundamental values, principles, and ideals that have motivated the larger community to establish this profession with these norms. For it is these very reasons, at least ideally, that have motivated the individual to make his or her professional commitment to these norms in the first place.

Suppose an elderly patient of long standing calls around lunchtime on Friday afternoon to say that he is still feeling some tenderness in the quadrant where a large, old amalgam restoration that had fractured had been replaced two days earlier. He is not really in pain, he says. It's just tender and uncomfortable. But the dentist knows the patient and realizes that he is very worried that something has gone amiss with the treatment. Under ordinary circumstances, the dentist would invite the patient to drop in later that afternoon to have the area examined. But that afternoon is the occasion of a music recital in which the dentist's thirteen-year-old daughter will perform. The dentist knows that his presence at his daughter's recital will not only be pleasing to him but is also an important moment in their relationship. Unfortunately, it is Friday afternoon, and seeing this worried patient on Saturday rather than putting him off until Monday would conflict with another commitment.

The accepted norms of a profession cannot provide clear answers to every such situation, but that does not mean that they provide no guidance at all. At the very minimum, as previously mentioned, they identify important questions about the values, principles, and ideals at stake. They also offer a way to evaluate their relative priority in clear-cut cases and thus assist the thoughtful decision maker in ethical deliberation.

THE OBLIGATION TO ACCEPT RISK AND ITS LIMITS

For many centuries, indeed up until about seventy or eighty years ago, becoming a health professional meant accepting a significantly higher risk of contracting a life-threatening infectious disease than was faced by the average person. During the mid-twentieth century, however, it was medical science's successes in controlling fatal infectious diseases that received attention, not caregivers' risk of infection. But the arrival of HIV and AIDS changed this. Both the health professions and the community at large began to realize that the permanent defeat of lethal infectious diseases was a myth—and a dangerous one at that. With regard to HIV and AIDS, the "Universal Precautions" of the US Centers for Disease Control and Prevention (CDC) were developed to provide health care workers with a high level of protection against HIV infection. But since then, additional outbreaks—of SARS and Ebola, to name just two—have further reinforced our awareness of the risks that health care workers can face. Dentists' exposure to these risks is often greater because even the simplest oral assessment can expose a dentist to blood-borne and other pathogens.

What did not change during the era when fatal infectious diseases seemed to have been controlled was the conviction that those who become health professionals make a commitment to accepting a greater-than-ordinary risk to life and health if this is necessary for the proper care of their patients. This chapter has stressed that in addition to their obligations to the patients in their care dentists also have obligations to other people, and weighing these different obligations can become complicated. Among these obligations is the obligation for dentists to protect themselves from life- and health-threatening risks in order to provide care for future patients who will need their assistance. How should this obligation be weighed against the needs of a dentist's current patients?

One important but partial answer to this question is provided in the ADA Code:

> PATIENTS WITH BLOODBORNE PATHOGENS: A dentist has the general obligation to provide care to those in need. A decision not to provide treatment to an individual because the individual is infected with Human Immunodeficiency Virus, Hepatitis B Virus, Hepatitis C Virus or another bloodborne pathogen, based solely on that fact, is unethical. Decisions with regard to the type of dental treatment provided or referrals made or suggested should be made on the same basis as they are made with other patients. . . . The dentist should also determine, after consultation with the patient's physician, if appropriate, if the patient's health status would be significantly compromised by the provision of dental treatment. (Advisory Opinion 4.A.1)

That is, the dentist's obligation to provide appropriate oral health care to a patient is not ordinarily outweighed by the fact that doing so involves risk to the dentist's life or health. Under ordinary circumstances—which include the dentist's taking precautions against the spread of infection that medical science has identified as appropriate, such as the CDC's "Universal Precautions" in the case of HIV or AIDS—the only exception is if providing appropriate oral health care would significantly compromise the *patient's* General Health. But what the ADA Code does not mention is if the risks to the caregiver are great enough and are not the product of the caregiver's lack of appropriate caution, then there can sometimes be good reasons for the larger community, in dialogue with the dental profession, to oblige dental professionals to limit their caregiving for certain classes of patients.

Similarly, if providing a certain form of care does not yield sufficient benefit to the patient when compared with the extent of the risk it involves for the caregiver, and thus the community at large, then again it can be reasonable for the larger community, in dialogue with the dental profession, to judge that the dental professional's obligation to care for current patients is outweighed by the risk to the practitioner as a provider of care for future patients.

To understand these limits on the obligation to provide care, it is necessary to try to articulate the reasoning process that goes on in the community at large, in the dental profession, and especially in their dialogue with each other as dentistry's professional norms are formulated. Consider for a moment the account of the Greek historian Thucydides. In the second book of his *History of the Peloponnesian War*, he writes of a plague that struck Athens in about 430 BC: "A pestilence of such extent and mortality [as] was nowhere remembered." Neither "human art," he tells us, nor "supplications in the temples" were of any avail against it. Nor were the physicians "of any service, ignorant as they were of the proper way to treat it." But the physicians continued to care for those who were infected. In fact, the physicians "died themselves the most thickly, as they visited the sick most often."

Now, no thoughtful community would want to have its health care providers dying "the most thickly" like this. No thoughtful community, lay or professional, would accept professional norms that would place the lives of health care professionals at such great risk that the community would soon have to do without them, nor would a provident community let them face grave risk when even by doing so they could achieve very little good for their patients. Instead, the community and its health professions would establish norms of professional practice that would preserve the ranks of health professionals so that they may provide needed services to those who survive the crisis, and they would also weigh the risk the health professionals ought to face against the benefits they could effectively bring to their patients. Thus, they would take a long-term, whole-community approach to the weighing of risks and benefits as they examine alternative ways of understanding the obligations of health professionals in the face of risk.

Consequently, it is very unlikely that any society's view of the obligations of its health professionals, in regard to facing risk to their own lives and health, is that this obligation is unlimited. It is likely, to put the same point another way, that if the AIDS virus were able to pass far more readily from patient to caregiver, then the community and the health professions would quickly begin to regulate contact between caregivers and patients so that the ranks of caregivers would not be wiped out and other people in need of health care would not be left without assistance.

The presumption in this thought process, as has been pointed out, is that the health professional has already made a commitment to accept greater-than-ordinary risk for the sake of proper care of the patient. But other considerations, having to do with the long-term well-being of the whole community, may indicate limits to this obligation and even identify cases in which the health professional should not be bound by that obligation. While the health professional's relationship to the individual patient remains one of care for the patient's needs, he or she is still professionally committed to attending to the needs of the whole community over the long run as well. Sometimes the latter consideration may take precedence over the former.

This is why the judgment of the Centers for Disease Control and Prevention (CDC)—and of other organizations whose judgments have agreed with the CDC—about the degree of risk of HIV transmission to caregivers when the CDC's recommended "Universal Precautions" are being observed is so important. This is essential data for the professions and the larger community in weighing the risks to caregivers against the short-term and long-term benefits of care for HIV-positive patients in order to determine the types of situations in which a health professional's ordinary obligation to accept risk should be overridden. In general, the judgment of the CDC is that the "Universal Precautions" are sufficient to keep the risk to providers in ordinary treatment situations minimal. The clear implication of this judgment is that, when "Universal Precautions" are employed, health care professionals are obligated to provide all ordinary treatments that patients need unless providing these treatments would place the patient at unacceptable risk.

How does this reasoning translate to dental care? Dental professionals only rarely provide direct life-saving treatment to patients. It might seem to be in the community's interest, then, to exempt dental care providers from the obligation of accepting greater-than-ordinary risk to their lives for the sake of their patients on the basis that the benefit to patients is not worth the risk. But the dental community frequently provides patients with relief from intense oral pain and enables patients to maintain forms of oral functioning that are of great psychological importance, not to mention nutritional importance, to most human beings. In other words, although a patient's life is rarely directly at stake in dental care, dental professionals still serve patients in ways that people value greatly.

If a dentist failed to treat a patient's severe oral pain, then, out of concern that doing so would place the dentist's life at a slightly increased risk of possible lethal infection from that patient, even when employing appropriate barrier techniques, the community at large, and most health professionals today, would find that dentist guilty of unethical and unprofessional conduct. But if the risks were far greater or if the benefit to the patient was far less important, then it is likely that the community's long-term interests would be better served if the dentist's obligation to accept risk was overridden in such circumstances.

Of course, a patient with active AIDS, for example, is a patient who is immunosuppressed. This patient may, therefore, need treatment of a special sort or in a special location *for the patient's own protection*. There may also be dental procedures that would not be performed for such a patient because the benefit to the patient does not outweigh the risk of the procedure *to the patient*. Such patient-centered reasons for not treating a patient or for referring a patient elsewhere for treatment are not central to the issues under consideration here.

For a time during the 1980s and early 1990s some dentists (as well as some professionals in other health fields and some members of the larger community) expressed serious doubts about the adequacy of the CDC's and other institutions' judgments about providers' risk of HIV infection from patients. If the judgments of the CDC and of the other researchers who supported them were to be proven inadequate, then the question would obviously have to be reopened—that is, whether ordinary dental diagnosis and treatment involves sufficient risk such that a dentist's obligation to face that risk should be more limited. But the weight of scientific evidence rests with the CDC and the other scientific organizations and institutions that support its judgments in these matters. The burden of proof that there is sufficient scientific evidence to reopen the question regarding limiting dentists' obligations to provide ordinary dental care would, then, certainly rest on anyone challenging it.

It is worth stressing again that a specifically *social* kind of ethical thinking has been employed here to sort out the extent and limits of the dentist's obligation to face personal risks to life and health. The focus has been on the overall long-term negative effects on the *community as a whole* as these are weighed against the overall long-term benefits for the community because the community will depend on dentists for its dental care in the future. Weighing losses and benefits to all affected parties and comparing alternatives in terms of such losses and benefits is precisely how reasonable people judge the details of social roles and social policies of all sorts; this includes weighing the relative merits of alternative patterns of professional practice and alternative ways of conceiving of the professional obligations of a given group, such as dentists.

The principal reason why we have social roles and social institutions in the first place is to help us all live together and respond to life's challenges together more effectively over the long run. But to shape and reshape these roles and institutions so they meet our needs, we have to be able to *think socially* in the sense just described.

Health professionals, for the most part (i.e., excepting those who specialize in public health) serve most of their patients one at a time and face to face. When dentists think of their professional obligations, they tend to think first and foremost of their obligations to each individual patient, probably imagined most often as an individual patient in the chair before him or her. Social ethical thinking requires us to ask our questions in a different way.

The point here is not that the dentist is supposed to think socially about each patient in the chair. If the dentist acts professionally and ethically toward that patient in accord with the ethical standards of the dental profession, which are already intended to be based on careful social thinking in dialogue with the larger community, then the patient will be properly served. But when the questions at issue are about *what* those ethical standards *ought to be* and whether they can be made more precise and better suited to the circumstances at hand, *then* the thinking must be explicitly *social*. It must be conducted in terms of the well-being of the whole community over the long run.

CONSCIENTIOUS DISOBEDIENCE OF PROFESSIONAL OBLIGATIONS

The fact that professional obligations can conflict with obligations based on other commitments raises an important question, the answer of which must be stated clearly. This is because the rhetoric of the professions could easily seem to imply that when such conflicts arise, responding to some other commitment would involve a clear violation of one's professional obligations, that one's professional obligations must always "win." In other words, it might seem that the only time a member of a profession may morally privilege other obligations is if there is no clear violation of his or her professional obligations.

But this claim is surely false. Situations will sometimes arise in the life of almost every professional in which the professional is certain, after careful deliberation, that acting according to some other moral commitment would involve violating a professional obligation but in which the *other* obligation is the weightier under the circumstances. In such a situation, something very important will be lost either way, but life is sometimes like that. If the other obligation is, on conscientious reflection, the weightier, then the moral action is the one that favors it rather than the professional obligation with which it conflicts.

What this fact about professional obligations reminds us of is that professional obligations are "made" obligations. First, they are made in their being accepted through the ongoing dialogue of the expert group and the larger community that creates and defines the profession and its norms in the first place. Second, they are made significant in the life of each dentist by his or her commitment to become a member of a profession and to abide by its ethical standards. "Made" obligations are made, as has been said, for *reasons*. These reasons can be summarized in terms of the benefits to be secured and the harms to be avoided by establishing this particular profession with these particular norms of practice. It is important to remember that these *reasons* are more important than the norms of the profession, for they are the basis of these norms' importance. If a profession's accepted norms somehow came into conflict with these reasons, then obviously the norms would have to be set aside in that situation and would have to be changed if the situation were common. Another possibility, though, occurs more often. It is the situation in which one's professional obligations are in conflict with *other* benefits and with the avoidance of *other* harms. In such a situation, morality requires the decision maker to ask whether the *other reasons*, the other benefits and harms, the other principles and ideals at stake in the situation, are weightier than the *reasons* behind the profession's norms. If they are, then the profession's requirements must take second place and the dentist must *conscientiously disobey* what is professionally required.

It may seem a very strange thing to say in a book on professional ethics in dental practice that sometimes one must conscientiously disobey one's professional obligations. Certainly such situations should not come up very often. Ordinarily, if a person found situations requiring conscientious disobedience to arise regularly, it would be time to ask whether he or she were in the right profession. Still, it should not be news that after careful and conscientious reflection a person ought to do what he or she sincerely judges to be ethically required in the situation, even if this means violating professional obligations. Saying this does not demean and should not undermine professional commitment. Instead, it affirms an essential element of professional obligations—that they are "made" obligations—and reminds us of what being responsible for acting ethically means, at the deepest level, in the first place.

THINKING ABOUT THE CASE

Moral decision makers rarely follow the steps of the model proposed earlier in this chapter in the order presented. Instead, as was noted above, they move back and forth between the steps, finding in reflections on Step Three something crucial for completing Step Two, and so on. But in this commentary on this chapter's case, "How Much Sacrifice?" the steps of the model will be followed in order to demonstrate how the components of deciding/choosing connect and work together.

It turns out, however, that Dr. Sullivan actually has two very different sets of facts to deal with and, therefore, two very different decisions to make. One of these concerns Edith Blake's potentially high risk of being HIV-positive. Dr. Sullivan must determine whether that possibility should affect her decisions about Ms. Blake. Three points about this aspect of the case have been made in this chapter. The first is that dentists and other health professionals undertake an obligation to accept a greater-than-ordinary risk of infection, even fatal infection, when they become health professionals. The second is that the risk of contracting HIV when universal precautions are being followed is low enough that it is within the range of risk that, from the point of view of the larger community, health professionals are obligated to accept. In this respect, the case as described does not provide any reason to believe Ms. Blake's possibly being HIV-positive lessens Dr. Sullivan's obligation to treat her. The third point asks whether providing the dental care that the patient needs would significantly compromise the *patient's* General Health, but additional facts about Ms. Blake and her dental needs would be needed to know if this question is relevant. So, the following commentary will focus on the other decision that Dr. Sullivan has to make—namely, how to deal with Edith Blake's financial situation, given her need for extensive dental care.

Step One: Identifying the Alternatives

Theoretically, Dr. Sullivan could have just told Ms. Blake what she needs and left the decision of how to handle it up to her, whether the patient could afford it or not, including the restorative work on the upper-left second bicuspid. In that case, perhaps Dr. Sullivan would simply have provided Ms. Blake with pain medication and referred her to some place where she could get the emergency restoration on the upper-left second bicuspid for free or where her $30 would cover it, if there were such a place in town. But Dr. Sullivan has already foreclosed that option by telling Ms. Blake that she will do the restoration and by trying to refuse her $30.

But Dr. Sullivan still has a number of other options. She could simply accept a major financial loss and do everything Edith Blake needs in the best way possible with little compensation. Or she could try to meet all of Ms. Blake's dental needs but provide only the minimum acceptable level of treatment for each problem. As mentioned above, this might mean composite buildups instead of crowns, for example, and other minimum treatments for the other problems. In that way, Ms. Blake's needs would be met within the standard of care, but the work would involve less financial loss for Dr. Sullivan. Or Dr. Sullivan might only provide the emergency treatment that Ms. Blake needs today at a loss—namely, a cleaning and the restoration on the upper-left second bicuspid—and then wait on additional treatment until Ms. Blake can pay for it, either as it is provided or by some sort of payment plan. Or Dr. Sullivan might provide the emergency treatment and cleaning and then wait until Ms. Blake can pay a certain part of the cost of remaining treatment, with Dr. Sullivan taking the rest as a loss. There are probably other alternatives, but these seem to be the most important ones.

Step Two: Determining What Is Professionally at Stake

Dr. Sullivan is certainly professionally required to address Ms. Blake's emergency condition, even at some sacrifice to herself. Moreover, since she has (1) responded with diagnostic procedures and X-rays that the patient has accepted, (2) proposed cleaning and restorative treatment on the upper-left second bicuspid that the patient has accepted, and (3) proposed not charging her usual fee for these services, Dr. Sullivan is obviously both professionally and morally obligated to do what she has said she will. But since Ms. Blake has again offered her $30 in at least partial payment for the treatment, Dr. Sullivan could change her mind without fault about taking it, at least from the point of view of the commitments the two parties have made to each other. But these are not the issues that Dr. Sullivan most needs to address. The more important question is how she should deal with Ms. Blake's need for additional care when the patient has so little money to pay for it.

Since Dr. Sullivan already offers payment plans to her patients to help them get the dental care they need, we can assume that she believes she has an obligation to assist patients in obtaining dental care. As was mentioned, this seems an unavoidable obligation of dentists who practice in a society that does not provide its citizens with secure, universal access to needed dental treatment. But this obligation also has limits, as was noted and will be discussed more fully in chapters 11 and 12. But the fact that Dr. Sullivan acknowledges this obligation and has responded by providing needy patients with payment plans does not tell us whether she is obligated to make additional and perhaps greater sacrifices for Ms. Blake. Some principle of consistency might suggest that Dr. Sullivan should at least provide a payment plan to Ms. Blake, and, in fact, Dr. Sullivan has already offered that. Yet, even that might be above and beyond the call of professional duty if she is already carrying a lot of unpaid patient accounts and accepting considerable financial loss as a result.

Our society's understanding of the extent to which dentists are obligated to accept financial loss to secure dental treatment for patients unable to obtain it in other ways is far from clear. Most assuredly, dentists are not obligated to risk the solvency of their practices (provided they are otherwise well managed). They surely would be acting wrongly if their efforts to provide care to the needy deprived their other patients of record of needed care, at least if those other patients had no convenient alternative for treatment (and maybe even if they did since there are important values in an established dentist-patient relationship that the dentist is obligated to consider). Dentists are also not required to deprive themselves and their families of a decent standard of living. Our society's standards in this regard are hardly precise, but it certainly seems acceptable to the larger community, at the present time, for dentists to have secure standards of living in the middle to upper-middle class, so it would not seem that a dentist should be professionally obligated to sacrifice so much that this level of earning would be placed at serious risk. Since dentists must also provide for their own savings for retirement in our system, they may also legitimately reserve some portion of their earnings for this purpose.

Nevertheless, in a society like ours, a dentist is still professionally obligated to make some sacrifices for patients who need care that they cannot pay for. Most dentists acknowledge this obligation and provide some degree of charity care, either free care or care provided at a loss, to needy patients. Most dentists provide some measure of such charity care after the fact in the form of treatments that are not paid for. Sometimes, however, if the reasons for nonpayment are other than a patient's financial circumstances, these "write-offs" should probably be viewed as a business loss rather than as the fulfillment of the dentist's professional obligation to assist needy patients with access to care. But awareness of all these facts about her professional obligations still does not automatically resolve Dr. Sullivan's ethical question about how to deal with Edith Blake's need for additional treatment. (Some dentists provide charity care by working in clinics for those who lack access to the oral health care they need or by supporting such organizations in other ways, and others do so through programs in the third world where unmet oral health needs are typically much greater. Chapter 12 will discuss such effort and some cautions that the ethical dentist should keep in mind regarding them.)

One line of thought for Dr. Sullivan to pursue is the idea that Ms. Blake is not her only patient in need of charity care and that Ms. Blake's needs are considerably more extensive than most patients of this sort in her practice. Would she be fulfilling her professional obligation better if she declined to provide extensive treatment for Edith Blake in order to provide a greater quantity of less-expensive charity care for a larger number of other patients? Or is there something professionally inappropriate about counting people and dollars in this way?

Suppose Dr. Sullivan were to follow this line of thought—that is, considering her charity care in terms of trade-offs among her charity patients. Since there is a limited amount of financial leeway in her practice, such trade-offs are actually very likely, if not inevitable. One reasonable approach would be for her to figure out a set amount of charity care that she would be able to provide per year or, more effectively, per quarter. In a well-managed practice she would, for example, already have calculated her regular costs and what she needs to save to replace and improve equipment. She would also have to determine what would be a just payment to herself for her services, including saving for eventual retirement; this might require some thinking about, and perhaps some consulting with, her family and other dependents. What is left after these matters are covered is profit, and one appropriate use of profit, it would seem, is to fulfill a dentist's obligation to provide charity care. On the basis of such thinking, Dr. Sullivan could then set the upper limit of the amount of charity care that she would be able to provide each quarter. One benefit of planning for charity care in this way is that when a patient needs charity care Dr. Sullivan would be able to quickly determine if the needed care was within the range of the sacrifices that she professionally owed her patients or if doing the case for delayed payment, partial payment, or no payment would take her beyond that amount. In addition, if she were over that amount for a given quarter, she could honestly say to a patient that she couldn't afford to help just now. She could be more forthright about it and more confident that what she communicated to patients about it had been carefully thought out. She might also be able to tell them that they could return in the next quarter, at least for treatment that could wait, since, if she didn't borrow too much from future quarters, there would always be some resources there that a patient could utilize later. Of course, Dr. Sullivan would not have time to work out all of these details as she raced back and forth between operatories, trying to finish Edith Blake's restoration while taking care of the other patients scheduled that afternoon. But these are the sorts of professional-ethical considerations, including determining whether some patients might be more deserving of charity than others, that should be part of her thinking about the financial question when she did have time to think it all out clearly.

There are, of course, many other aspects of Dr. Sullivan's obligations as a dental professional that might have bearing on this case. But only one other set of questions seems especially pressing at this point: How should Dr. Sullivan act in order to respect and enhance Edith Blake's autonomy and bring their relationship as close to the ideal of an Interactive Relationship as possible?

The conversations between Dr. Sullivan and Ms. Blake have been open and straightforward. There is no reason to think that Ms. Blake is not participating as fully as she can in the treatment decisions that are being made. But she is a person who has, until only very recently, spent a long time thinking of her life as something out of her control and not worth controlling. Therefore, Dr. Sullivan ought to pay special attention to these aspects of their relationship as well as the aspects specifically focused on treatment in order to see if she is helping or hindering Ms. Blake's now-growing sense of positively controlling her own life.

One important candidate for these reflections concerns the decisions yet to be made about finances—but this time from the point of view of Ms. Blake. She has already expressed fairly strong convictions about not wanting to take unfair advantage of Dr. Sullivan's generosity. It might not be very respectful of Ms. Blake's current efforts to be choosing her own path in life if Dr. Sullivan unilaterally determines how the financial arrangements should be handled. In this instance, the dentist probably has a professional obligation to involve the patient not only in choosing whether or not to accept a particular payment plan that the dentist offers but also in the thought processes necessary to devise it. For by doing this, Dr. Sullivan will do the most to support and enhance her patient's Autonomy and the possibility of them working together as interactively as possible, even on narrow treatment plan and payment issues.

On the other hand, the reader may doubt that this last concern is properly part of the dentist's professional obligation in the situation. This will depend on how strongly one believes that the several areas of decision-making that go on between dentist and patient can be separated and on how broadly one understands the reach of the dental professional's obligation to enhance Autonomy as one of dentistry's Central Practice Values and work toward the ideal of an Interactive Relationship. The authors' view is that it is very difficult to separate the various kinds of decisions that dentist and patient together must make and that, under the special circumstances of such a case as this, the dentist's professional obligations do extend to such matters.

Step Three: Determining What Else Is Ethically at Stake

Even if the considerations discussed in the last two paragraphs are not properly part of the dentist's obligations as a professional, the values and moral principles at stake in them are still of unquestionable moral importance. For respecting and enhancing people's autonomy is an important standard of moral conduct in almost every modern culture and almost every theoretical description of morality. Perhaps even more important is a person's ability to see himself or herself as valuable and worth taking care of, which is a necessary condition of most relationships and achievements that make life worthwhile. Consequently, Dr. Sullivan cannot be satisfied that she has attended to everything that is morally significant in this case until she has asked herself how to best support Ms. Blake's autonomy and sense of self-worth, whether doing so is, at least to some extent, part of her professional obligations in the case or not.

In addition, there are other broad moral standards besides those deriving narrowly from her professional commitments that bear on whether Dr. Sullivan may be obligated to make sacrifices for Ms. Blake, as a fellow citizen and as a fellow human being, when Ms. Blake is in significant need. These concern the justness of a society's systems for distributing its resources, especially in response to people's basic needs, and the extent to which Dr. Sullivan's (and her family's) resources are more than, less than, or equal to her (and their) fair share within those systems. It is possible that Dr. Sullivan gives far more than she is professionally obligated to in charity care and yet falls short of what she ought to be doing for the needy of our world when good fortune, the gifts of parents or an inheritance, or even good investments or hard work have given her so much. If such is the case, it ought to be taken into account.

These are examples of the kinds of additional, and in truth more fundamental, ethical concerns that have bearing on a case of this sort. There could well be others, but these are the most obvious. It is also important to reemphasize a point made earlier, that sometimes the additional, not specifically professional, moral concerns will outweigh even the clear-cut professional requirements (with which they conflict or which they may reinforce). In such cases, morality requires the dentist to act on the most significant of his or her obligations, even if—as was mentioned above—this would require conscientiously disobeying professional norms. The additional concerns in the case at hand, though, do not seem to be in direct conflict with what Dr. Sullivan is professionally required to do. They either reinforce her professional obligations in the case or they require her to go beyond what she is professionally required to do.

Step Four: Determining What Ought to Be Done

Even with this much detail about the case and about the professional and additional moral considerations that Dr. Sullivan ought to consider, we are not in a position to say without qualification that she ought to resolve the financial issue about Ms. Blake's future treatment in such-and-such a way. It has still not been specified how much charity care she already provides or the extent of her own and her family's financial resources. Nor is there any convenient way to provide this information here without writing a novel—or at least a sizable short story.

But the authors can say this much for sure: Both Dr. Sullivan's professional commitment to respect and enhance her patients' autonomy and to work for as interactive a relationship as possible and her obligation to Edith Blake as a fellow human being who is trying to find her way back to a life of self-respect and self-determination require Dr. Sullivan to find a way to work with Ms. Blake so that she can obtain the needed treatment if she is willing to do that. Unless doing so would somehow be an extreme hardship for Dr. Sullivan or require her to break very important commitments or violate very important relationships of other sorts, we do not believe she may merely say to Edith Blake (in effect), "Here is what you need, and I will provide it if you can pay for it, period." Moreover, if working out a way for Ms. Blake to receive the needed treatment would involve such extreme "costs" for Dr. Sullivan, then we believe Dr. Sullivan is obligated—again by the importance of Ms. Blake's now-growing potential for self-respect and self-determination and for related professional reasons as well—to explain enough of the relevant circumstances to Ms. Blake that she will understand that Dr. Sullivan is not rejecting *her*, even if Dr. Sullivan cannot offer her all the help that she needs.

Suppose, finally, that Dr. Sullivan and Ms. Blake have a careful conversation about a long-term care plan for Ms. Blake, including various possible financial arrangements. Let us say that Dr. Sullivan is not able to offer all the treatment that Ms. Blake needs at no cost but offers it at a reduced rate, with a payment plan as a possibility or even the possibility of Ms. Blake paying for the treatment in work, either directly for Dr. Sullivan or for some charitable organization. But suppose Ms. Blake views this offer as too generous to be acceptable. Suppose she sees, in her growing sense of her own worth and ability to choose her own way, a need to refuse such generosity in order to take care of her needs by her own efforts, without special assistance. Suppose she thanks Dr. Sullivan sincerely and promises to come back once she has a real job, even though she knows that her teeth may be considerably worse for it, because she is strong enough in her sense of caring for herself to see her self-determination as a priority at this point. How should Dr. Sullivan respond to this refusal?

This question obviously takes the case to a new point, with different alternatives and many additional facts in place. But it is worth posing because, first of all, it challenges the reader to ask whether Dr. Sullivan's effort to maintain an Interactive Relationship would now have to be thought of as a failure because the patient is choosing to delay needed treatment. Or should this effort and Ms. Blake's response be thought of as indicating two important truths about the dental profession that have already been stressed at several other points in this chapter? First, the Central Practice Values that dentistry is committed to bringing about for its patients are clearly not the only values in human life, so sometimes they will be outweighed by other concerns. Second, dentistry exists for the sake of these values, not these values for the sake of dentistry. Or more broadly, the dental profession and the practice of dentistry exist for the sake of enhancing people's well-being, not the people or their well-being for the sake of preserving the profession or its norms. It is important to stop and recall, from time to time, that this profession and its practice, honorable and worthy though it truly is, is only a part of a larger and considerably more important whole as humans work individually and together to live their lives the best they can.

After Judging: Choosing a Course of Action

Moral reflection concludes when a judgment is made about what ought to be done or not done. But after a person has come to such a judgment, there is always another, different kind of activity needed before any course of action is carried out, and that activity is *choosing*. Other people can contribute to someone's moral reflection and judgment in many ways, by invitation or unbidden, directly or indirectly. Other people can also form their own judgments of the action that the person eventually chooses, either before the fact or in retrospect. But no one can choose for another. Dr. Sullivan is a fictional person, but if she were a real person, there would be no one who could choose her actions but Dr. Sullivan herself.

Moreover, judgments about what ought to be done, even very carefully deliberated judgments, do not automatically determine choices. It is always possible for a person to choose a course of action different from that which the person judged he or she ought to take. It is also possible for a person to choose a course of action when his or her judgment about what ought to be done is not fully formed or when the best judgment that he or she can form is that two (or more) alternatives are superior to all others but are themselves of equal moral significance. If Dr. Sullivan were a real person, the authors would hope that she would choose the course of action she judged morally superior to the other possibilities.

But she could do otherwise.

Finally, if Dr. Sullivan were a real person, it would be important for her to recall that often when a human being chooses a course of action, choosing is not simply over and done with once the action has been carried out. In addition to its other effects, every act of choosing has a specific kind of impact on the chooser, a kind of momentum so that it is easier and more likely that he or she will perceive the situation the same way the next time, more likely that he or she will conceive alternatives in the same way the next time, will value in the same way the next time, and will prioritize and act in the same way the next time. Choosing, in other words, habituates. Each choice sticks with us, predisposing us slightly more each time to perceive, conceive, value, prioritize, and act similarly the next time. This is something to take account of as one chooses and to keep track of as patterns of predisposition, and eventually habits, are built up over time.

Patients with Compromised Capacity

CASE: MRS. MORRIS'S WONDERFUL TEETH

Dr. John Benedict has agreed to offer dental services to residents at Riverside Retirement Center and Nursing Home who do not have their own dentist. Recent changes in state law require that a dentist examine every nursing home patient at least once a year. Martha Morris, a seventy-eight-year-old widow who has lived at Riverside for eight years is one of his first patients in this new role. Dr. W. C. Elbinger, who died five years ago, was her previous, longtime dentist, and she has not had a dental examination since before he died.

Mrs. Morris's forty-eight-year-old son visits her regularly and now brings her to Dr. Benedict's office. He knows enough about the previous dentist to say that Mrs. Morris liked the man and his work very much; she takes great pride at still having all her natural teeth. The son says she received periodontic scaling on several occasions since she first came to Riverside because, at least twice, she needed repeat visits to Dr. Elbinger's to complete the treatment. Mrs. Morris never mentioned a desire to see a dentist to her son or to the nursing home staff after Dr. Elbinger died, and her son never thought about it. Mrs. Morris has suffered increasing memory loss and other mental deficits over the last four and a half years—caused by a continuing series of TIAs (transient ischemic attacks) during that time.

When Dr. Benedict talks with her, Mrs. Morris recognizes that she is in a dentist's office and that Dr. Benedict is not her former dentist. She cannot remember Dr. Benedict's name, though, and asks him what it is every few minutes. With each telling, many details of her report about her last dental visit vary, including when it was. She repeatedly expresses, though, her great satisfaction in having never needed a prosthesis, crediting it to her previous dentist and her own lifelong oral hygiene.

Unfortunately, it is clear that Mrs. Morris's oral hygiene has not been maintained for some time—perhaps since her mental functioning began to wane four and a half years ago. Many nursing homes, otherwise quite well run, do not adequately emphasize daily oral hygiene for their patients. Dr. Benedict suspects that Riverside may be one of these and makes a mental note to forcefully press this matter with Riverside's medical director at their next meeting.

But that will not help Mrs. Morris's current condition. The periodontal involvement of the upper and lower posterior teeth is so advanced, bilaterally, that Dr. Benedict sees no alternative other than maxillary and mandibular partial dentures. Even major periodontal treatment, including surgery, bone grafting, and selective implants will not save the teeth; all have class III mobility and would need transitional stabilization to delay discussion of full upper and lower dentures. Dr. Benedict even wonders why Mrs. Morris is not experiencing considerable pain.

Dr. Benedict, after explaining his findings to Mrs. Morris and her son, asks her, "Does it ever hurt when you chew?"

"No, my teeth are wonderful," she answers. "Dr. Elbinger and I made sure of that."

"Is she on a regular diet," he asks the son, "or on a soft diet? A soft one would put less strain on her teeth."

"She started complaining a while ago that the dining room was serving tougher meat than they used to," says her son. "She may have been having a problem chewing, but institutional food is never terrific, so I never thought about her teeth being the problem."

"My teeth have never been a problem," says Mrs. Morris, "and I take good care of them. I intend to take every one of them to the grave."

"I'm afraid, Mrs. Morris," says Dr. Benedict once again, "that your back teeth are all very loose because the gums and bone have become diseased. There is no way we can correct the problem without removing a number of those teeth and giving you a partial denture to wear, one for the top and one for the bottom."

"Do you mean false teeth?" asks Mrs. Morris in horror.

Dr. Benedict shows her samples of upper and lower partials and, with a diagram, points out which of her teeth cannot be saved.

"I don't want those things," she says adamantly. "I'll never ever wear false teeth! After all my years of taking care of them and all of Dr. Elbinger's good work, you're not going to take my good teeth out and give me false ones!"

What should Dr. Benedict do and why?

TREATMENT DECISIONS FOR PATIENTS WITH COMPROMISED CAPACITY

For patients unable to participate at all in a treatment decision, two notions are widely accepted as the best guidelines for making ethically correct treatment decisions both within the health care community and in American society more broadly. In addition, for patients who are best described as being "partially capable" of participating in treatment decisions—rather than "not capable at all"—these two guidelines are a good place to start the discussion as well. The first of these guidelines is to *do whatever the patient would choose in the situation if he or she could choose.* This guideline is sometimes called the principle of "substituted judgment"—that is, another person's decision substitutes for the patient's but precisely in choosing *what the patient would choose if he or she could do so.* Obviously, however, the judgment that a patient *would* choose a certain course of action, if he or she could, is a hypothetical judgment. It is a hypothetical judgment about what would be the case and is, in fact, based on a hypothesis that is contrary to the facts of the case, for the fact is that the patient is *not* able to choose his or her treatment. This means that the judgment that a patient *would choose a certain course of treatment if he or she could* must always be accompanied by another judgment—a judgment about how *dependable* the first judgment is. That is, the evidence that supports the first judgment, about what the patient would choose, must continually be tested to make sure the first judgment has strong enough support for it to be reasonably used to guide treatment decisions for the patient.

Some writers propose that the moral basis for using this guideline is respect for autonomy. That cannot literally be the case, however, because the treatment in this kind of case is for a patient who is *incapable* of choosing autonomously. There is no autonomy, in the strict sense, for us to respect. What is being respected instead, in this guideline, is a different feature of human beings—that is, the value that most human beings associate with acting *consistently* over time and living by a fairly consistent set of values over the course of one's life. For most human beings, one of the most important values is achieving a sense of being one within oneself—of what in the 1960s was called "getting it together," of what might quite accurately be spoken of as *integrity*. This is the value that the guideline of *choosing what the patient would choose if he or she were able* tries to preserve for the patient, the value of *living consistently* according to a set of values over his or her lifetime.

In some instances, patients provide sufficiently detailed directions about their health care ahead of time so that, although they are incapable of decision-making when the decisions must be made, those who make the decisions for them can be fully confident that they are doing what the patient would have chosen if he or she were able. Medical Advance Directives are often not detailed or specific enough, however, to guide decision makers and caregivers, and detailed Advance Directives specifically about dental care are almost unheard of. So decision makers and caregivers must frequently interpolate what treatment the patient would choose in the present situation on the basis of other sorts of data from other situations in the patient's past. For example, family members or friends, or perhaps the health care provider personally, may have had conversations with the patient about conditions the patient wants to avoid or treatments the patient would never choose under any circumstance. Or these individuals may have a fairly clear understanding of the values, goals, or ideals of conduct that guided the patient during his or her past, and they may be able to use this information to judge what the patient would choose in this situation if he or she could do so.

But, obviously, many patients will not have given signals as helpful as these. Even then, if enough data about a patient's previous choices or values is available (although none of the items is clearly indicative alone) a total picture may still emerge that could support a judgment that the patient would choose a certain course of action if he or she could. Often, though, there is not enough data, the data available is not clear enough, or there is contradictory data from different sources and a dependable judgment about *what the patient would choose* is not possible. In such a case, when the judgment about *what the patient would choose* is not well supported or is doubtful for some other reason, then this first guideline cannot determine treatment decisions, and a second guideline must be used.

The second guideline is to *do whatever is in the patient's best interest*—that is, what maximizes the patient's well-being. This is the guideline to follow when the first guideline—*doing whatever the patient would choose if he or she could choose*—cannot be followed because we do not have strong enough evidence to determine what the patient would choose. This second guideline is also the guideline to follow with regard to patients who have never been able to make their own choices—for example, small children and those who have had severe mental deficits from birth. For these are patients who have had no opportunity to exhibit the kind of commitment to certain values, ideals, and ways of life that we need to look for as evidence for judging what they would do if they could.

Note that *best interest* necessarily refers to the best *net* well-being of the patient; this is therefore what is to be sought according to this second guideline. This is because every course of action for every patient involves both benefits and burdens—such as losses, costs, and pains. Note also that *whatever is in the patient's best interest* is not necessarily what the patient would choose if he or she could choose in the situation. That is, the first guideline preserves the patient's option to possibly act in a way that is not in his or her own best interest. A patient, for example, may choose for the sake of some other person or group or for some other reason. Consequently, the second guideline will not necessarily pick out the same action to be performed for a patient that the first guideline would pick out—provided there is sufficient evidence that the first guideline can be used at all. When the second guideline is used, though, the range of alternative actions to be considered narrows because only courses of action that are arguably in the patient's best interest can be considered.

Sometimes people are uneasy with a guideline that tells them to do something in another person's best interest because, they say, they are not necessarily privy to *what the patient would consider* to be in his or her best interest. But the second guideline does not instruct us to do *what the patient would consider* to be in his or her best interest. If we had enough data to determine what the patient would judge to be in his or her best interest, we probably could reasonably judge *what the patient would choose* in the present situation. In that circumstance, we should act according to the first guideline because the first guideline should be applied first if it can be applied at all. (That is, in technical terms, these two guidelines are "lexically" ordered because the second guideline comes into play only when the first cannot be used because sufficient data about the patient's interests and values is not available). Therefore, the person or persons judging *what would be in the patient's best interest* must use their *own* best judgment, taking into account whatever information about the patient and about human beings generally is available to them. In such an analysis, they must simply make the best judgment about the patient's best interests that they can.

THE ROLE OF PARENTS AND LEGAL GUARDIANS

Dentists in the United States know that a minor child's parents have a legal right to choose dental treatments for their child and that court-appointed guardians have the same legal right to choose treatments for their wards. The presumed moral justification for such legal structures is that, ordinarily, parents are the parties most concerned about their child's best interests and are, therefore, most likely the best judges of what will maximize their child's overall well-being. The sense of obligation that accompanies the role of a court-appointed guardian, plus the courts' efforts to select, in each case, the best person for this role, presumably provides a similar likelihood that the guardians' treatment decisions will best serve their wards' interests. Yet there are many cases where parents or legal guardians make choices to the greater or lesser detriment of a child's or ward's health.

Many health care providers want to argue that, in matters of health care, dentists, physicians, nurses, and other professionals are at least as committed, by their professional roles, to the well-being of the incapable patient as are parents or guardians and that, in health care matters, they are almost always better informed about the child's or ward's best interests. Instances of children or wards being ill served by their parents or guardians, then, make many health care professionals doubt the wisdom of current legal structure. When, however, health care providers believe a particular child or ward is being harmed by parents' or guardians' treatment decisions, the only recourse under current law, except in emergencies, is to make use of the legal system.

Of course, dentists and other health professionals may still ethically decline to act as a parent or guardian chooses; it is simply a fact of dental practice that dentists' obligations, as health professionals, sometimes point them toward a course of action different from what appears to be required by law in its determination that parents and guardians are to make the final decisions about treatment. Simply declining, however, will sometimes leave the child or ward in serious need of dental intervention; the dentist's refusal to treat, then, will ordinarily require—both ethically and legally—that the dentist help parents or guardians find another dentist to care for the patient. (In chapter 10, the section titled "Firing the Extremely Uncooperative Patient" provides a more detailed look at dentists' refusal to treat.)

In extreme cases, a dentist's professional obligation may require using the courts to try to override the law's presupposition in favor of a parent's or guardian's judgment of a patient's best interest. In addition, laws about reporting child abuse or elder abuse may be relevant. Such laws have grown stronger in recent years, and it might be argued that the presupposition in favor of parents and guardians is becoming more qualified in American society. Such changes in the law have not made dentists' choices any easier, though, when their judgment of what is best for a patient runs counter to the judgments of parents or guardians about what ought to be done for the patient. (Court-mandated reporting is discussed in chapter 10.)

A question asked in chapter 6—how much sacrifice of time, effort, or other interests does a dentist's professional commitment require?—is relevant to the amount of legal risk that a dentist is professionally committed to face for the sake of his or her patient's

well-being. On this matter there are no clear statements anywhere in the ethical literature. The larger community continues to support, however, the general presupposition
of current law that favors parents and guardians, even when bad judgments on their
part are known to occur. This continuance of legal support for parents and guardians
can also be taken as evidence, then, that dentists and other health professionals are not
considered to be under obligation to face extreme legal risks when the risks to the incapable patient's health are not extreme. Dentists, because of their commitment to their
patients' dental and general health, will often feel quite guilty in such situations; they
become concerned that the failure is theirs for not successfully educating the patient or
guardian who makes a bad choice for a patient. But there are limits, both human and
professional, in how much a dentist is required to try to change a parent's or guardian's
choice, provided the risk to the patient is not one of extreme harm. When the risk of
harm is extreme, however, the dentist may well be obligated, as stated above, to try using
the legal system to prevent harm, with all the sacrifices (and possible legal risks) that this
might involve.

At the other end of the spectrum, many patients and guardians happily collaborate
with the dentist in the decision-making about the dental care of their child or ward. Obviously, it is not possible for a dentist to establish an Interactive Relationship with a patient
who is incapable of autonomous decision-making. Still, in addition to the two guidelines
explained in the previous section, the dentist should also strive to attain the professional
ideal of an Interactive Relationship with the patient's parent or guardian when making a
treatment decision for a patient incapable of participating in that decision-making process. (Some patients, arguably a great many of them, are capable of *partial* participation
in treatment decisions; their situation will be discussed in detail below.) Nevertheless,
the final decision-making role assigned by the law to parents and guardians—and the
dentist's dependence on parents and guardians for information about the patient that
a dentist needs to act on the two guidelines discussed above—are excellent reasons for
dentists to use their relational skills to develop as interactive a decision-making process as
possible in dealing with the parents and guardians of incapable patients.

THE CAPACITY FOR AUTONOMOUS DECISION-MAKING

This chapter has focused, up to this point, on patients who are wholly unable to participate in treatment decisions. The most clear-cut examples of such patients are infants and
patients who are unconscious. But most dentists rarely treat patients of either of these
types, and there are many people in the larger health care system who fall neither into
the category of *wholly incapable* of participating nor into the category of *fully capable* of
participating.

In other words, the simple division of patients into those who are fully capable and
those who are wholly incapable is inadequate. Our thinking about patients must be
replaced with a finer-tuned set of concepts, and additional ethical guidelines must also be
identified about treatment decisions for those patients who are neither wholly incapable

nor fully capable. These norms will be examined in the next section. As indicated above, such patients will be referred to here as partially capable patients.

In order to make determinations about patients' capacity to participate in decision-making, however, it is necessary to identify the characteristics that we attribute to someone who is capable of autonomous decision-making. This section will identify five distinct sets of such characteristics and, along with these characteristics, it will describe some of the corresponding ways in which the capacity for autonomous decision-making can be diminished.

Before proceeding, however, it is important to stress that when a dentist is judging a patient's capacity for autonomous decision-making, the focus should be on the decision at hand; it is the patient's capacity for *that* decision that is at issue. Patients whose capacity for autonomous decision-making is significantly compromised in some areas of their lives may still, nevertheless, be quite capable of making a decision about a particular treatment that the dentist is recommending or of deciding between possible treatments that are within the standard of care for the patient's condition. In the same way, a patient who is able to make decisions about many other areas of his or her life may, nevertheless, be compromised when it comes to making a decision about a needed dental treatment. The core components of the human capacity for autonomous decision-making fall into five fairly distinct categories:

1. The ability to understand the relationship of cause and effect

2. The ability to recognize the alternative courses of action that are available for choice and to choose between them (as indicated in chapter 6, we take for granted that the activity of choosing among alternative courses of action is distinct from the activity of reasoning and judging about alternatives, whether before or after choosing one of them)

3. The ability of a person to conceive of himself or herself as one who can choose between the alternatives in a given situation

4. The ability to reason comparatively about alternative courses of action in order to reach a moral judgment about them

5. The ability to form and choose values, principles of conduct, and personal ideals to guide one's moral judgments and shape one's moral reflections and conduct accordingly

Two different perspectives are useful in discussing each of these categories, although a detailed analysis of each category from both perspectives would be a major undertaking and is well beyond the scope of this book. One is to focus on what abilities a growing child must develop for adults to think of him or her as a fully capable decision maker. The other focuses on the kinds of deficits observed in those who have developed a fuller capacity for autonomous decision-making but who then experience some loss or diminishment in that capacity.

Understanding Cause and Effect

For the first category, consider a child's developing ability to understand the relationship of cause and effect—both in general and in matters affecting the child's body and health, the oral cavity, and the child's oral health. At some point, a child starts to understand a cause-effect connection between tooth brushing and healthy teeth, for example, or between a dentist's removal of a carious lesion and placement of a restoration that leads to the cessation of pain in chewing.

There is developmental evidence, however, that until the age of five or six, most children retain a "magical" view of the relation between their health and various other factors in their environment rather than understanding, even rudimentarily, the relevant cause-effect relationships. Young children who understand cause and effect in some situations may not understand it in others—for instance, the relation of dental interventions to oral health and function or even to limiting pain (see Perrin and Gerrity, "There's a Demon in Your Belly: Children's Understanding of Illness"). In a similar way, some developmentally disabled people and those with certain neurological deficits—for example, persons with certain kinds of senile dementia or Alzheimer's disease—may not be able to understand the relationship between their own or a dentist's actions and the condition of their oral cavity, their oral comfort and functioning, and other aspects of their oral health.

Recognizing Alternative Possible Actions and Choosing between Them

The second component is the general ability to imagine alternative courses of action, recognize their availability for choice, and choose between them. The child learns that he or she may direct his or her actions in any of several different ways in a given situation, according to his or her own choice. In the authors' observations, the general capacity for choice seems to develop sometime between the ages of four and six, but reliable psychological research to support this or any alternative account of the matter has not been located.

For some whose development is delayed, this ability is not achieved until later in their lives, and some developmentally disabled persons do not achieve it at all. In addition, certain neurological conditions can destroy the neurological structures on which the activity of choice depends, and certain severe forms of emotional or mental illness seem to render their victims generally unable to recognize the possibility of different courses of action and/or to choose between them.

Viewing Oneself as a Chooser in the Situation

The third category concerns the ability of a person to see himself or herself as a chooser in a given situation, as contrasted with the general ability, just described, of recognizing alternative courses of action as available for choice and making choices at all. Some psychologists call this third ability "locus of control." Just because a child has learned he or she can make choices between alternative courses of action does not guarantee that the child will be aware that this ability is relevant to himself or herself in a particular situation or category of situations. The child may attribute the controlling power to some other party or to other circumstances beyond the reach of his or her own choices. That is, depending on the facts of a situation or type of situation, and the child's understanding of the situation and of his or her own abilities in relation to it, the child may or may not view himself or herself as a "locus of control" regarding that situation. The question is whether the child perceives that the matter at hand depends, at least partially, on her or his own choice rather than solely on the choices of others or on other kinds of factors that are not influenced by the child's choices and actions.

The developmental evidence for this ability suggests that, in matters potentially controlled by adult authority figures, children's sense of themselves as effective choosers seems to wax and wane during various stages of late childhood. Many nine- to eleven-year-olds, for example, are apparently more aware of their capacity to control matters affecting them than many twelve- to fourteen-year-olds, who tend to consider adults in positions of authority to be more controlling of events affecting them than the young persons are themselves. In addition, persons who are delayed in their development or are developmentally disabled and persons suffering from neurological conditions and severe emotional and mental illness may also lack an awareness of themselves as capable of making choices in certain kinds of circumstances they face.

Once a person matures and fully develops the general sense of himself or herself as being able to affect events beyond the self, the principal deficits to a person's sense of self as an effective chooser are primarily the particularized effects of the actions of others. Others' actions may severely limit the range of a person's alternatives in a given situation, perhaps eliminating all of the alternatives from which the person hoped to be able to choose. In situations in which this occurs it can be difficult for even very independent individuals to retain a strong sense of being in control of their lives. Natural conditions may have the same effect on the range of a person's available alternatives, but learning that one is an effective chooser ordinarily includes learning that there are many natural limits to effective choice, as well as many imaginable and desirable alternatives that are, nevertheless, not available at all. The realization that these limitations are not truly a lessening of one's genuine capacity as an effective chooser but rather a limit on the alternatives available for a person to choose from is itself a mark of maturation.

The most dramatic form of such adverse influence by other people is coercion, where a chooser's range of significant alternatives is narrowed drastically by another party's threat of harm. People's emotional connections to one another are so powerful and so diverse, however, that there are many ways to manipulate a person's emotions in order to diminish their sense of themselves as choosers without resorting to the level of coercion that formally threatens harm. Children and others whose general awareness of themselves as choosers is either not fully developed or is precarious for other reasons are even more susceptible to the destruction of this awareness as a consequence of others' coercion, emotional manipulation, or—depending on how it is employed—others' exercise of social authority.

One particular deficit that belongs under this heading and with which dentists are unfortunately all too familiar is excessive fear. Fear in its most extreme forms is capable of rendering some individuals completely incapable of choice in a given matter, most likely by preventing them from seeing themselves as capable of influencing their situation in any choosable way. It would be a serious mistake, though, to assume that fear routinely renders patients incapable of choice if they are capable of choice in other areas of their lives and are aware of themselves as choosers in the same or similar situations. For there are many situations in life where some measure of fear and an awareness of potential harm is not only reasonable but even a necessary source of input for judgment and action. In other words, the dentist's judgment that a given patient is so fearful that he or she is thereby rendered incapable of autonomous choice should be a very rare one, made only under the most extreme of circumstances.

Reasoning Comparatively and Judging What Ought to Be Done

The fourth category is a person's ability to reason comparatively about alternative courses of action in order to reach a comparative judgment from among them. Neither of the first three abilities alone, or in combination, necessarily implies that a child has the ability to understand specific cause-effect systems or the ability to examine the actual alternative courses of action presented by the situation at hand, nor does it imply that the child has the ability to rationally compare the alternative courses of action in terms of relevant values, rules, ideals, and so forth in order to form a moral judgment about them. As chapter 6 explained, these cognitive activities are considered by the authors to be necessary for forming moral judgments about alternative courses of action and to constitute a category of human activity distinct from the activities and abilities discussed in the three previous categories.

Exercising the ability to reason comparatively about alternatives requires, as a precondition, the child's development of the ability to suspend judgment from a course of action presently under consideration in order to examine and compare additional alternatives. It also requires, for its fullest development, growth in the ability to compare alternatives in terms of more general standards, such as a set of values, rules of conduct, ideals, virtues, and so on. This ability depends in turn, for its fullest exercise, on the child's having developed the ability to reason both inductively and deductively (and to employ other forms of reasoning if, as some philosophers claim, these two categories of reasoning do not exhaust the field), as well as to conceive of future states of affairs, to predict (or comprehend a prediction of) their likelihood, and to hypothesize. Some of these capacities have been closely associated with the emergence of what Piaget called the "formal operational stage" of cognitive development, which he saw typically appearing at about twelve years of age. But a more important point for present purposes is that the many component abilities that are requisite for the fullest exercise of moral judgment do not develop at the same rate.

The most obvious form of partial incapacity that falls under this heading is the inability of a patient to make an autonomous choice by reason of his or her having only incomplete information or understanding of the alternatives that are available for choice. Obviously this form of incapacity can come in varying degrees, for a person might have all the relevant information to make a judgment about some of the available alternatives, either more or fewer, but in any case not about all of the alternatives that are important. Or a person might know of the possibility of each of the most important alternatives but lack key information about the nature of the consequences of, implications of, or likelihood of some of them, either more or fewer. Most patients, for example, are initially unable to make an autonomous choice about dental treatment because the information they have about the condition of their mouth and the alternatives available to choose between are incomplete. Fortunately, this deficit can be rectified by proper education and the capacity for autonomous choice restored for most dental patients. But even with dentists' careful efforts to educate their patients, some will continue to be unable to understand the information that is essential to making a carefully reasoned choice about treatment.

Another form of incapacity that falls into this category is the condition of a person who is making a logical error in reasoning about the alternatives he or she is facing. Sometimes what appears to be an error in logical reasoning is more correctly described as a conceptual mistake or, perhaps, simply a conceptual misunderstanding. That is, the parties involved may not be reasoning with the same set of concepts, and the deficit can be corrected by establishing a consensus about the meanings of key terms and the implications of key ideas. Like deficits in the necessary information, logical and conceptual errors can often be corrected with careful instruction.

A more radical kind of incapacity exists if the person's ability to grasp information or to reason logically is impaired for physiological reasons. This could include the effects on the person of otherwise appropriate medications or by reason of emotional or mental illness. In such cases, determining the extent of the deficit in logical ability, if it extends beyond a particular piece of reasoning, can be an especially difficult task.

The reasoning involved in making a treatment decision is moral reasoning—that is, it consists of judgments concerning a person's values, principles of conduct, ideals, and so on. Reasoning about the obligations of the dentist that arise from the dentist's professional role as well as obligations derived from the other roles and commitments of decision makers are also matters involving moral judgment. But there is no reason to assume that logical reasoning and conceptual clarity are less relevant when making moral judgments than in any other area of human reflection. One obvious presupposition of this book is that conceptual clarity and logical reasoning can take a thoughtful moral reasoner a long way toward good moral judgments. The dentist seeking to judge a patient's capacity for making an autonomous choice or wanting to judge the effectiveness of his or her efforts to enhance a patient's autonomy in decision-making should, then, pay as much attention to logical reasoning and conceptual clarity in matters of values, rules, principles, and ideals as in any other matters.

Having Formed Values, Rules, and Ideals to Guide Moral Thinking

The fifth component of the capacity for autonomous decision-making is a person's ability to form and choose values, rules of conduct, and personal ideals to guide his or her moral reflections and moral judgments and to shape his or her conduct accordingly.

It might seem that as soon as a child is able to judge and compare alternative courses of action and to make choices according to his or her judgments the child is capable of the full exercise of autonomous choice. But autonomy implies more than judgment and control regarding only the present set of alternatives. It also implies that present judgments and choices are part of a pattern that extends across specific situations and, in the mature person, includes judgments about the kind of person one aims to be. That is, present judgments and choices are the work of a self who is not only making decisions in each instance but also connecting them and, especially as habits form, makes them repeatedly and coherently across (at least a part of) a lifetime.

Consequently, the fullest exercise of autonomy requires a person to be aware that he or she is a self with a particular history and with a distinct identity shaped by that history and by the impact of his or her previous judgments and choices. But factoring into such an awareness of oneself is the understanding that he or she has developed (or is at least developing) a particular set of values, principles, and ideals that motivate actions consistent with them—that he or she is moving toward a future that will be significantly shaped by present values and choices both in external fact and in the contents of the self that he or she will then be. Without these elements of awareness, the person cannot be said, in any strong sense, to be forming and choosing values, principles of conduct, and so on, nor can that person be said to be shaping moral reflection, moral judgments, and his or her conduct according to them.

The older child, who can exercise the abilities described under the first four headings, has still rarely had enough experience exercising his or her judgment to support saying that he or she has already formed and chosen a set of values, principles of conduct, or ideals. At best the process is just beginning and even then only in an unusually mature older child or young teenager. But as a person approaches the end of his or her teens, we ordinarily expect to see signs of a chosen set of values, principles of conduct, and personal ideals. There will often be much naiveté to such choices at this point, but if this process were not at least under way, a late teen would be considered morally immature and lacking in any really important sense of who he or she is and what should guide his or her actions. We would, in other words, not attribute a developmentally appropriate capacity for autonomous choice to such a person.

When this capacity is more fully developed in adults, we often speak of it in terms of integrity or authenticity because what is developing is a person's sense of who he or she is over a lifetime. In terms of virtue and character, this capacity cannot be effectively exercised unless the key values, principles, ideals, and patterns of perception, reflection, judgment, and action become habituated so they can be operative in most situations without self-conscious attention. Another way to speak of this component is in terms of the notion of consistency in one's values and commitments, which was mentioned in the discussion of the first guideline for making treatment decisions for patients who are wholly incapable of participating in the decision-making process.

Mature adults who have developed this component of autonomous decision-making do not ordinarily lose it altogether except as a consequence either of a severe neurological deficit that attacks the parts of the brain on which its exercise depends or of an extreme psychological disruption of the personality. But persons who suffer from serious phobias, addictions, or compulsions do have the experience of performing actions or experiencing needs or desires that are alien to their formed and chosen values in the affected areas of their lives. This is why those who suffer from such maladies are not held fully responsible for the experiences they have—although, depending on the circumstances, they may be held responsible for their actions—that are driven by their phobias, addictions, or compulsions because the person's chosen, choosing, self-forming self cannot be fully identified with these elements of their makeup.

Less dramatic in their effects are desires to act, and possibly actions as well, that are simply inconsistent with the person's own chosen values, principles of conduct, and so on. Such desires are common in human experience, and their presence is not in itself a sign of any lessening of the capacity for autonomous decision-making. But if a person acts on such a desire and does so knowingly (i.e., there is no deficit of understanding, as described under the fourth category above), we may ask if the act was autonomous precisely because it is "out of character." In other words, it is in violation of the pattern of values, principles, and so forth that the person lives by. But it is always possible that the person has conscientiously acted in a contrary way, or perhaps that the person has decided to live by a changed set of values, principles, and so forth and the unusual choice is a mark of this. For these reasons, it is rarely possible to determine that an individual's capacity for autonomous decision-making is seriously impaired, much less destroyed, solely on the basis of a single judgment, choice, or action that is contrary to his or her usual pattern.

Finally, as was noted above, a person can have a deficit in the capacity for autonomous choice not only in the sense that one or several of the five sets of characteristics just described is compromised but also in the sense that only decisions regarding a particular subject matter, possibly only the subject matter at hand, are affected. A person may, for example, be able to conduct (the first three categories) quite sophisticated business affairs with full understanding (the fourth category) yet be unable to comprehend (the fourth category again) adequately enough for autonomous decision-making the relationship between his or her oral structure and his or her oral function and values, principles, and so forth that could motivate choosing between his or her current treatment alternatives. Or a person may act with complete confidence and see himself or herself as an appropriate "locus of control" (the third category) in all other areas of his or her life but find it psychologically difficult to see himself or herself as a chooser in matters of dental treatment when drilling or other feared operations are involved.

The effort to identify the nature of a patient's deficits therefore involves three judgments, not just one. The dentist must try to identify the specific components of the capacity for autonomous decision-making that are affected by the deficit and also the degree of the shortfall from full functioning for each. Third, the dentist must also determine whether the aspects of the patient's experience that are affected by the deficit(s) include matters crucial to the decisions in which the dentist hopes the patient will participate. For, as was noted above, a deficit in another area of the patient's life may not make any significant difference in his or her ability to participate in a treatment decision about the matter at hand. If the deficit does not affect matters crucial to decisions about the patient's dental care, then the dentist should deal with the patient in regard to those decisions just as he or she would deal with any fully capable patient under the same circumstances.

Unfortunately, many people have a tendency to assume that a deficit (or incomplete development) in one component of autonomous decision-making justifies dealing with a patient as if he or she were wholly incapable. But this simply is not so. A dentist who acted in this way would be in violation of the norms of dentistry that make Autonomy an important Central Practice Value for dental practice and that identify an Interactive Relationship as the ideal that the dentist should always be striving for. Therefore, whenever there is a suspicion of a deficit in the capacity for autonomous decision-making, whether partial or complete, the dentist must determine if it affects matters crucial to present dental treatment decisions or other important aspects of this dentist-patient relationship.

The dentist must also be on his or her guard not to move too hastily from one or two pieces of evidence that a patient is not fully capable to the conclusion that this is certainly the case, much less to actions based on this conclusion. While evidence of a patient's incapacity may, in some cases, be simply obvious and overwhelming, the importance of Autonomy as one of dentistry's Central Practice Values and of the ideal of an Interactive Relationship in dental practice places the burden of proof on the one who would judge a patient either partially or fully incapable.

PATIENTS WITH PARTIALLY COMPROMISED CAPACITY

It seems clear that if a person cannot grasp cause-effect relationships at all or cannot grasp them specifically in regard to his or her health, we must consider that person simply incapable of participating in decision-making about health care interventions, be that dental or any other sort. The same is true if the person is wholly incapable of choosing between alternatives or of recognizing that alternative courses of action are available and similarly if the person is wholly incapable of reasoning comparatively about alternatives and reaching a moral judgment about them. Such complete deficits render a person incapable of autonomous decision-making. The two guidelines explained earlier in this chapter articulate how the ethical dentist will make treatment decisions regarding patients who are completely incapable of participating.

But there are many kinds and degrees of *partial capacity* for autonomous decision-making. The dentist should not ethically deal with a partially compromised, partially capable patient as if that patient were wholly incapable any more than he or she should rightly treat such a patient as fully capable. What, then, can we say about the obligations of dentists toward partially capable, partially compromised patients when it comes to treatment decisions affecting their oral health?

The short answer to this question comes from what has already been discussed about the hierarchy of Central Practice Values and about the ideal of an Interactive Relationship between dentist and patient. Both norms of professional dental practice require that the dentist work to maximize the patient's exercise of Autonomy, provided the patient is not choosing interventions contrary to his or her Oral or General Health. Therefore, if a patient's capacity for autonomous decision-making is compromised, but not wholly compromised, the dentist is obligated to try to correct whatever it is that is lacking—in other words, to eliminate the deficit if that is possible so that, together with the dentist, the patient can make a choice about treatment with full autonomy.

Exactly what a dentist is called on to do to rectify a deficit in a patient's capacity for autonomous decision-making will depend on the nature of the deficit. This is why the dentist must first try to determine which component ability (or abilities) of the five that constitute the capacity for autonomous decision-making is (are) affected. We can begin here with examples of some of the simplest deficits to correct.

It has already been noted that, if the patient lacks some understanding of what alternatives are available, or important information about any of them, the dentist obviously must determine where the gap in understanding lies and then address it with relevant information or education. For example, a patient may have all the relevant information to make a judgment about some of the available alternatives but not about all of the alternatives that are important. Or a patient might understand the availability of each of the most important alternatives but lack key information about the nature of some of the potential consequences or their likelihood. In a similar way, if the patient can understand cause-effect relationships but does not understand the cause-effect connections between the available treatments and the outcomes for his or her oral health, comfort, and function, the dentist needs to carefully explain these connections, perhaps drawing on analogous connections of cause and effect that the patient might already understand.

Such defects in understanding are generally the easiest deficits of autonomous decision-making to correct, provided the dentist can determine what is missing and then can either teach it to the patient who lacks it or guide the patient to learn it in some other way. But such deficits can sometimes prove less easy to correct because of a patient's lack of ability to grasp the relevant facts, either because the patient is of a mind-set that will not permit new learning on the subject or for some other reason. The question of how a dentist ought to proceed when a deficit proves uncorrectable will be addressed later in this section.

Dentists are also familiar with fearful patients. Many dentists have developed or learned special techniques—beyond just saying, "these are the facts and the choice is yours," which treats this deficit as if it were a deficit of understanding—for comforting fearful patients and helping them make autonomous choices in spite of their fear. Sometimes, however, the patient's fear not only compromises his or her capacity for autonomous choice but it extends beyond the dentist's ability to address it. A referral may be needed, unless emergency care is called for. Then the question of how a dentist should deal with an uncorrectable deficit arises again. For example, if the patient's fear of endodontic therapy in the case in chapter 4 was interpreted to be a serious compromise of his capacity for autonomous decision-making, then, unless Dr. Clarke has techniques for addressing it that she has not yet tried, she will be faced with exactly this question of possible referral for the nonemergency aspects of his treatment and how to deal ethically with the emergency aspects if the patient's fear-induced deficit proves to be uncorrectable.

Patients can also be affected by other powerful emotions or other psychological states, such that they cannot accept the fact that they have certain alternatives and not others or that their alternatives are limited in certain ways. This may seriously limit their ability to consider relevant treatment alternatives or to view themselves as choosers—as the locus of control—in the treatment decision situation. Patients might also have powerful feelings or other psychological states that make them unable to fully evaluate their alternatives in terms of their own values, principles of conduct, and so on.

Depending on the severity of the underlying cause of the deficits, a dentist may be able to correct the deficit with a friendly chat, a bit of personal reflection, or a story about another patient facing similar challenges. But even though the relevant decision concerns dental treatment, more severe deficits might require the tools of psychotherapy and so may be well beyond the dentist's ability to correct. As in the example from the case in chapter 4, the dentist might need to refer the patient and postpone nonemergency aspects of care, but she will still be faced with how she ought to deal with needed emergency care when the deficit of a partially compromised patient proves to be uncorrectable. But the dentist is obligated, nevertheless—as when the deficit is one of information and understanding—to make an extra effort to try to bring the patient as much as possible to an affective state in which autonomous decision-making is possible. The dentist should not say, "This patient's problems are not my concern. I am only concerned about the functioning of the oral cavity."

The same conclusion is required when the focus is on a dentist's obligations toward children who are patients. Because of the importance of the dentist's commitment to patients' autonomy and to the ideal of an Interactive Relationship, the dentist is obligated to work proactively to assist the development of each child's capacity for autonomous decision-making. At whatever stage of development of the five component abilities in which a dentist finds a youthful patient, the dentist is obligated to work to enhance the child's growth in this regard. This is not the dentist's first obligation, for the child's Oral Health and General Health and Life take precedence. But the dentist should not say, "I am only concerned about the oral cavity. The development of this child as an autonomous decision maker is not my concern."

In fact, the dentist's obligation specifically to support and enhance every child's Oral and General Health also has implications for how the dentist deals with children and their developing capacity for decision-making. The relationship between a dentist and a child can have a powerful impact on the child's ability to deal with future health care providers cooperatively and without great fear, both within dentistry and in health care generally. The dentist must consider whether the way he or she interacts with a child might yield more negative health effects for the child in the long run by the impact of these actions on the child's future ability to relate to health care providers effectively rather than consider only the specific oral benefit that is currently the focus of the dentist's attention. Many children will be in the chair who are well developed for their age in autonomous decision-making but who are still functioning only partially in regard to oral health care decisions. But circumstances will also arise when children sit in the chair who have sufficient developmental or other deficits in decision-making that cause the dentist's efforts to enhance the child's autonomous decision-making regarding his or her oral health to come up short. When either of these circumstances is the case, the question arises again about how to deal with patients with partially compromised but uncorrectable capacity for autonomous decision-making regarding the dental care they need.

Before addressing that question, a comment is also in order about the amount of time and effort that a dentist is obligated to expend in trying to correct partially compromised patients' deficits. Dentists are certainly obligated, as was argued in chapter 6, to sacrifice their own self-interest and their other commitments to some extent for the sake of their patients' well-being, and this chapter has argued that enhancement of partially compromised patients' capacity for autonomous decision-making counts as part of that well-being. But there are no clear guidelines about this in the most obvious components of the ongoing dialogue between the dental profession and the community at large about dental professional norms. The dentist must surely balance such efforts for each particular patient against the effort needed to provide adequately for that patient's Oral and General Health since these outrank Autonomy in the hierarchy of Central Practice Values. A dentist must also balance efforts of this sort for each patient against the needs of other patients in other operatories and the waiting room and in the dentist's practice at large. But these considerations do not address the still harder question—of the sort raised in chapter 6—of how much sacrifice of other considerations a dentist is professionally obligated to accept to assist patients in this way.

It seems clear that the attitude of Dr. Prentice, in the case in chapter 2, is subject to serious challenge. Dr. Prentice told Jack Williamson that if patients want education beyond what is essential information about proposed treatments they can have it, but only "with the meter running"—in other words, in return for additional charges to the patient. The discussion in this chapter supports the view that a dentist's ordinary dealings with a patient ought to include *some* additional assistance for a patient's partially compromised decision-making capacity if it is needed.

At the other end of the spectrum, a dentist is surely justified in limiting his or her efforts in this regard to what will not *seriously* jeopardize the dentist's own well-being and the dentist's other justifiable commitments in his or her nonprofessional life. Thus, a dentist may be justified in telling a patient that additional assistance in dealing with the patient's fears or other difficulties in reaching treatment decisions is available but that the extra time and effort involved on the part of the dentist will involve an additional charge. Similarly, a dentist's special efforts to assist developmentally compromised patients may deserve an additional charge. Absent a more clearly formulated guideline, the most important point to stress is that assisting the partially compromised patient with a view to the patient making a fully autonomous treatment decision, in as fully an interactive a relationship with the dentist as possible, is most certainly an ordinary requirement of ethical dental practice.

Now, finally, let us consider the issue of treatment decisions for partially compromised patients whose deficit proves to be uncorrectable because of the limits of the dentist's ability to assist or appropriate limits, as just discussed, on the dentist's expenditure of time and effort in trying to do this. This is a very subtle matter that has been discussed very little in the literature of health care ethics, and those who consider it carefully may well differ in their solutions. The authors' proposal is to follow the same two guidelines proposed earlier in this chapter regarding patients who are wholly incapable of participation but with an important modification to the first guideline.

First, then, a dentist who concludes after appropriate effort that a patient's partial incapacity for autonomous choice is uncorrectable must ask whether he or she has (or can obtain within appropriate limits of time and effort) enough understanding of this patient to allow the dentist to identify and then act on the choice that the dentist reasonably believes the patient *would have* made if the patient were fully capable. In other words, can the dentist—ordinarily by taking account of those components of autonomous decision-making that the patient is still capable of carrying out effectively—along with the help of others who may know about the patient's previously held values, principles of conduct, ideals, fears, hopes, and so forth—"make up the difference" for the patient's partial incapacity?

Answering this question will be difficult in almost every instance, especially because dentists often do not have detailed understanding of their patient's larger systems of value and so forth, even when they are long-term patients. But if a dentist can answer this question conscientiously in the affirmative, then the authors propose that the dentist act on the choice that he or she judges the patient *would have* made if the patient had not been partially incapacitated. As was explained earlier in this chapter, when doing this, the caregiver enables the patient to function, if not autonomously in a strict sense, then at least in a manner consistent with his or her own values, principles of conduct, or personal ideals to the maximum degree possible. This is the closest conformity to the norm of the value of the patient's Autonomy and the ideal of an Interactive Relationship that the patient's circumstances permit.

But if the dentist judges that he or she does *not* have (and cannot get with the appropriate help of others) enough understanding to "make up the difference" for the patient in this way, then the authors propose that the patient—even if not actually incapable—must be viewed as being *functionally incapable* of autonomous decision-making, "functionally" because the partial deficit cannot be corrected by the dentist and cannot be "made up for" by determining what the patient hypothetically *would have chosen* if capable. In such a case, since such a patient cannot be cared for according to the first guideline, decisions about the patient's care should be made under the second moral guideline that is appropriate in care of patients who are wholly incapable of autonomous choice—namely, to act in the patient's best interest, as was explained previously.

In some cases, as has been indicated, it may be possible to provide a partially compromised patient with assistance that the dentist can't personally offer in the form of an appropriate referral. When this is what ought to be done, then the dentist ought to provide only emergency dental treatment, using the two guidelines just explained to determine the nature of that treatment. But the patient may refuse this referral effort. If the patient refuses, wanting to proceed with treatment in spite of the dentist's judgment that the patient's decision-making capacity is impaired, the dentist should try to determine if there is any other way that a delay in nonemergency treatment might assist the patient in overcoming the deficit. If not, then the dentist is professionally justified in proceeding with the nonemergency treatment as determined in accord with the two guidelines just explained.

Finally, there is the situation in which the dentist is unable to determine with reasonable confidence whether the patient is functioning with full capacity or with partially diminished capacity. Suppose the dentist tries with questions, visual aids, or other means to determine whether the patient really understands the treatment alternatives and really sees himself or herself as a chooser in the matter, is really judging the proposed treatment according to his or her own values, principals, ideals, and so on, but the dentist is still not confident that the patient is capable enough to participate in the needed decision-making process. At the same time, the dentist is not certain that the patient's capacity is significantly diminished either. How should the dentist proceed in a case like this?

Once again, if the dentist has any resources left to try and has not yet reached the appropriate limits of sacrifice of other interests for the sake of this patient's well-being, then clearly the dentist should try again or try something else to resolve the issue. For the differences between how a dentist deals properly with a capable patient and how a dentist deals properly with a patient with diminished capacity are morally significant, and the one approach should not be substituted for the other without good reason. But if the dentist is at the limit of his or her resources and is justified in not expending further effort to determine the patient's condition in this respect, then he or she must treat the patient as if the patient were functionally one way or the other, since precisely what cannot be determined is how capable the patient actually is.

Some readers may take the view that, under such circumstances, the patient should be treated as if he or she were capable of autonomous decision-making out of respect for dentistry's Central Practice Value of Autonomy, provided important Oral Health needs were not going unmet, even if the patient were declining some beneficial forms of treatment. But the authors' judgment is that the alternate view is correct, that the dentist should deal with such a patient as the dentist would deal with one who is not capable of autonomous decision-making, applying the two guidelines already discussed above. The authors' reason for this judgment is the ranking of the patient's Oral and General Health above the patient's Autonomy in the hierarchy of Central Practice Values for dental practice.

THINKING ABOUT THE CASE

Mrs. Morris's inability to remember Dr. Benedict's name and the variations in her account of her last visit to Dr. Elbinger's office are strong evidence of memory deficits. But they do not point necessarily to any deficit in her ability to make a decision about the treatment proposed to her. This is a situation in which the dentist must be careful to ask, of each of the deficits in capacity that are present, whether that particular deficit is relevant to the dental treatment decision at hand.

But Mrs. Morris does seem to suffer from deficits that are relevant to this treatment decision, for she seems to believe that her posterior teeth and gums are actually in fine shape. She is capable of some components of autonomous decision-making regarding dental care, for she still seems able to recognize the relevant cause-effect relationships— that is, that dental treatment can have beneficial effects on oral comfort and functioning, and she has a long-standing value commitment to hygiene and proper dental care and appears to grasp that there are alternatives to choose between and that she can be a chooser regarding it. But she seems unable to understand important facts about her situation—that is, the serious problems with her posterior teeth, and her lack of key facts means she is not applying these values and principles to her actual situation but is instead attempting to choose a course of action that is incompatible with her values.

Dr. Benedict should always mentally pause long enough to ask if the evidence he has confirms the presence of a partial deficit. In the present case, however, the answer to this question seems clear, for the conversation reported in the case contains a number of indications that Mrs. Morris does not understand the condition of her posterior teeth. One of these, her reported attribution of her difficulty in chewing to the institution offering tougher cuts of meat, is not implausible in an institutional setting, as her son reasonably concluded. But Dr. Benedict has observed mobile teeth and advanced periodontal disease in all four quadrants. While it is possible, if unlikely, that Mrs. Morris has experienced no serious pain or discomfort from her periodontal disease, the existence of the disease is a matter of demonstrable clinical fact in this case. Given what he has observed and Mrs. Morris's repeated claims that nothing is amiss, Dr. Benedict would be perfectly justified in concluding that she is suffering from a significant partial deficit in capacity. What, then, ought he to do about it?

His first priority, in relation to the norms of respecting patients' Autonomy and striving to bring about an Interactive Relationship to the extent this is possible, ought to be to try to correct the deficit. Dr. Benedict should therefore try again to explain to her that her posterior teeth are in serious trouble. Perhaps by using mirrors he could help her see the affected gum tissue. Perhaps by gently manipulating the mobile teeth or having Mrs. Morris do this herself he can bring her to understand that there is a problem.

Here, unfortunately, he might face a difficult dilemma of competing values. Mrs. Morris's conviction that her teeth are in excellent shape is clearly very important to her. It may be an important element of her self-esteem at a time when she can sense that other faculties are weakening. Therefore, Dr. Benedict needs to proceed cautiously in educating Mrs. Morris about her periodontal disease. At some point he may conclude that it would be better, in terms of her overall psychological health, not to press the reshaping of her understanding and imagination any further and to leave her with her deeply embedded view that her teeth are in excellent shape, treat her as someone with an uncorrectable deficit, and apply the two guidelines explained above. This might be the best trade-off of valued elements of her well-being that the dentist can identify in the situation.

Let us assume that after a bit more conversation Dr. Benedict justifiably concludes that Mrs. Morris is uncorrectable in her conviction that her teeth are in fine shape. She suffers, in other words, from an uncorrectable partial diminishment of her capacity for autonomous decision-making that is clearly crucial to participating in the treatment decisions that need to be made. The values of Mrs. Morris's Oral and General Health, not to mention the fact that Dr. Benedict has accepted Mrs. Morris as his patient, mean that Dr. Benedict cannot ethically step aside from the case at this point. He must now determine how he ought to deal with this incorrectibly diminished patient.

The proposal made earlier was for the dentist first to try "making up" for the deficit from what he or she knows of the patient's other functioning capabilities. In this case, Mrs. Morris has a long and articulate history of valuing dental health and good dental treatment. It is quite reasonable to propose that *if* she could understand that her oral structures are severely impaired and she is at serious risk for deteriorating oral function, she would choose appropriate dental treatment to address the situation. Although such a choice would conflict with her conviction that her teeth are in excellent shape, it is precisely that conviction that is false and needs to be "made up for" by the dentist's interpolations. It is therefore reasonable to propose treating Mrs. Morris with extraction of the affected teeth and fabrication of removable partials to replace them.

This course of action also seems, from one point of view, to be supported by the second guideline discussed earlier—namely, to act in the patient's best interest. On the other hand, Mrs. Morris might be so resistant to using the partial dentures and so distraught that her "perfectly healthy" teeth have been extracted that her oral function, her psychological condition, or at the very least her nutritional situation might be affected negatively by this course of action. If the impact of this course of action on her Oral and General Health were going to be great enough, concern for these values would take precedence over the effort to respect her autonomous decision-making capacity. So Dr. Benedict has a difficult judgment to make in this case. He may well need to get further information from the nursing home about Mrs. Morris's eating patterns, comfort in chewing in her present condition, and so on before he can make a careful judgment about the likelihood of the possible negative effects of extraction and fabricating partial dentures. Only then can he weigh these effects against the positive effects for oral function and comfort, appropriate nutrition, and respect for her Autonomy in its diminished degree that extraction and the dentures might produce. Unless Dr. Benedict has a fair amount of confidence about these matters, he may have to delay treatment of the posterior teeth until he can make a more confident judgment.

Patients with uncorrectable partial deficits in capacity that are crucial to the treatment decisions at hand can raise very difficult professional-ethical judgments for dentists. It is the very nature of the situation that the dentist does not have everything he or she needs in order to respect the patient's Autonomy and to work for an Interactive Relationship with the patient, and, especially at the outset, the dentist also often lacks important information even for determining what course of action will be in the patient's best interest. The best path for a dentist to take, both professionally and to reduce the anxiety and frustration that invariably accompanies such cases, is to enhance his or her skills at facilitating autonomous decision-making and assisting patients in overcoming partial deficits in their capacity for autonomous decision-making. This is also, obviously, the very path recommended by the ideal of making relationships with patients, whatever their abilities, as interactive as possible.

8

XXXXXX

Working Together

CASE: TWO SETS OF GUMS

Dr. Jesse Watkins is a soft-spoken, personable man. Though few dentists fail to quickly notice his intelligence and technical skills, it is his humility that is most impressive. His patients recommended him warmly for his skill but especially for his gentleness and compassion. He graduated several years ago from the state university's graduate periodontics program. It was a gutsy choice on his part to enter the program; he gave up a solid, five-year-old middle-class general dentistry practice in his old family neighborhood and knew he would be dependent as a periodontist on referrals from general dentists of many different backgrounds. But in addition to his desire to meet the intellectual and technical challenges of specialized practice, this was also his way of partly repaying his personal debt to those who had given him the opportunity to receive an education when many of the talented youth with his background did not get one.

He located his specialty practice in a near suburb of the state's largest city, close enough to the city's middle-class minority neighborhoods that he might get referrals from the little group of minority general dentists who served them. But he also knew he needed referrals from the majority of dentists in both the city and the suburbs if his practice was to survive.

During the first lean years, he and his wife made ends meet with her position as an account executive at a local television station. Dr. Watkins spent a lot of time visiting general dentists throughout the area and teaching continuing education classes on periodontics for general dentists through the local dental society so that he would become known. Now, in its fifth year, Dr. Watkins's periodontics practice is solidly established, with a lengthening list of faithful patients and a large number of referring dentists from many ethnic backgrounds.

At present, two patients sit in Dr. Watkins's operatories. Alonso Nelson was referred by Dr. Jack Chong, whose practice serves patients from a dental program for the city's transit

149

workers union. Many general dentists would not refer Mr. Nelson, preferring to trust their own skills and keep Mr. Nelson from having to bear costs, travel inconvenience, and additional time spent traveling to a specialist. Dr. Chong is not overly cautious about treating the more common forms of periodontal diseases, but he has found his past collaborations with Dr. Watkins to be very constructive. So Dr. Chong is confident that Dr. Watkins will not only do a good job for his patients but will contact him if anything about his own work needs attention before talking with his patients about it and that Dr. Watkins will encourage his patients to continue working with Dr. Chong as their general dentist. Dr. Watkins has given Dr. Chong useful information and helpful advice about a few patients in the past, and Dr. Watkins, in turn, has always taken Dr. Chong's comments and insights seriously. So, rather than performing a procedure for Mr. Nelson that Dr. Chong has done only a couple dozen times since dental school and that he would need to reschedule for a later date in any case, he prefers to send Mr. Nelson to a specialist who does these procedures twenty or thirty times a week.

Mr. Nelson enters Dr. Watkins's operatory well informed about his periodontal condition and the procedures that Dr. Watkins will likely discuss with him. Mr. Nelson suffers from diabetes mellitus and self-administers a daily regimen of insulin injections. In spite of a daily oral hygiene routine carefully developed by Dr. Chong and his dental hygienist, Mr. Nelson's diabetes is obviously beginning to take a toll on his gums.

After reviewing Mr. Nelson's medical and dental history and examining his mouth, Dr. Watkins notes several indications for possible full-mouth periodontal surgery. But he is also concerned, taking everything into account, that full-mouth surgery for Mr. Nelson at this time might do more harm than good. He thinks it may still be possible to buy Mr. Nelson more time before that step would be needed. If this second path is followed, Mr. Nelson will need to work even more closely with Dr. Chong and his dental hygienist and also make regular visits to Dr. Watkins's office to assure things don't quickly get out of hand. But putting off the risks of full-mouth surgery, even for one year, are worth the effort in Dr. Watkins's judgment.

Before discussing these thoughts with Mr. Nelson, Dr. Watkins calls Dr. Chong's office. Dr. Chong is finishing up with a patient at that moment, so Dr. Watkins asks Mr. Nelson if he can wait a few more minutes until Dr. Chong is free. When Dr. Chong comes to the phone, Dr. Watkins explains his thoughts and asks Dr. Chong if there is anything he may have missed. When Dr. Watkins determines that he and Dr. Chong are in agreement and that Dr. Chong's hygienist will also be on board, Dr. Watkins and Mr. Nelson speak via speakerphone with Dr. Chong and his hygienist, and the four of them go through the treatment plan in detail. Mr. Nelson agrees with every step and is grateful to have the surgery postponed for a time.

Meanwhile, Kathleen O'Gara is in Dr. Watkins's other operatory. She recently moved to the area from the town where she was born and now works at the same television station as Watkins's wife. Kathleen began noticing some pain when chewing, and because of the distance, she does not think it reasonable to go to the dentist who had treated her since she was a teenager, Dr. Herbert Schmidt, whom she liked a lot. So she has gone to a local clinic where she has been informed that she has severe periodontal disease and periodontal surgery is advised. She can't believe it; Dr. Schmidt never mentioned such a thing. So, having heard from someone that Sarah Watkins's husband is a periodontist, she found him in the telephone book and made an appointment.

On examination, Dr. Watkins confirms that Ms. O'Gara has an advanced form of periodontal disease. Ms. O'Gara gets very angry when she hears this and tells Dr. Watkins she expected the husband of a friend to say something less frightening. (Dr. Watkins has never heard his wife mention Ms. O'Gara, and his wife later confirms that she barely knows her.) Dr. Watkins gently acknowledges the emotional response, bypasses the familiarity comments, and simply asks Ms. O'Gara if Dr. Schmidt had ever spoken with her about gum disease.

"He would look at my teeth and then clean them with that little rubber thing on the drill," she answers. "The last couple of visits, he said he found some deposits or something and that he would scrape it off. But it made my gums bleed. I really didn't like it. Once in a while he would have to do a filling. But he said my teeth were very strong. He said that every year, twice a year, since I was fifteen. That's seventeen years of strong teeth. Now I move away and I'm told my teeth are in wretched shape. I want to know what's going on."

"I'm a specialist, Ms. O'Gara, but I did practice as a general dentist for five years before going into periodontics, so I think Dr. Schmidt was quite justified in saying you have strong enamel and a good bite. I don't see any signs of active decay and only a few small fillings. All of these are signs of excellent teeth. That's why I asked if Dr. Schmidt ever specifically talked about the health of your gums. Strong teeth need healthy gums to do their work. The scraping on your last two visits might well have been aimed at treating a periodontal condition, especially if Dr. Schmidt was going down below the gum line."

"He's a very good man. I can't imagine that he would have forgotten to tell me anything important about my teeth. He's the only dentist I ever went to who was kind and considerate. The dentists my parents took me to when I was little were like dictators—they had no compassion. I used to cry and scream every time I had to go, until I went to Dr. Schmidt. My girlfriend's mother recommended him when I was in high school. I went to him and never went anywhere else after that. He certainly would have told me if something was wrong with my gums. Couldn't all of this have happened since I last saw him?"

"How recently was that?" asks Dr. Watkins.

"I moved here eight months ago. I had a checkup and cleaning about six months before that. I was due for another when I left there, but I figured I would wait until I found a new dentist here. Then I never got around to it. I guess I was nervous about starting with a new dentist, since I had so many bad experiences before Dr. Schmidt."

"There are exceptions, but it's rare for a periodontal condition like yours to sneak up on a person," says Dr. Watkins gently. "May I ask if Dr. Schmidt took X-rays of your teeth at your regular checkups, especially after he started that scraping? X-rays can help show if a periodontal condition exists—even if it's not obvious just by looking in the mouth."

"I don't like X-rays, doctor, and Dr. Schmidt and I had an understanding about that," says Ms. O'Gara. "He used to take them when I was younger, but once I heard of the risks, I told him I was opposed to them. He wasn't happy about that, and the more he explained the more I felt like I was being pushed into something I didn't want. I told him so and he stopped."

"Have you noticed bleeding around your gums?"

"Yes, but that's what happened when Dr. Schmidt did the scraping, and I didn't like it."

"Has that been going on for a while?" asks Dr. Watkins.

"Yes."

"Did you ever discuss that with Dr. Schmidt?"

"It didn't happen very often until recently, maybe last spring. Before that it was just now and then. I don't remember being worried about it, but I suppose I might have mentioned it to him. Like I said, his scraping made my gums bleed, so I might have mentioned it then. Are you saying he should have been paying more attention to my gums?" asks Ms. O'Gara.

"Your periodontal disease has undoubtedly progressed since you last saw Dr. Schmidt, if that was fourteen months ago," says Dr. Watkins. "But it's unlikely there were no signs then. Dr. Schmidt probably thought the scraping plus your regular oral hygiene would be enough to keep it under control. He probably didn't want to alarm you unnecessarily. Perhaps he figured keeping a close eye on the condition—because you were so regular with your checkups—was enough. Did he show you how to brush and floss as part of your daily care?"

"No, he never mentioned using dental floss or I would have gotten some. You are saying he would have found something fourteen months ago if he had looked, aren't you?" asks Ms. O'Gara.

"Well, I wasn't there, obviously, and I haven't spoken to him or seen his records. I can certainly say that for someone of your age and history the disease in your mouth is far enough advanced that it would be unusual for the more common kinds of periodontal disease to go from being unnoticeable to this point in only fourteen months."

"Then what are you going to tell me to do?" asks Ms. O'Gara, clearly upset.

"You obviously had a very positive relationship with Dr. Schmidt," says Dr. Watkins, "and that is something to build on now. Dr. Schmidt did a fine job with the small fillings you needed. If you wouldn't mind, I want to contact him to see what he noted about your periodontal condition back then and whether he had any plans in mind regarding it. I can offer better care when I'm able to work closely with a patient's regular dentist. Dr. Schmidt cared for you the longest and was the most consistent with you until now. But since he's quite a distance away, I would still recommend you contact a general dentist in this area. Hopefully we can help you establish a good long-term relationship like the one you had with Dr. Schmidt.

"As for your periodontal disease itself," continues Dr. Watkins, "I understand how disappointed you must feel, learning about all of this so suddenly. But there is plenty that can be done. It's also not so far advanced as to be a serious threat if you begin to take action now. I would be happy to develop a treatment plan for you if you would like. It will involve medications and other periodontal treatments, including some surgery, and also working closely with my dental hygienist. We will need to help you develop a pattern of self-care to prevent the condition from worsening now or recurring later. I would also work closely with your general dentist here when you get one."

Ms. O'Gara silently studies Dr. Watkins's face for a few seconds, then stands up from the chair, takes her purse from the counter, and heads for the door. "I don't think I can ever trust any dentist again," she says, and she is out of the office before Dr. Watkins can say another word.

Ms. O'Gara never returns to Dr. Watkins's office and declines to speak with his receptionist when she calls to ask how Ms. O'Gara is doing and if she has additional concerns or questions. Several weeks later, though they barely know each other, Ms. O'Gara goes out of her way to tell Sarah Watkins, "I have nothing to say to you." Hearing of this strange incident from his wife, Dr. Watkins becomes more concerned about Ms. O'Gara's final words as she left his office. Though Ms. O'Gara did not give him clear permission to contact her previous dentist, her expressed lack of trust in all dentists and her history of dental fear prompt Dr. Watkins to carefully consider the next step. Ms. O'Gara still needs proper follow-up, whether from the clinic that referred her to his office or another local dentist or periodontist or perhaps a special counselor for her dental phobia.

Having little else to go on, Dr. Watkins makes a call to Dr. Schmidt. He tells him that Ms. O'Gara has visited his office and about her severe periodontal disease. Dr. Watkins explains that she left suddenly and without treatment, although its importance was explained to her. He wants Dr. Schmidt to be aware of this in case he hears from Ms. O'Gara or perhaps wants to take the initiative of calling her about getting treatment.

Dr. Schmidt tells Dr. Watkins that he remembers Ms. O'Gara very well and that he had been treating her for a periodontal condition when she was his patient. "It was completely under control at that time," he explains. "As usual, a little scaling and regular use of the toothbrush was all that was needed. I sometimes wonder how you periodontal specialists stay in business."

Dr. Watkins wishes Dr. Schmidt well and politely ends the conversation without saying anything more or trying to answer his question.

COLLABORATION VS. THE MYTH OF THE LONE RANGER

Many strands of American culture, and many aspects of dental training as well, conspire to inculcate a picture of dental practice—and of human life in general—as something that is principally accomplished alone. Many important and undeniable facts about dental practice give the lie to this picture. Besides the obvious contributions of the members of their office staff and, for most dentists, a chairside assistant, all dentists continually depend on the work of dental and biomedical researchers, and all researchers, in turn, depend on dentists and others in practice to share their experiences and data. Together they can better articulate the needs of patients and how their research efforts and treatment recommendations affect patients' oral health needs. General dentists are also unavoidably dependent on specialists for cases they can't or do not want to handle;

specialists, in turn, depend equally on general dentists to refer patients to them and for maintaining the continuity of patient care. The specialist's work, like that of the generalist's, is carried out within the context of patients' lives, basic home care routines, and the possibility of other complex medical and oral conditions. All dentists also depend in a number of ways, then, on the educational and therapeutic initiatives of public health dentists; public health dentists, in turn, depend on the educational and preventive activities of dentists in office-based practices.

Every dentist's success in practice, in other words, depends on collaborating effectively with many individuals and institutions, as well as on working together through formal dental organizations and informal groups of many sorts. Nevertheless, these facts can fade in significance under the influence of our cultural perception of dentists as single-handedly confronting the challenges to patients' dental health—the picture of dentists that most often dominates both the profession's and the public's imagination.

Because of this perception, the most underdeveloped of the nine categories of professional norms described in chapter 3—not only for dentistry but for all our society's professions—is the category of Ideal Relationships Between Co-professionals and Others Assisting in Care. Many readers may even be surprised that the authors consider this a category of professional norms for dental practice; guidelines for conduct in this area may well seem more like rules of etiquette among dentists than norms of ethical professional conduct. But some guidelines for conduct of relationships between co-professionals do clearly state that these are matters of professional obligation for dentists, and there are important reasons for seeing a general ethical commitment to effective collaboration as part of dentistry's ethics.

First, some of the more familiar categories of professional norms that have already been mentioned have clear implications about the relationships of dentists with their co-professionals. For example, the norm of Competence obviously requires that dentists not practice beyond their expertise; hence, referring patients whom they cannot adequately care for in their practices to other professionals who can care for them is a form of professional competence. The Central Practice Value of Autonomy and the Ideal Relationship between dentist and patient both require that this referral not undermine the patient's relationship with his or her general dentist. In addition, if dentists believed that how they viewed and treated one another made no professional difference, then this and many of dentists' other obligations to their patients would be almost impossible to fulfill.

Suppose that both the general dentist and the specialist viewed themselves as "lone rangers," responding to patients' dental needs without acknowledging their dependence on collaborators. Each would work to strengthen his or her own relationship with the patient and connect with the other practitioner only grudgingly when the limits of his or her expertise had been reached rather than trying to bring the patient the greater benefit of two heads and two lives of rich professional experience working together. The authors submit that this is only one of many aspects of dental practice in which the relationships of co-professionals are not matters of professional indifference. The picture of the dentist as a "Lone Ranger" is a myth. The provision of appropriate care for patients is dependent on dentists working together and, as chapter 15 will stress, a dentist's ability to grow in professionalism also depends on his or her development of positive, collegial relationships with other dentists.

Because this component of the professional-ethical practice of dentistry has been so little examined, this chapter will survey a number of areas of dental practice in which, in the authors' judgment, a self-conscious commitment to effective collaboration can make an important difference.

COLLABORATION BETWEEN GENERALISTS AND SPECIALISTS

The most obvious example of professionally required collaboration is the one emphasized in the introductory case and in the examples used so far—namely, collaboration between the general dentist and the specialist. On the other hand, general dentists might send their patients to specialists only after they have realized, through experience, that they have practiced beyond their ability, and specialists might simply treat the patients and send them back to the generalist without a spirit of collaboration. But where collaboration is highly valued and where working with another dentist is viewed as a positive component of good patient care, the general practitioner's temptation to practice up to or even beyond the limits of his or her current expertise is lessened. Thus, fewer errors occur as the result of a dentist practicing at or beyond the capabilities of his or her technical skills and knowledge, and patients are likely to receive better overall care. General dentists are also not afraid that the specialist will fail to support, or may even undermine, the general dentist's relationship with and work for the patient. For when the care of the patient is viewed collaboratively, then the specialist has a clear obligation to support and strengthen the patient's relationship with the general dentist. Nor will the specialist begrudge "returning" the patient to the general dentist. For in the specialist's view, if care of the patient is genuinely collaborative, the patient has never "left" the generalist's care. At its best, in fact, collaborative care of a patient is team care. The generalist and specialist view themselves as caring for the patient with combined knowledge and combined skills, each respecting the contributions of the other and each working to integrate his or her own contribution with the positive contribution of the other (rather than working to have the patient view his or her own contribution as the one that is the most important).

This picture of collaborative practice is, admittedly, somewhat idealized because of the often competitive nature of dental practice in today's society and because of the demands of daily practice on each dentist's time and energy and also because of the social and economic history of American dentistry as a profession which was previously practiced almost exclusively solo. A dentist can say to the larger community, "Our society has created pressures that draw us into competition and conflict. Therefore, that is how I shall live and practice." But this is not necessary, and it is certainly not the best way for dentistry to serve its patients, individually or collectively. Instead, dental care can be viewed as being inherently collaborative, and dentists can affirm this reality about their profession in their actions and in their education of the larger community about dental care.

There is, of course, one respect in which every professional does practice alone. For to be a professional is to be independently capable of making expert judgments about clients' needs and the means to redress them or fulfill them, and in every professional-client interaction, there is a moment—or many moments—when the professional makes a judgment about the client's need, determines possible interventions, and chooses to support (or not, for the client's sake) the client's choices. Even when the practitioner is on a team and even within the most interactive of relationships with a client, these moments of professional judgment and choice must still precede—for every professional involved—what the team, or the professional(s) and the client as a unit, then judge and choose together. This is a moment that belongs to the individual professional in the exercise of his or her own expertise and best ethical judgment, even if the fruit of this moment will not become effective until it is blended with the fruits of other practitioners' similar exercise of their expertise, along with the judgments and choices of the client, and even if much will be reconsidered and reevaluated as a result of those exchanges. At that moment of judgment and choice for one's client, one practices one's profession singularly, no matter how interactive and collaborative the larger setting of one's practice.

This aspect of professional practice involves a high level of individual responsibility. The dentist at chairside must pull together all the relevant information about the circumstances of the given situation for the sake of the well-being of a unique person and make a human decision that will influence and affect that person's life. But this fact about professional decision-making is in no way in conflict with the fact that the larger setting of one's professional practice necessarily and absolutely should be genuinely collaborative. Nor should social and economic accidents that once made dental offices places where just one dentist serves patients be taken as defining circumstances for what it means to practice dentistry at its best.

Particularly as economic and other pressures in the surrounding environment may try to pull dentists apart, these professionals ought to think carefully about the real nature of dental practice and the real nature of its ethical roots, and they should reaffirm and reemphasize in word and action that it is a collaborative enterprise. Admittedly, this picture of dentistry as collaborative also needs to take account of the demands such collaboration places on dentists' time and energy: It takes extra time and extra phone calls and the special effort of communication among equals—experts with differing areas of expertise and different practice experiences; it takes compromises in planning and subtlety in communication about disagreements to work things out together without giving up; and it requires more effort to properly communicate with the patient how the dentists and others involved in the patient's care are working together.

Many dentists, both general practitioners and specialists, may find themselves asking who is going to pay for this extra time and effort. But no ethical dentist would ask who is going to pay for the time and effort needed for him or her to practice competently. The commitment to practice competently comes with the commitment to practice dentistry at all. Our proposal here is that a commitment to collaboration is equally fundamental to the proper practice of dentistry. The myth of the dentist as lone ranger is just that, a myth, and dentists ought to practice according to the correct ideal and ought to represent their practice and educate the larger community by presenting the image of dentistry as a collaborative endeavor. (This does not answer the question about who will pay for the changes in practice patterns that upholding this commitment would require, but it does place the question in its proper context.)

WORKING WITH OTHER PROFESSIONAL COLLABORATORS

The examples up to this point have focused on dentists working together with other dentists. But dentists are not the only co-professionals that dentists work with, so collaboration with other dentists is not the only implication made by the norm of Ideal Relationships Between Co-professionals. Admittedly, as the range of possible collaborators extends, there may be a tendency to view relationships with these collaborators as merely business relationships. But the collaborative nature of the best dental practice, both in its technical aspects and in its relational aspects, means that these relationships are also significant from a professional point of view. (The ethical issues involved in managing a dental practice and dealing with its business relationships will be examined in chapters 10, 12, and 13.)

The larger community, with whom the dental community has a dialogue to determine the contents of its professional commitments, quite reasonably views the members of other health professions with whom dentists work in the care of patients to be professionals in their own right. So the larger community would be surprised if they learned that a dentist viewed any of these relationships to be solely business relationships. But the ethical standards appropriate to dentists' relationships with their patients' physicians, mental health professionals to whom they refer patients, and others to whom they entrust a share in their fiduciary responsibilities toward patients are rarely expressed in the dental literature. Yet for each one of these practitioners, their professional obligation to work for the patient's good clearly includes a requirement that they coordinate their efforts, and these obligations require both an attitude of respect for each other's expertise and standing as a professional and whatever practical actions are needed to work effectively together. Dentists ethically should not relate to other professionals simply in whatever ways are convenient, mutually agreeable, or profitable. The nature of dentists' relationships to these collaborators is a matter of professional obligation.

To begin with physicians, there are many pressures that can make the ideal of collaborative practice between a patient's dentist and his or her physician difficult to achieve. Limits of time and energy, already noted in discussing the relationships of general dentists and specialists, are obviously relevant here—so, too, is the questionable cultural assumption that longer education yields a more valuable form of expertise. Another contributor to some dentists' feelings that they are viewed as subordinates when working with physicians is the questionable cultural assumption that death is the worst evil, along with the assumption that preventing death is the physician's principal professional goal.

There are good reasons to believe that physicians share a professional obligation to maintain collaborative relationships with their co-professionals and that they should therefore be working against these challenging assumptions in order to practice collaboratively

with dentists as professional peers. But other than the occasional opportunity to educate physicians about their mutual obligations through common patient experiences and
effective collaboration in practice over time (for which task hospital-based dentists may
have the most frequent opportunity), dentists will generally only be able to manage their
own house in this matter. For their part, then, dentists are obligated to practice collaboratively with physicians when the latter's role in patients' care is important and to
work against the pressures that tend to cast either party into a subordinate professional
position. One particular pitfall that dentists should watch out for is any defensiveness
that feelings of being—and especially actually being treated as—a subordinate can easily
prompt, for this reaction can mar the relationship with a collaborating physician and
become harmful to the patient as well.

Similar reflections about collaboration with mental health professionals are also in
order. Each profession's obligation to practice collaboratively requires efforts on both
sides to work together effectively and with mutual respect for each professional's distinctive expertise in order to benefit the patient through their combination. Often enough,
the challenge to collaborative practice regarding mental health professionals will run
in the reverse direction from the challenges vis-a-vis physicians. For the professional
whose expertise is based in the "hard" biological sciences may consider professionals in
psychology, social work, and related disciplines to be practitioners of the "soft" sciences
and hence inferior in importance, decision-making ability, and capability to help the
patient. Cultural biases in favor of the "hard" sciences can be challenged on theoretical
grounds and all the more so when the goal is to help the patient deal with his or her oral
health needs and when doing so is especially difficult for some reason. In any case, the
dentist's obligation, grounded in the patient's need for the integrated expertise required
to respond best to his or her needs, is to practice collaboratively with the mental health
professional.

WORKING WITH DENTAL HYGIENISTS

The theme of working together is very important in the relationships between dentists
and dental hygienists, and there can be no doubt that both have important obligations to
work collaboratively for the sake of providing the best patient care. But the specific character of these relationships is unavoidably affected by the social status of dental hygiene
in a given society—that is, whether that society considers dental hygiene to be a distinct
profession or not. Determining whether dental hygiene is considered a distinct profession
in a given society requires us to look at the actual social arrangements of that society.

As was explained in chapter 2, professions have four characteristics that differentiate
them from other occupations: (1) A profession possesses a distinctive expertise that consists of both theoretical knowledge and skills for applying it in practice. (2) This expertise
is exclusive to the profession and is a dependable source of important benefits for society.
(3) Because of this expertise, the larger society grants professionals, both individually
and collectively, extensive and exclusive decision-making authority in matters of their
expertise. (4) Professions adhere to a set of professional ethics—that is, professions and

professionals have special obligations that other members of a society don't necessarily have and that require their expertise to be employed primarily for the benefit of those they serve, which is in turn the basis of trust in professionals by those they serve and the larger society as a whole.

Dental hygiene does possess expertise that consists of both theoretical knowledge and skills for applying it in practice, and this expertise is a dependable source of important benefits for the patients hygienists serve and for the larger society. In addition, dental hygienists commit to practice in accord with a set of ethical standards and primarily for the benefit of those they serve, and this, in turn, grounds the trust of those they serve. In all these ways, dental hygiene is exactly like other professions and, most hygienists believe, should be considered a distinct profession.

But at the same time, dental hygienists' expertise is possessed equally by dentists and is therefore neither distinct nor exclusive to the discipline of dental hygiene, and dentists' knowledge and skills in applying this expertise are much more extensive than those of most dental hygienists. In practice, dentists whose offices include the services of a dental hygienist may leave all exercise of the kinds of expertise specific to dental hygienists to that hygienist and may well grow less adept at their exercise than the hygienist because of this. But, it is stressed when these points are argued, the dentist *could* provide the same services to patients that the dental hygienist does and has been just as well trained in those kinds of expertise as the hygienist. On the basis of considerations of this sort, the proposal that dental hygiene is a distinct profession can be challenged.

At the time of this writing in American society, however, a much stronger challenge to the proposal that dental hygiene is a distinct profession is available. The third characteristic of a profession is that the larger society grants professionals, both individually and collectively, extensive and exclusive decision-making authority in matters of their expertise. The matter is under challenge, and changing patterns of professional practice and professional authority in other professional groups suggest that relevant changes could also occur in the ways that oral health care is provided within American society. But at the time of this writing, dental hygienists are permitted by law to provide services to patients only under the supervision of a licensed dentist. In practice, this supervision ordinarily accords a practicing hygienist a great deal of opportunity to make independent judgments about a patient's condition and the best way to address it within the scope of the dental hygienist's expertise; when this is the case, the relationship between dentist and dental hygienist more closely mirrors the relationship between a dentist and another oral health professional. But as long as there is a legal requirement in American society for supervision by a dentist, dental hygienists' employment of their expertise in the service of patients, no matter how independently they may actually practice in a given situation, lacks the social authorization for independent practice that is typical of a profession.

It is, of course, an ethical question, whether, within the specific limits of their expertise, dental hygienists could practice without supervision without significant risk of harm to those they serve. But this is an ethical question to be resolved by the relevant representatives of the larger society (e.g., state licensing boards and legislative bodies), and the examination of this issue is beyond the scope of this book. But since exclusivity on the one hand and independence on the other are commercially beneficial, it is not surprising that this issue is energetically contested on both sides. What do these things tell us about the ethics of the relationship between dentists and dental hygienists and their respective obligations to work collaboratively together? Even though the issue of dental hygiene's status as a profession or not is complex, and social determinations of whether dental hygienists' practice should be supervised are contested, yet there is no doubt that both dentist and dental hygienist would have obligations to work collaboratively because the good of patients requires it, and the first duty of each in his or her respective role is to act for the good of his or her patients. But these social factors, along with the typical employer-employee relationship, can make the achievement of a collaborative partnership more difficult.

Dentists' and dental hygienists' efforts to collaborate will be most beneficial to patients if they are built on mutual respect for each other's expertise. The fact that a dentist's training and expertise includes that of the hygienist's is no reason for the dentist to view the contributions of a hygienist to patient care as being unskilled or less valuable. Their contributions to the patient's well-being are based as much on appropriate training and experience as the dentist's, even though their training covers a smaller range of presenting conditions. Nor should the social requirement of supervision decrease the respect due to the hygienist as a fellow human being and a caring and committed colleague in the provision of oral health care.

Collaborative practice between a dentist and a dental hygienist can also be hindered by episodes of political conflict between their professional organizations and by stories of personal wrongs and enmity that, even when true, can easily get generalized and acquire the status of legends. But dentists, we propose, are obligated under the norm of Ideal Relationships with Co-professionals and Others Assisting in Care to seek collaborative relationships with the dental hygienists with whom they work and to work together with them against these challenges to collaborative practice. For their part, dental hygienists have the same obligations because of their role in providing expert oral health care. In all such collaborations, however, the dentist, whose expertise covers the whole range of general dental care, should have the principal relationship to the patient in order to integrate the contributions of all those involved with the patient's care, both for clarity in the patient's decision-making and again for the sake of the best oral health care outcomes.

WORKING WITH NONPROFESSIONAL COLLABORATORS

Finally, there are the nonlicensed collaborators with whom, in spite of their nonlicensed status, the dentist shares important fiduciary responsibilities in the care of patients. This group can include dental assistants, office managers, receptionists, and many other kinds of staff members, depending on the particular responsibilities they are assigned in a given office or institution. The relevant question is whether the duties assigned to such a person put that person in a fiduciary relationship with the patient. That is, is this person asked to make judgments and engage in actions in relation to the patient that are extensions and expressions of the dentist's professional judgments and interventions on behalf of the dentist's professional relationship of commitment to the patient's well-being?

The distinction here may be a subtle one in practice. There may be dentists who make it clear that, even if staff interact effectively with patients and make them comfortable, the staff member's actions are his or her own; the relationship between the dentist and the staff member is a business relationship, and the staff member is carrying out a job that is not part of the dentist's caregiving relationship to the patient. But many dentists assign duties to their staff in such a way that the staff understand, and communicate in word, manner, and deed to the patients, that they represent the dentist to the patient and, in carrying out their tasks, are extending the dentist's expert care and professional commitments to the patient. Such staff members, precisely because they represent and extend the actions of the professional, have ethical fiduciary responsibilities to the patient (even if they do not have legal fiduciary responsibilities). If they fail in a task in this role, they have not only done a job poorly but have detracted from the relationship between dentist and patient and lessened in some measure the dentist's achievement of the values he or she is committed to securing for the patient. If they succeed, they directly actualize those values in some measure and contribute to the relationship between patient and caregiver.

We do not believe that dentists' obligation to practice collaboratively requires them to assign such fiduciary roles to all of their nonprofessional staff members. But the more directly a staff member deals with patients, the harder it is to separate his or her work from the overall care of the patient provided by the practice. For the judgments, actions, and relationships provided to a patient constitute for that patient a single, complex activity and cannot be separated into independently deliverable pieces. The dentist's obligation to practice collaboratively, then, requires that staff to whom fiduciary roles are assigned be considered, to an extent, genuine collaborators in the care of the patient and, therefore, be treated as genuine contributors to the practice's success in providing professional care to its patients.

The precise implications of this obligation in the daily life of an office or institution will depend on the actual fiduciary duties assigned. Dentists who act on this obligation will certainly view good professional care as the work of the whole team rather than solely as the work of the office's professionals, and they will share credit accordingly. They will certainly heed the insights of fiduciary staff about patients and may share certain forms of decision-making with them as well. The point is that good care of patients requires that those who are given the role of collaborators must be enabled to function in that role effectively and be respected for fulfilling that role.

This consideration of nonprofessional staff members is related to an obligation that a dentist would have as an employer in any case and is a matter of justice. That is, employers have an obligation to match employees' opportunities and relationships with their responsibilities so they have the opportunity to perform in the manner expected of them and to receive affirmation for doing so. But the present point is that dentists' obligation to practice collaboratively extends to the dentist's relationships to staff members who are functioning in fiduciary roles and relationships in regard to patients.

PREVENTING UNPLANNED OUTCOMES
AND BAD WORK

There is another reason for stressing the professional value of working together for collaborative dental care. For the most effective way to prevent unplanned outcomes and the possibility of bad work by the dentist is not simply for the dentist to pay closer attention to details and exercise greater caution; dentists habitually try to do this already. Instead, the most effective way to prevent unplanned outcomes is to view all dental care as care that is provided by a *team*. Even two-handed dentistry, when that is practiced, is ordinarily provided not by the dentist alone but by the dentist and a receptionist/office-manager who typically, except for some emergency calls, interacts with patients before the dentist sees them and/or after the dentist's direct work is done.

The key to reducing unplanned outcomes is to actively include the entire team in preventing them. This requires, first of all, a commitment to open communication within the team, where every member of the team is fully authorized to raise a question or ask about something out of the ordinary and to address such questions to every other member of the team, including the dentist. The receptionist who greets the patient or the assistant who seats the patient in the operatory may, for example, notice that the patient does not look well, when the dentist, moving from patient to patient, might overlook it. But staff members may not feel free to say something about this to the dentist unless the culture of the office is one of open communication.

A second requirement is that the whole team meets together to identify, in advance, where unexpected events might happen in order to have a plan in place if they do—a plan that the team has agreed upon as a group. Such plans, when they prove useful, will in time become standard practice. But the point here is to prepare in advance for each day's potential challenges. This is the ideal way to be ready for them as a team rather than hoping that whoever encounters the unexpected will figure out the most appropriate response on the spot. For example, the dentist or another team member may ask, "Mrs. Brown has a ten o'clock this morning for a routine checkup, but given how anxious she always is in the chair, what can we do to get her in and out quickly for her sake, and how should we manage things if her examination doesn't go smoothly and we're going to have to take more time with her?" It's far better to plan for such eventualities in advance, either at a team meeting before the first patient arrives or through some other system of continuous open communication.

The third requirement is to establish a "No Blame" attitude for the entire team. Even with a culture of open communication in place and team meetings that address the question of, "What could go wrong today?" and plan for it, unplanned events will still happen. When they do, when something does "slip through the cracks" despite the office's efforts at prevention, there may be a tendency to try to figure out who is responsible, who to blame. But if the team really is committed to viewing the care of patients as something they all do *together*, then the correct answer to the responsibility question is always "all of us." If the team's efforts failed to prevent an unplanned outcome, then it is the *team* that needs to rectify the situation, not one or two individuals. That is, shared responsibility for success in preventing unplanned outcomes entails shared responsibility for shortfalls when they occur.

The combination of these three team initiatives, especially when they become habitual within the team, are the most effective way to prevent unplanned outcomes and bad work, and every dentist should seriously consider incorporating them into his or her practice. But these initiatives will not take hold or be effective if the nonlicensed professional staff members are not viewed by the dentist and do not view themselves as genuine collaborators in the provision of professional dental care. The dentist's professional obligation to build as interactive a relationship as possible with nonprofessional staff does not require the use of error-prevention techniques like these. It strongly supports their use, though, and points to dentist-staff relationships where staff members are viewed as necessary and genuine contributors to patient care.

IMPAIRED DENTISTS

Very few dentists would view the plight of an impaired colleague with indifference or make their first response a punitive one. Most physical and many psychological afflictions are not within a person's power to control. Even substance addictions, though their victims retain an important measure of responsibility for their condition, can seem almost inaccessible to intervention in a person under the physical and emotional strains that are common in dental practice. Dentists impaired in their practice by any of these conditions are ordinarily viewed sympathetically and with the hope that they will be able to overcome their condition and continue to practice competently or return to competent practice after treatment, if treatment is necessary.

Such sympathy and hope could easily be considered mere sentiment among people who happen to share knowledge, skills, and a mode of occupation but who have no particular obligations to one another. But this view of these common sentiments fails to express an important component of dental professionals' obligations that binds every dentist to every other dentist in important respects: namely, it is an aspect of the commitment to collaborative practice that has not been evident in the examples discussed so far. It is clear from dentistry's obligation to assure the community that the profession will prevent dental expertise from being used inappropriately that every dentist's patient is, in some sense, every other dentist's patient. It is also the fact that the whole community is every dentist's Chief Client in more than one sense, which justifies the existence of peer review committees (which will be discussed in chapters 9 and 13) and promotes active support for public health educational efforts.

In the present instance, where the obligation to prioritize collaboration is under discussion, this relationship has a further implication. If every member of the community is my patient, from the point of view of securing at least a minimum standard of dental health for all patients and protecting patients from misuse of dental expertise, then every dentist is also my collaborator in these respects. In these aspects of dental care, we who are dentists practice together as a team, all of us. If any dentist is impaired in his or her practice, then it is my collaborator who is impaired. Just as I would react with sympathy if a close, more direct collaborator were impaired and work to protect our shared patient from bad work, I would also help my close collaborator correct the deficit and thus be restored to full and competent practice. So, too, should I respond to more distant collaborators.

The impaired colleague is not a distant loner in trouble; he or she is someone to whom I am bound by ethical ties. Ethically, I cannot be merely sympathetic; this collaborator's well-being is my concern, for his or her sake and for the sake of our common patients. Whether more specific action is in order—directed to a certain individual in need, to institutionalized assistance programs, or the like—or one chooses to make one's professional sacrifices in some other way, a dentist may not ethically view the impaired collaborator as someone with a problem that is only his or her own.

In addition, the term "impaired" can be read more broadly to include dentists who suffer from conditions that have not yet compromised their competence in practice but that have a natural progression that makes such compromise very likely. Those who collaborate closely with such persons and who see indications of a condition of this sort could not ethically stand by as the condition ran its course. Their obligations to patients and their obligations to their co-professionals would require them to look for ways to alert the practitioner to the problem and to help him or her recoup before the impairment actually compromised appropriate practice. The message here is that dentists are properly viewed as collaborators with all other dentists in the society, and they therefore have an obligation to attend to the signs and symptoms of such conditions and to alert those who suffer from them and help them take action before patients and the practitioner suffer significantly. Here again, concrete details of the situation will determine what course of action a person should take to act in accord with the commitment to collaborative practice regarding such conditions. But the obligation of collaboration, as the clearest directive of the norm of Ideal Relationships Between Co-professionals, most certainly applies.

THINKING ABOUT THE CASE

The case provides specific examples of professional collaboration and the lack of it. The first point deserving comment is an obligation of dentists that the larger community now requires of all professionals, as well as of persons in many other roles of society. This is well expressed in the American Dental Association's *Principles of Ethics and Code of Professional Conduct*: "Dentists shall not refuse to accept patients into their practice or deny dental service to patients because of the patient's race, creed, color, sex, or national origin" (4-A). This obligation is not only required of dentists in their role as health professionals but in their roles as citizens and as business people as well.

However, the literature of dental professional ethics rarely mentions the further point that it would be a strange irony if such discrimination were unethical in regard to patients but acceptable in regard to professional colleagues. Dentists and health care practitioners in almost every discipline and area of practice in the United States, not to mention around the world, now include members of every race, gender, and ethnic group. In a society like ours with a long history of many forms of unethical discrimination, it is not surprising that daily life in the dental profession has been touched by such discrimination and has only very recently begun to bear significant witness to its decrease. Dentists' obligations toward their co-professionals clearly disallow such discrimination and clearly require that professional relationships be based on professional qualities that will benefit the patient both directly and through the building of strong collaborative relationships among the professionals involved.

Therefore, a dentist's choice of collaborators ought to be determined solely by the kind of professional expertise, both technical and relational, that the patient's needs require. Particularly in large metropolitan areas, general dentists may have a wide range of special-ists from which to choose in each area of specialty care. In choosing specialists, dentists ought to pay attention to the technical expertise, communication skills, manner, and philosophy of dental practice that will benefit the patient most. They ought not pay attention to any factor that is irrelevant to ideal patient care or to effective collaboration between professionals to that end.

In the case at the beginning of the chapter, the collaboration of Dr. Chong and Dr. Watkins is intended to underline the ways in which mutual respect, trust, and close dialogue can benefit the patient and provide both professionals with a strong sense of support from a respected colleague. Mr. Nelson will receive his periodontal surgery, if and when needed, from a skilled specialist rather than a dentist with limited experience in the procedure and who feels he would be practicing close to the limits of his expertise. In fact, because of his more extensive training and experience in the area, Dr. Watkins is able to develop a treatment plan that actually postpones the surgery and its risks for a time.

In addition, by not waiting to refer until his own efforts prove inadequate and the case "blows up on him," Dr. Chong enables Dr. Watkins to enter the case when he is able to do the most good, rather than later when the worst has already happened. This is obvi-ously better for Mr. Nelson, but it is also a vote of confidence and professional respect for Dr. Watkins's expertise from a colleague who is knowledgeable enough to do more for the patient, though perhaps not as well.

By first contacting Dr. Chong and carefully discussing his findings and proposals with him, Dr. Watkins obtains another colleague's feedback to strengthen his clinical judg-ment about the case, again benefiting Mr. Nelson by having his case considered by two heads and two dentists' professional experience. At the same time, Dr. Watkins's consult-ing Dr. Chong affirms his positive judgment and respect for Dr. Chong's expertise and the latter's good relationship with the patient, thus providing the general dentist with the support of a respected colleague as well.

Further, by their active collaboration, the two dentists educate Mr. Nelson in the ways of professional expertise at its best, not as the work of lone rangers but as the joining of different skills and lives of professional experience for the patient's benefit. Even if a bad outcome would occur, their collaboration on the treatment plan is more likely to leave Mr. Nelson convinced that both dentists did everything good dentists could do. This is because he would know that each was there to strengthen the other's contribution and protect him from errors. This also correctly educates this patient, and others he might talk to, about how dental expertise is applied most effectively.

The degree of collaboration between Dr. Watkins and Dr. Chong described in the case may be fairly rare in practice. There are real challenges to collaboration between general dentists and specialists and between dentists and other professionals. But in many real practice settings, general dentists and specialists do overcome these challenges and even practice collaboratively on cases and learn effectively from each other over many years. In other words, the challenges to collaboration are real, but so is the possibility of achieving collaboration in daily practice.

The case also highlights Dr. Chong's respectful collaboration with the dental hygienist in his office with regard to Mr. Nelson's treatment. But, as presented, the case did not put emphasis on the role of nonprofessional staff members. But it is easy to imagine that the success of both dentists in dealing with their patients is also attributable in significant ways to their nonprofessional collaborators. Both dentists are presented as people who respect others and value others' contributions—whether they are professionals or not—in proportion to the value these individuals add to patient care.

The second story in the case, the story of Ms. O'Gara, is obviously less happy, in spite of a long, generally positive relationship between her and Dr. Schmidt and the efforts of Dr. Watkins to help facilitate the best outcome in the present situation. As chapter 9 will explain, Dr. Watkins is ethically correct in saying he cannot make a judgment about Dr. Schmidt's role in relation to Ms. O'Gara's advanced periodontal disease. Unless Dr. Watkins talks with Dr. Schmidt about this patient (and perhaps even after he has done so), he may not be able to piece together what evidence Dr. Schmidt actually had to indicate the condition's progress fourteen months earlier (or before that), nor would he be able to form a clear picture of how much Ms. O'Gara understood of what Dr. Schmidt told her about it (if anything) or her level of cooperation with recommended self-care or treatment (if there was any) or if there was a previous history of systemic disorders or other potentially relevant factors—such as indications of juvenile or early adult periodontal disease—and so on.

But the focus of this chapter is not on whether Dr. Schmidt did or did not perform bad work for Ms. O'Gara or on how Dr. Watkins should speak to that issue. Issues of that sort will be discussed in chapter 9. Dr. Schmidt is clearly a dentist of considerable competence and skill in relating to patients, even if his diagnosis and/or treatment of Ms. O'Gara's periodontal disease might have been lacking. He is portrayed here because he is an example of something else that is at the center of this chapter's attention: He is a lone ranger. He practices solo, not only in the sense of being the only professional in his office but in his view of dental practice. For him, the practice of dentistry at its best is the work of one person, the general dentist, who meets all the challenges of a patient's Oral Health by virtue of his own wits and professional expertise alone. He does not have the assistance of a professional dental hygienist to help him properly assess and treat the early stages of periodontal disease if his own routine attention to a patient's daily hygiene experiences is patchy in this area, and therefore he practices at the limits of his competence regarding it. He also looks doubtfully on the general need for specialists, trusting his own judgment and skills even at their limits.

The case does not provide enough detail about Dr. Schmidt to form a very careful judgment of his practice or even his care of Ms. O'Gara. But he can easily be imagined to embody the image of the dentist as lone ranger—that is, as the epitome of solo practice, going it alone instead of viewing dental expertise as collaborative from the start. Whether the circumstances provide Dr. Watkins with enough of an opening that he should try to educate Dr. Schmidt about a more collaborative view of periodontal care and of dental care in general is a close judgment call. Perhaps there is a question about whether Dr. Watkins should have ended the telephone conversation when he did; perhaps he should have made an effort to help his colleague overcome this deficit in his view of dental practice. But Dr. Watkins and Dr. Chong know something very important about dentistry in general that Dr. Schmidt may not—that it is the professional obligation of every dentist to collaborate effectively with his or her co-professionals.

A FINAL WORD: PATIENTS' OBLIGATIONS TO COLLABORATE

Finally, a word is in order about patients. The crucial ethical importance of the dentist fostering and supporting the dentist-patient relationship has been emphasized often up to this point. But so far nothing has been said about the patient's obligations within this relationship. Do patients have an obligation to collaborate?

Mr. Nelson interacts with the dentists in this case in a way that is very different from the interactions of Ms. O'Gara. Even though Dr. Watkins tells him something he did not expect and that seems to be at odds with the recommendation of his general dentist, Mr. Nelson does not become adversarial. He listens to the explanations offered and accepts the invitation to participate in the conversation between professionals that eventually leads to his acceptance of the professionals' proposals for him. Ms. O'Gara quickly moves from listening to attempting to manage the conversation with Dr. Watkins; she is surprised at his diagnosis because it is different from what she took away from her previous, general dentist's diagnoses. Does Mr. Nelson merely fulfill an obligation to collaborate, or is his response to the situation above and beyond what he owes these dentists? Is Ms. O'Gara's reaction to Dr. Watkins inappropriate or is it reasonable and justified?

Patients certainly take on a role when they seek a dentist's assistance. This role is not one that the patient can simply cut from whole cloth in each encounter with a dentist. This is because, in establishing norms for the dental profession, the larger community and dental community in dialogue have also, at least implicitly, established parameters on the conduct of patients. At one extreme, if capable patients are uncooperative enough, a dentist may "fire" such a patient, as chapter 10 will discuss. On the other hand, however, patients do not have a role-based obligation to undertake significant sacrifices for the dentist's well-being. So whatever commitments a patient can be said to have made in establishing a patient-dentist relationship, they certainly involve "less"—they are both less demanding of sacrifice and are less precise in what they require—than the obligations that dental professionals have toward their patients.

If patients do take on a role, then, it is not some sort of categorical mistake to say that an uncooperative patient is acting inappropriately. Patients act inappropriately by making it harder to maximize the benefits they receive; they act inappropriately in terms of the relationship that the patient has voluntarily entered into with the dentist but then hinders or renders ineffective by their conduct. However, people change course often in life. The mere fact that a person has started on one path by seeking a dentist's assistance and then changes to another path is not automatically a moral fault. It happens frequently in the commercial marketplace. So what, if anything, justifies the conviction of so many dentists that something morally significant is at stake in patients' conduct? Why should a capable patient who refuses to collaborate with the dentist without good reason be considered morally at fault?

The reason for this conviction, we propose, is not some social role of "being a patient" that is analogous to the health professional's special role, with its sizable set of norms governing the professional's conduct. The moral significance of the patient's cooperation derives from a more fundamental, nonconventional set of obligations between human beings that is related to justice and is most naturally summarized under the word "reciprocity." This is the aspect of justice in human relationships that pertains to a fair or equal distribution of burdens within those human relationships.

When a social arrangement requires one group of people to bear all or most of the burdens of a relationship while others bear none or few, many people would declare that distribution of burdens unfair or unjust. The provision of dental care requires considerable sacrifices on the part of dentists, in particular sacrifices for the sake of patients' well-being that are required by the professional norms that the dialogue between the profession and the larger society have determined. Admittedly, dentists make these sacrifices by their own choice to become professionals. But from the point of view of the distribution of burdens, how one came to have certain burdens is not as important as who shoulders which ones.

Thus, being a patient involves some burdens, beyond the burden imposed by disease, most pertinently the burdens of cooperation and resisting the fears and desires that may lead to uncooperative behavior. Admittedly, some patients' fears, apprehensions, and desires are so great that they effectively cannot help but be less than cooperative, but the ordinary patient does not have this much trouble bearing the burden of cooperation. However, dentists typically view the patient's burden of cooperation as significantly less burdensome than the dentist's burden of professional sacrifice. Thus, a patient who is unwilling to accept his or her burden of cooperation but still expects the dentist to bear his or her full burden of professional sacrifice is often judged to act unjustly and therefore to earn, rightly, the moral criticism of the dentist. That is, it is not that the patient has a social role–based obligation to be cooperative but rather that this obligation is a matter of justice and reciprocity.

How can dentists facilitate patients' acceptance of this burden? The first answer to this question is the same as the first answer to every other "how to" question in this chapter: The dentist facilitates collaboration by viewing the enterprise as collaborative from the start and speaking, acting, and regarding the patient accordingly. If the dentist treats the patient as a collaborator, the patient is more likely to act like one; if the dentist treats the patient as a passive recipient of services—or worse yet, as simply a consumer of services in the marketplace—and especially if the dentist views himself or herself as the lone possessor of the relevant values, understanding, judgment, and so on, then the patient is likely to follow the role assigned him or her in this model or perhaps to resist it energetically. The lesson here is the same lesson proposed many times in the preceding chapters: The most effective and appropriate relationship between dentist and patient is an Interactive Relationship in which the patient and dentist emphasize their standing as moral equals, as collaborative judges of the best courses of action, and as co-choosers of the path they will follow together. The ethic of collaborative practice—which is the best guide in a dentist's interactions with other professionals and with nonprofessional staff members who contribute to patient care—is rightly seen as also being the best guide for dentists' relations with patients.

9

✕✕✕✕✕✕

Bad Outcomes and Bad Work

CASE: DR. SINGER'S VACATION

Sandra Stuart, a thirty-six-year-old corporate loan officer for a large bank, feels discomfort around a three-unit bridge placed by Dr. Frances Singer eight weeks earlier. Ms. Stuart calls Dr. Singer's office. A recorded message says Dr. Singer is on vacation and another dentist is taking her calls and gives a phone number. There is no answer at that number, however, and no way to leave a message either. So Sandra opens the telephone book and calls the first female dentist she finds, Maria Alverez, DMD, to explain her discomfort and concern that the bridge seems to be moving.

Upon examination, Dr. Alverez finds that the bridge is loose and also has open margins. The gums are inflamed around the abutment teeth and under the pontic; there is no other inflammation anywhere else in the mouth or any signs of carious lesions or other restorations. Dr. Alverez asks Ms. Stuart, "Was this bridge permanently or temporarily cemented? Do you know?"

"I had a temporary bridge in there when it was being made," says Ms. Stuart. "After Dr. Singer put it in, I didn't think I needed to come back about it unless it gave me problems. Up until a week ago it felt fine. She certainly didn't tell me it was temporary, and I've completely paid for it."

"Then it was probably permanently cemented," says Dr. Alverez.

"Is that a problem?" asks Ms. Stuart.

"Sometimes a dentist will temporarily cement a new bridge to see if it causes any problems before cementing it permanently. It depends on the situation and how the dentist wants to handle it. Both approaches are acceptable. So, there's no problem in Dr. Singer's having cemented it permanently. That's one standard way of doing it."

"But why is it moving around? If she intended it to be permanent, why is it loose?" asks Ms. Stuart. "And why am I feeling soreness right in the same spot?"

171

"The gum tissue is inflamed along that whole section," says Dr. Alverez. "It's very likely that the bridge is causing the inflammation, especially since you don't have any gum inflammation elsewhere in your mouth. I'd like to try removing the bridge—it looks like I easily can—to see if I can figure out what's going on there, if that's OK with you. Once I know more about what's going on we can talk a bit more about various options. I can then re-cement it, permanently or temporarily, depending on what I find when I am done. Would that be all right?"

"Yes, please do whatever you think will help," says Ms. Stuart. "I've been avoiding chewing on that side for nearly a week and I really want it fixed. Does it look like it was made right?"

"A lot goes into making a three-unit bridge," says Dr. Alverez. "At first look, I think some minor adjustments may help eliminate the inflammation. It might fit better if it were a bit snugger near the gums. That may seem strange, but the gums can actually get irritated when there's a gap between the bottom of the bridge and the gum tissue. They're much happier when there's no gap. I may or may not be able to fix that right here this afternoon. First, I need to remove the bridge to see how it fits onto the teeth that are holding it in place. The irritation and mobility could also be coming from some cause I haven't seen yet. Some people, for example, are allergic to the materials used to make the bridge."

"That's fine," says Ms. Stuart, "go right ahead."

Dr. Alverez easily removes the bridge and quickly determines that the preparations are nonretentive, extremely conical with overprepared interproximal walls; she sees no signs of congenitally deformed teeth or previous extensive carious lesions. The buccal wall is underprepared, making the abutment overcontoured at the gingival margin. The anterior abutment is also very short, and the relief spacing for cementation seems excessive. She considers whether newer bonding cement might help compensate for the tooth preparations and bridge fabrication but also notices the tooth shade is brighter than the surrounding natural teeth.

It seems to Dr. Alverez that Dr. Singer did not do the best job with this bridge. Dr. Alverez assumes the bridge was fabricated at a lab rather than by Dr. Singer or someone in her office. But even if some of the overcontouring and any interproximal impingement are laboratory fabrication issues, she thinks to herself, if Dr. Singer cemented this inadequate bridge, the responsibility is hers, and there's certainly no blaming the lab for the inadequate preparations. She ponders what to do about it. Should she tell Ms. Stuart outright that Dr. Singer made a bad bridge? And what should she do clinically, regardless of what she says about Dr. Singer? Dr. Alverez decides to first find out if Ms. Stuart can tell her anything more about the bridge than what she has already said. "Did Dr. Singer say anything more or give you any special instructions about the bridge?" asks Dr. Alverez.

"Well, she did talk to me about brushing carefully in that area and flossing regularly. I didn't use floss before, but I've been brushing faithfully since I was a kid. So I started brushing in that area more carefully and flossing too. I don't think I did anything to disturb the bridge though. It just started feeling like it was moving around one day, and pretty soon it started feeling sore there. Could I have done something to cause the problem?" asks Ms. Stuart.

This is as good an opening as Dr. Alverez is likely to get if she wants to get Dr. Singer off the hook. Should she take it, finding some way to make the problem appear to be with Ms. Stuart's self-care? Should she just re-cement the bridge temporarily and tell Ms. Stuart to chew carefully for another ten days until Dr. Singer returns? Should she ask Ms. Stuart why she needed the bridge, what caused the tooth loss? Should she try to reach Dr. Singer to discuss the case before taking any action, including re-cementing the bridge? What ought Dr. Alverez do?

APPLYING PROFESSIONAL NORMS TO BAD OUTCOMES

Just as everything about a profession depends on its ethical commitments, so everything about a profession depends on its expertise, which is demonstrated in the ability of its members to dependably produce good outcomes. As a consequence, when an unplanned, undesirable, less-than-adequate, or bad outcome occurs, determining what ought to be done about it can be very difficult. It is difficult enough when a dentist's own work has an undesirable outcome, which will be discussed later in this chapter. It is even more difficult when the unplanned, undesirable, less-than-adequate, or bad outcome is the result of another dentist's work. For our purposes here, we will first focus only on *bad outcomes*. We will say more later in this chapter about the differences between *bad outcomes* and *bad work*.

Most of the nine categories of dental professional obligation described in chapter 3 are relevant to determining how dentists ought to act when they are faced with another dentist's bad outcome. The most obvious category for such a situation might seem to be Ideal Relationships between Professionals because two practitioners are involved, and the bad outcome complicates their relationship with each other and with the patient. But because a patient is also involved, the categories of dentistry's Central Practice Values and the Ideal Relationship between dentist and patient are just as significant. The most important of the Central Practice Values in such a case will be the patient's Oral and General Health, followed by the patient's Autonomy. The patient's Oral Health is important in terms of the seriousness of the bad outcome and the complexities of its correction. It is also important in that the "second dentist"—that is, the one who concludes that another dentist, the "first dentist," has had a bad outcome—may need to provide the patient with emergency treatment, specialty treatment, or possibly even continuing treatment as the patient's general dentist, depending on the circumstances. The patient's Autonomy is important because both dentists must figure out how to deal with the patient in a manner properly respectful of his or her Autonomy despite the difficult situation. In a similar way, both dentists are obligated to develop as interactive a relationship with the patient as possible, an effort that is complicated because two dentist-patient relationships are involved.

The category of Ideal Relationship to the Larger Community is also involved in such a situation because of the dental profession's commitment to the larger community that it will supervise the practice of its members so that the profession's expertise is not misused in ways that harm patients. The profession fulfills this obligation partly by making sure dental school programs graduate well-trained practitioners, requiring practitioners to maintain and improve their skills through continuing education, and, to some extent, educating the public about good professional practice patterns. But when a bad outcome occurs, another side of this supervisory role comes into play. The second dentist must determine whether the bad outcome is the result of bad work by the first dentist.

If it is, then the second dentist must consider whether the bad work is symptomatic of a potentially harmful pattern on the part of the first dentist. When the second dentist judges this is the case, the appropriate response will ordinarily require further action, possibly contacting a dental organization's peer review body (depending on what is legally allowed within the second dentist's civic jurisdiction). Such professional organization peer review bodies (sometimes, but not always, independent of state-appointed "boards of examiners") would then examine the facts of the situation and ask the same questions about the first dentist's work that the second dentist needed to ask. The larger community would certainly judge the dental profession to have failed in its obligations if the dental profession and its individual members did not raise these questions and then follow through with appropriate action. More will be said about peer review and the supervisory role of the dental profession in chapter 13. The difficult ethical challenges involved in asking these questions about a bad outcome will be examined in the following pages.

Obviously, the norm of Competence is also involved. It applies to the first dentist, who may have practiced beyond his or her level of competence, who may have been competent to practice in a manner appropriate to the patient's clinical situation but failed to do so, or who may have practiced in a fully competent manner but had a bad outcome occur in spite of this. The norm of Competence applies to the second dentist in two ways. The second dentist will have to determine whether the bad outcome is the result of the first dentist's failure to practice competently—that is, whether it is an instance of bad work— as well as how serious the bad outcome is, whether it is part of a pattern of bad work and so on. In addition, the second dentist must provide competent treatment as required by the circumstances of the case. This may be emergency care or specialty treatment (if the second dentist is a specialist receiving the patient for that purpose) or temporary care for the condition resulting from the bad outcome or continuing general dental care (if the second dentist is the patient's new general dentist of choice).

The norm of the Chief Client is relevant here because cases of this sort remind the dental community that no patient is simply a patient of one dentist. Every patient is, in a certain way, a patient of every other dentist and of the whole dental profession. This is clear not only in the supervisory role that the whole profession exercises by noting and responding correctly to bad outcomes, and especially to serious or continuous bad work, but also in connection with public health and public education considerations and the obligation to provide emergency care to those who need it.

The norm of the Relative Priority of the Patient's Well-Being is also involved. For the second dentist must also determine how much of his or her time and effort are owed to the patient with the bad outcome, as well as how much are owed to the first dentist and what other interests may need to be set aside in the process. This norm is also involved for the first dentist, who must determine what, if anything, he or she owes the patient who has experienced the bad outcome.

The principal relevance of the norm of Integrity and Professionalism is that these sorts of situations test both dentists' commitments to staying committed to the well-being of the patient rather than focusing on either their own needs or focusing on their respective relationships with one another. The second dentist must now deal with all these extra issues, along with a patient who is certainly going to be upset and possibly angry at what has happened. The first dentist may become upset at the suggestion that he or she has performed bad work, even if the second dentist's judgment is that they are only dealing with a bad outcome and especially if the second dentist concludes that bad work is probably involved. It will take both dentists more than usual effort to stay true to dentistry's ethical standards as they work through situations of this sort.

WHEN IT'S ANOTHER DENTIST'S PATIENT

A dentist's observation of another dentist's bad outcome arises in two situations: (1) When the patient is chiefly another dentist's patient and (2) when the patient is either returning to a general dentist after a second dentist has done emergency or specialty care or is first coming to a new dentist and presenting with the work of previous dentists. In the second type of situation, the second dentist—that is, the one identifying the bad outcome—is either already considered to be the patient's regular dentist or is being considered for that role by the patient. In the first situation, however, the patient's chief relationship is with the first dentist rather than the second dentist; the second dentist—the one who identifies the bad outcome—must therefore treat the patient as the *first* dentist's patient in every respect except for the patient's need for emergency or specialty care. This and the next four sections will focus on the ethical complexities of the first situation, when it's another dentist's patient. Situations of the second kind will be examined after that.

Most dentists see other dentists' patients when those patients present for emergency treatment or come to a specialist for specialty treatment. In both cases, there is an accepted set of obligations regarding the relationships between the three parties. The American Dental Association's *Principles of Ethics and Code of Professional Conduct* (hereafter ADA Code) expresses one part of this obligation very well: "If [emergency] treatment is provided, the dentist, upon completion of such treatment, is obliged to return the patient to his or her regular dentist unless the patient expressly reveals a different preference" (4.B); "The specialists or consulting dentists upon completion of their care shall return the patient, unless the patient expressly reveals a different preference, to the referring dentist, or, if none, to the dentist of record for future care" (2.B).

The second dentist should treat the patient as the first dentist's patient in other respects as well. The second dentist must also actively work to support the relationship between the patient and the first dentist. A subsequent comment in section 4.C of the ADA Code, that the second dentist should not make "disparaging comments about prior services," identifies the bare minimum of such support. The second dentist should also encourage the patient to connect with the first dentist regarding the patient's contact with the second dentist and for the necessary follow-up care. The second dentist should encourage the patient to develop appropriate programs of self-care and to schedule regular visits with the first dentist. The second dentist also, ordinarily, reports to the first about treatments given, conditions observed, and so on.

This obligation of the second dentist to support the patient's relationship with the first dentist is not just an example of mutually self-serving professional etiquette. There are sound professional-ethical reasons for this requirement. First, the patient's Oral and General Health are better served through continuity of care by a single general dentist. Second, the Central Practice Value of Patient Autonomy is respected by supporting the patient's choice of a primary dental caregiver along with the plan of care that the patient and the primary dentist have previously worked out. Third, the goal of achieving as interactive a relationship as possible is supported by efforts to maintain and strengthen the patient's established relationship with his or her general dentist; this norm also supports the second dentist in making his or her relationship with the patient as interactive as possible within its limited scope.

But the presence of a bad outcome complicates this situation. This is because a bad outcome puts the achievement of each of these three benefits for the patient into question. First, an outcome would not be considered bad if it did not involve the absence or failure of a needed dental treatment or put the patient's oral or general health at some risk. Second, the patient's plan of care surely would not include choosing a bad outcome as such. In such a situation the first dentist may have fully informed the patient about possible bad outcomes and the patient may have consciously chosen the treatment with this risk in mind. A few moments of conversation with the patient will usually reveal if this is the case. When this is the case, the bad outcome involves no direct conflict with the patient's Autonomy. But when it is not, then something has happened that the patient has not chosen. A subtle question then arises about how each dentist is to properly respect the patient's Autonomy.

Supporting and enhancing an interactive dentist-patient relationship when an unchosen bad outcome occurs is now an ethical requirement for the second dentist as much as it is for the first. This is because the second dentist must now deal directly with the patient though the occurrence of a bad outcome does not automatically terminate the patient's relationship with the first dentist. The second dentist's first effort, for the reasons given, should be to maintain and strengthen the patient's relationship with the first dentist unless doing so seriously conflicts with achieving these benefits for the patient. To determine if this is the case, the second dentist must decide early on, as clearly as he or she can, whether the bad outcome is the result of the first dentist's bad work and then, if it is, determine how serious the bad work is. The dentist's obligation to consider these difficult questions requires careful examination.

Some dentists will immediately say, "You never know for sure. You never have all the facts." They conclude, therefore, that the second dentist is never able to legitimately judge that the first dentist did bad work.

Absolute certainty about the cause of an event is rarer than most of us think, even for an eyewitness. This is especially so when time has passed and one of the crucial players is not available. Still, many situations in life provide enough evidence about the cause of an event—even at a distance and with some points of view missing—that warrants a reason-able person to make judgments about the matter based on the evidence available. Other explanations of what happened are always possible, but sometimes the evidence available is strong enough to make those other explanations too unlikely. When this is the case, a reasonable person will have enough evidence to conclude that an error in judgment, technique, or communication on the part of another person has taken place. Therefore, while there are good reasons, as will be explained, for the second dentist to give the first dentist some benefit of the doubt, it would be intellectually dishonest to hold that the evidence of bad work is never sufficient. In sum, while we may never know all the facts, sometimes we know enough of them to know that we must judge that a bad outcome is the result of another dentist's bad work.

It is unfortunate that the two phrases "bad outcome" and "bad work" sound so much alike. The word "bad" in the first phrase refers to the well-being of the patient. A *bad outcome* is an outcome that fails to accomplish some benefit of treatment for the patient or possibly involves some harm or risk of harm to the patient's Oral or General Health. The same word, "bad," in the second phrase refers to the minimum norms of dental care. Bad work is a diagnosis, treatment, or communication with the patient that fails to meet the norms developed and practiced within the dental profession.

This means that not all bad outcomes are bad work, because two different standards of judgment are involved. Unfortunately, in contemporary society—and in many dentists' conversations with patients—the distinction between these two ideas is often overlooked. Rather than educating patients about the difference, most dentists—like most people in our society and like most patients themselves—prefer to say very little to their patients about the possibility of bad outcomes. The conflation of these two ideas is a serious mal-ady of contemporary culture. A widely accepted myth of contemporary society holds that the technologies, techniques, and support systems for them within contemporary health care are as infallible as the science that developed them is imagined to be. It is part of this myth to ignore the fact that all our technologies, techniques, and support systems, and even "infallible" science itself, are the work of fallible scientists and other fallible human beings rather than coming from some truly infallible source.

The myth of infallible science has enhanced the status of physicians and dentists who employ these techniques and technologies to address patients' ills. It has also shaped patients' expectations to the point that many of them accept the dubious corollary of this myth—namely, that all bad outcomes must be the product of human error (that is, that they must be bad work). As a result, for example, much in malpractice law and insurance liability products is a response to this myth. Physicians, dentists, and professional orga-nizations who use this myth to promote or defend their practices and professions, then, contribute to this cultural malady and its consequences. In such an environment, it is not surprising that dentists don't talk to their patients very much about bad outcomes.

Every dentist knows, though, that even the most expert dentist practicing most care-fully on a "textbook" mouth of a fully cooperative patient can still have a bad outcome. The myth of infallible science and its corollary of treating all shortfalls as instances of human error are false. A bad outcome is not necessarily a sign of bad work.

To judge whether a particular bad outcome is an instance of bad work, the second dentist needs information. In some instances, the bad outcome involves dental work that is physically defective, like the nonretentive preparations, poor marginal fit, and overcontouring of the bridge in the case at the beginning of this chapter. But often the second dentist will have to make a judgment on the basis of physical evidence that is less clear. When a patient presents with significant periodontal disease, for example, the patient may state that the first dentist never informed him or her of either the first incipient signs or the continuing progression of any kind of periodontal involvement. This may be a defect in the patient's memory, in the patient's attention to the dentist's words, in the patient's comprehension of those words, and so on. In addition, some bad outcomes occur without anyone being at fault, simply because human knowledge and human technology is limited in the face of complicated natural processes.

The second dentist cannot justifiably conclude that a bad outcome probably is, or is not, the result of bad work without carefully considering the clinical facts, the patient's comments about the situation, any available evidence that the patient has received, and whether the patient has understood the first dentist's comments correctly. Even then, however, the most a second dentist will ordinarily be able to conclude—without obtaining information from the first dentist about the clinical circumstances in which he or she operated—is that the bad outcome *probably is*, or *probably is not*, an instance of bad work. The separate question—whether the second dentist may, or ought to, communicate such a judgment to the patient—will be examined shortly.

Most dentists ordinarily give another dentist the benefit of the doubt, even when there is considerable evidence that a bad outcome is the result of bad work. This may appear to be mere professional face-saving or an example of inappropriate loyalty. Giving the benefit of the doubt may appear, in such a matter, contrary to the obligation of the dental profession to the larger community—that is, the obligation to watch for and eliminate avoidable bad work as much as possible.

There are two good reasons for presuming, however, that another dentist has attempted to do good work in spite of a bad outcome. First, most bad outcomes have many possible explanations that do not involve errors by the first dentist. If there is no strong evidence of bad work in the clinical facts and the patient's reports, it is more likely than not that bad work was not involved. Second, the technical education provided in accredited dental schools is carefully monitored, as is that of many of the dental profession's continuing education programs. This is to assure the larger community that, when new dentists are licensed, they have the knowledge and skills they need to practice capably. Their continual practice, furthermore, ordinarily enhances dental expertise rather than weakens it, and the same is true in general about dentistry's continuing education programs. All things being equal, then, it is most likely that a given dentist will conform to the relevant professional norms in any given clinical situation.

Situations will arise, nevertheless, in which the second dentist must conclude that a bad outcome *probably is* the result of the first dentist's errors in judgment, technique, or communication with the patient. Other situations will arise where evidence is not conclusive but is still strong enough to outweigh the benefit of the doubt favoring the first dentist. In such a case, a dentist would have to conclude that bad work *might be* involved, even though the evidence does not resolve the question either way.

THREE SITUATIONS

There are, then, three ethically distinct situations of potential bad work that a second dentist might face. Situations where (1) the second dentist judges that bad work is probably not involved, (2) the available evidence in the clinical facts and patient's reports cannot resolve a question of bad work, and (3) the second dentist judges, on the basis of available evidence, that bad work probably is involved.

The dentist is clearly obligated, in all of these situations, as 4.C of the ADA Code puts it, to inform the patient of his or her "present oral health status." This obligation derives from the Central Practice Values of Oral and General Health and also from the value of Autonomy. It is also required by the ideal of an Interactive Relationship between the dentist (either dentist) and the patient. All of these professional standards require that a capable patient receive sufficient, accurate information about his or her oral condition so the patient can make appropriate—and, it is hoped, interactive—decisions about it. (This chapter will limit its discussion to patients who are capable of participating in treatment decisions. See chapter 7 for the discussion of how to provide dental care for those not capable of participating or who have only diminished capacity to participate in the decision-making process. Obviously, bad outcomes and potential instances of bad work are likely to raise even more complex ethical questions when experienced in the care of these patients than they do for capable patients.)

Describing a patient's "present oral health status" necessarily includes describing the facts of the bad outcome; the dentist's professional obligations clearly require this of the second dentist. Additionally, there are no reasons to possibly override this requirement based in the dentist's professional commitments. The second dentist does have obligations to the first dentist as a co-professional. Yet, even if these include an obligation to protect the co-professional from certain kinds of harm, the values at stake for the patient in this situation—especially that the patient understand his or her present oral health status—take priority over those at stake for the co-professional.

Might the second dentist support the first dentist's relationship with the patient most effectively, perhaps, by not mentioning the bad outcome to the patient at all? If the patient is not aware of the problem or if the patient is led to believe that it is less important to oral health and function than it is, then the first dentist might deal more effectively with the bad outcome within his or her own relationship to the patient. Would this be a legitimate way, and sometimes the best way, for the second dentist to support the patient's relationship with the first dentist?

Here the ethical complexity of the second dentist's situation becomes clear. The second dentist is not simply the agent of the first dentist; the second dentist has a professional relationship with the patient as well. That is, the dental profession's requirement to respect the patient's Autonomy applies to the second dentist, as does the obligation to work for as interactive a relationship as possible with the patient regarding any matters the second dentist and patient must decide together. The second dentist should not violate the patient's Autonomy or accept an alternate kind of relationship with the patient, then, for the sake of not weakening the first dentist's relationship with that patient. This is another way that the norm of the Relative Priority of the Patient's Well-Being is relevant. The patient's Autonomy and the present dentist's relationship to the patient take precedence over the first dentist's relationship when these come into conflict even though the second dentist remains obligated to support the first dentist's relationship with the patient in every way when no such conflict occurs.

In a former era in which the Guild Model of dentist-patient relationships seems to have had much more normative force in US society, it might have been considered professionally appropriate to refrain from fully informing a patient about a bad outcome so the first dentist could let the patient know in the context of his or her own dentist-patient relationship. As already stressed at several points, though, there is no question that the understanding of dental professionals' obligations—in today's ongoing dialogue between the dental community and the community at large—is that the Central Practice Value of the patient's Autonomy and working for an Interactive Relationship with the patient take precedence over all other competing considerations, except direct risk to the patient's Oral and General Health.

Therefore, in all three of the situations under consideration here the dentist is obligated to inform the patient about the condition of his or her mouth, including giving an accurate description of the facts of the bad outcome. However, this conclusion does not imply anything about what more the second dentist may or may not say, or ought or ought not to say—either to the patient or to a relevant peer review authority—about the role of the first dentist in regard to the bad outcome.

Regarding what the dentist might say to the patient, there are two different sets of circumstances that need to be distinguished. First, the patient may ask the second dentist whether the bad outcome is the result of the first dentist's bad work. Under what conditions is the second dentist professionally obligated to respond to this question by saying that the bad outcome probably is the result of the first dentist's bad work? Are there any other circumstances in which the second dentist *may* ethically say this, even if he or she is not professionally obligated to do so?

Second, even though provided with accurate information about the condition of his or her mouth, the patient still might not ask about the role of the first dentist. Are there any circumstances in which the second dentist is, nevertheless, required to broach the subject and offer a judgment about the first dentist's role? Are there any other circumstances in which the second dentist *may* do so even if it is not professionally required? This last pair of questions will be examined below in the section titled "When the Patient Doesn't Ask."

If the patient directly asks the second dentist for his or her judgment about the first dentist's role regarding the bad outcome, how ought the second dentist deal with this question? We begin with the third of the three kinds of situations distinguished above because it is the most complex.

If the Patient Asks When Bad Work Seems Probable

The third situation is the one where the second dentist judges—on the basis of the clinical evidence and the patient's reports—that bad work probably *is* involved. It will shortly prove necessary to make two further distinctions about this situation that will divide it into four subcategories. We should first examine the strongest reasons for holding that the dentist in this situation should, however, always answer the patient's question truthfully and accurately according to his or her best judgment.

First, as has already been noted, the Central Practice Values of the Patient's General and Oral Health and the patient's Autonomy as well as the obligation to work for as interactive a relationship with the patient as possible all argue for the dentist to fully inform the patient of the facts the patient needs for treatment decisions. The second dentist's judgment regarding the first dentist's responsibility in relation to the bad outcome would seem to be one of these facts, so an honest statement by the second dentist about the responsibility of the first dentist would seem to be required.

Second, every dentist has an obligation to carry out the dental profession's commitments to the larger community. This means that the actions of individual dentists—though regulated and supervised only by other members of the profession—should nevertheless serve patients' well-being both technically and ethically. A dentist who refrains from accurately answering patients' questions about a first dentist's role in a bad outcome—when that bad outcome is judged to probably be an instance of bad work—seems, then, to fail in this obligation both personally and in the name of the whole profession. Thus, in some measure, the profession's privilege of self-regulation is placed at risk.

Third, the norm of Integrity and Professionalism requires that dentists' actions be guided by the values that the profession professes to uphold. As an expert group, the dental profession professes that its members always act in accord with clinical facts and place the well-being of patients ahead of their own (though within certain limits, as noted previously). A dentist who does not accurately answer patients' questions about the causes of a bad outcome—when these are judged to be probable instances of bad work—misrepresents the profession by, first, setting aside fact and, second, placing a co-professional's well-being above a patient's, thus misrepresenting the values for which the dental profession stands.

However, these normative considerations apply to different subcategories within this third situation in different ways, which leads, then, to different ethical conclusions about them rather than to the generic conclusions that may have appeared to follow from them so far. The first distinction that needs to be made is between, on one hand, instances of bad work that involve significant potential for future bad work (and possibly worse harm to the patient) by the first dentist and, on the other hand, instances of bad work that are merely the minor and/or occasional errors that inevitably occur in all expert practice simply because humans are fallible beings.

The ADA Code identifies a relevant distinction in section 4.C, where it says the dentist must determine whether the first dentist's bad work is an instance of "gross or continual faulty treatment." The authors interpret this to imply that some bad outcomes are only instances of the occasional and isolated technical errors that even the best of professionals inevitably make now and then. Obviously, concluding that a bad outcome is an instance of *continual* faulty work requires evidence from other occasions and almost always from other patients of the same dentist. The judgment that an instance of faulty treatment is *gross* does not require such a body of comparative evidence; it is less difficult to make the judgment of *gross* faulty treatment in practice, then, than the judgment of *continual* faulty treatment. The judgment that a bad outcome is probably the result of gross faulty treatment is the judgment that the error is so serious or harmful that it must be considered potentially symptomatic of a serious lack of caution or of proper training or of some other problem that the first dentist is not addressing. In both instances, since the second dentist is judging the bad work as gross or continual faulty treatment, the second dentist is also judging that the patient is at some risk of further bad work, and possibly longer-term harm, if he or she returns to the first dentist.

The dentist who never makes an error in clinical judgment, especially on a close call, and who shapes every restoration, makes every preparation, and takes every impression utterly flawlessly, leaving every patient happy and fully satisfied, is extremely rare, if such a practitioner can be found at all. Most such shortcomings from the theoretical ideal of perfect technical practice do not, though, cause discomfort or harm to patients, or they are brought back to the same dentist who was responsible for them for adjustment or redoing. Thus, when they occur, they are mostly resolved within a single dentist-patient relationship, without the involvement of a second dentist.

Few dentists would fault a dentist who makes an occasional error of this sort. But most dentists would fault a dentist who is unconcerned about an error; who makes an error so serious or harmful that it seems symptomatic of a serious lack of caution, lack of proper training, or some other deeper problem (i.e., gross faulty treatment); or whose work gives evidence of a pattern of errors that the dentist is not addressing (i.e., continual faulty treatment); or who fails to deal properly with the patient regarding it. (The question of how a dentist should deal with his or her own bad outcomes and bad work will be discussed later in this chapter.) The chief reason that dentists do not fault one another for occasional technical shortfalls is that these are not evidence that patients are being placed at risk of future bad work or possible harm. They are truly minor (as compared to gross) and truly occasional (as compared to continual).

This view—that dentists and experts in almost every field rightly take of each other's minor occasional mistakes—is, unfortunately, countercultural. Just as many people apparently accept the myth of infallible health care technology, many also seem to assume that flawless human technical behavior is invariably possible. From this point of view, however, the only ethical alternative to flawless technical performance by a professional would be for the practitioner to withdraw his or her care for the patient, presumably in favor of a technical performer who is flawless. Such thinking also assumes that the determination of whether one can perform flawlessly in a given situation is always clear-cut. Consequently, the distinction between occasional, minor bad work and gross or continual bad work is not widely accepted. Yet this distinction is crucial to understanding a second dentist's professional obligations when he or she must determine whether another's bad outcome is probably an instance of bad work.

The second distinction that is needed here is culturally most evident in certain kinds of legal settings. It concerns the amount of evidence needed for a person to publicly offer a negative judgment of another person's conduct, especially in a setting where relevant expertise appears to be involved. The way US society deals with people's negative public judgments of others' conduct—especially in suits for defamation of character and the like and also in ordinary discourse—indicates that as a society we believe a great deal of evidence is needed to support a negative public judgment of another's conduct. This is especially the case when relevant expertise appears to be involved (rather than when the judgment appears to be casual, uninformed, or purely gossip, for example). The amount of evidence required to support such a negative public judgment is ordinarily considered to be greater than that needed to publicly assess another's actions positively.

It is therefore necessary to distinguish situations where (1) the second dentist justifiably judges but *only in his or her own mind* that the bad outcome is probably an instance of bad work (based on evidence of clinical facts and the patient's reports) from situations where (2) the evidence is strong enough to support a *public* negative judgment of the first dentist by the second dentist by informing the patient that the first dentist probably performed bad work (and doing so even if the patient was completely unaware of it up to this point). For communicating a judgment to the patient must be considered a *public* act. Communications from patient to dentist are private and therefore subject to the restrictions of professional confidentiality. Communications from the dentist to the patient, however, may ordinarily be repeated by the patient at will without violating his or her relationship to the dentist. The second dentist's judgments about the first dentist's work, when communicated to the patient, must therefore be considered *public* judgments, and it is obvious that professional expertise is involved in relaying them.

Consequently, a greater measure of evidence is needed for the second dentist to tell the patient that the bad outcome has probably resulted from the first dentist's bad work than is necessary for the dentist to conclude privately, in his or her own mind, that this is probably the case. Thus, section 4.C of the ADA Code states: "Dentists issuing a public statement with respect to the profession shall have a reasonable basis to believe that the comments made are true." (The authors are not claiming that dentists are under a legal obligation in this regard, rather that there is a widely applicable social rule about the amount of evidence needed to publicly judge another's conduct negatively—a rule that is applied formally in certain legal contexts but applies more broadly—and that it is directly relevant to the professional-ethical issue under discussion here.)

Even though dentists sometimes protest that there is never enough evidence, it was argued above that situations do arise where the second dentist has sufficient evidence to privately judge that bad work probably has occurred. But the evidence needed for this private judgment is often not sufficient for a *public* judgment to this effect, and the dentist would not be justified in communicating *to the patient* that it probably is bad work because that would be a public judgment. A dentist will frequently, in fact, lack sufficient evidence to meet this burden of proof unless he or she has communicated about the circumstances of the work with the first dentist, and even then, the second dentist might still lack sufficient data unless the communication with the first dentist was careful and detailed. Most dentists who observe another dentist's bad outcome, however, do not have the opportunity to communicate with the first dentist before being asked about the bad work with the patient. Therefore, dentists are frequently not in a position to answer a patient's question about whether, in their judgment, the bad outcome is probably the result of the first dentist's bad work. This is because they often lack the evidence needed to make a *public* statement, which includes statements to the patient, to that effect.

There is one notable exception in US society to the social rule about the degree of evidence needed for a negative public judgment, especially where expertise is involved. If a person is called to testify in court, he or she is required to publicly state his or her negative judgment there—together with the evidence for it—just as it is and without first determining whether the evidence meets the standard under consideration here. The restriction about speaking without sufficient evidence is lifted, then, in this special setting. This is because the judge, jury, and other participants are considered capable of evaluating the evidence offered for the witness's judgments, in relation to other evidence provided within the court situation, for themselves; actually, they are required to do so by their special roles in the court.

Let us now return to the situation where the second dentist must deal with a patient's question about the role of the first dentist in a bad outcome when the second dentist's private judgment—justified by the clinical evidence and the patient's reports—is that this probably *is* an instance of bad work. We now have four subcategories of this situation to examine.

Only a Private Judgment and Not Gross or Continual

The first subcategory is for those circumstances where two things are true: (1) the available evidence is strong enough to support a dentist's *private* judgment that this is probably bad work but not strong enough to justify a statement to the patient to this effect because this is viewed as a *public* statement and the standard of evidence for a public statement is not met, and (2) the dentist's personal judgment is that the bad work probably is *not* an instance of gross or continual faulty treatment. Under these circumstances, if the patient asks, the dentist is *not obligated* to communicate his or her private judgment on the role of the first dentist to the patient. The dentist may instead respond that there is not enough evidence for him or her to judge the matter. This is a truthful and accurate answer, given the standard of evidence relevant to making a public statement; it is therefore consistent with the dentist's obligation to respect the patient's Autonomy and work for as interactive a relationship as possible, for the relevant social standard of evidence qualifies the extent (that is, sets the limits) of the dentist's obligations under the Autonomy norm. If the dentist does answer in this way, however, he or she should inform the patient that the standard of evidence that has not been met is a fairly stringent standard; this is to avoid misleading the patient into thinking that some lower standard of evidence has not been met—especially the standard one would apply in forming a private judgment of the matter. The dentist would, moreover, certainly be acting unethically if he or she tried to intimate that the inadequacy of the evidence somehow suggests that the first dentist acted properly—especially since the second dentist's private judgment is that the bad outcome is probably an instance of bad work. Misleading the patient in this way would clearly violate the Central Practice Value of the patient's Autonomy and would also undermine the second dentist's commitment to an Interactive Relationship with the patient. Since the patient is not judged to be at risk of continued bad treatment or possible harm from the first dentist, the Central Practice Values of the patient's Oral and General Health and the requirement that the profession guard against harmful practice are not compromised by such an answer.

A typical answer in response to a patient's question under the circumstances of the first subcategory might sound like this: "That's a very reasonable question, Mr. Jones. Unfortunately, there are many factors involved in a bad outcome of this sort. A judgment on my part would require fairly strong evidence for me to tell you that the outcome was probably the result of some error on Dr. Smith's part. And the facts, as I can determine them, do not support that kind of judgment." As subsequent discussion in this chapter will indicate, we believe that the best resolution of such situations occurs when the second dentist can also say, "I would like to call Dr. Smith to tell him what I have seen, and I would recommend that you contact him yourself, at your earliest convenience, so the two of you can work together to deal with what has happened."

However, if the second dentist is not *obligated*—under the circumstances of the first subcategory—to communicate his or her private judgment of probable bad work to the patient, *may* the second dentist still do so? Or would that be a violation of professional obligation in some way?

The social standard of evidence, discussed above, argues against any negative public judgment on the part of the first dentist when that standard of evidence has not been met. There is one professional consideration, however, that might justify telling the patient of one's private judgment about probable bad work even if the evidence did not meet this standard. Suppose the second dentist had good reason to believe that doing so would significantly enhance the patient's well-being, either by producing a significantly better relationship between the patient and the first dentist or by bringing about a significantly greater realization of the Central Practice Values for the patient or something similar. Then the benefits to the patient might justify the second dentist communicating his or her private judgment to the patient. Under such circumstances—when the second dentist *may* ethically answer the patient's question, even though not obligated, the second dentist would be obliged to make it clear to the patient (1) that the ordinary measure of evidence required for this communication is not available and (2) that the second dentist's judgment is, for that reason, less certain than it would be if the ordinary standard for evidence had been met. But it must be stressed that the only consideration that can justify a dentist's communicating his or her private judgment to the patient—under the circumstances of the first subcategory—is a significant contribution to the well-being of the patient. It seems likely, however, that circumstances meeting this criterion would rarely occur.

Only a Private Judgment and Probably Gross or Continual

In the second subcategory are circumstances where (1) the evidence available to the dentist is again *not* strong enough to justify a public judgment (in other words, communication to the patient) that the bad outcome is probably an instance of bad work but (2) the dentist's judgment is that the bad work probably *is* an instance of gross or continual faulty treatment. Under these circumstances, if the patient asks, the dentist's answer must again communicate that the evidence available does not pass the threshold ordinarily required for him or her to make a public judgment on the matter. In this situation, however, because of the risk to the patient, we propose that the dentist must do two additional things.

First, the dentist must indicate to the patient that, though the evidence is limited, it suggests the patient may be at risk of future bad work or harm. Advising a patient that the bad outcome is to be taken seriously (gross or continual) and that the evidence is very limited is a subtle matter; that is, the advice being offered is based only on a "possible" or at most "probable" conclusion rather than something the second dentist is sure of. (Recall, in the second subcategory, the dentist does not have enough evidence to meet the standard of evidence for a negative public judgment—especially since expertise is clearly involved.) The genuine risk of future bad work or harm for the patient (evidenced by the probable presence of gross or continual faulty treatment), though, requires the second dentist to inform the patient about this risk, even if the patients does not ask about it. Not doing so would violate the dentist's professional obligations to preserve and enhance the patient's Oral and General Health, respect the patient's Autonomy, and play a part in the dental profession's supervisory activity to prevent inadequate practice. Second, Article 4.C of the ADA Code states that dentists must report probable instances of gross or continual faulty treatment "to the appropriate reviewing agency as determined by the local component or constituent [dental] society." If something probably indicates gross or continual bad work where the patient is at risk of further bad work and possibly harm in the hands of the first dentist, then other patients of the first dentist are at potential risk as well. Reporting the matter to the peer review organization introduces a group that, collectively, is more capable of determining if bad work—specifically gross or continual faulty treatment—did take place. They are also in a position to take further action, if needed, to protect this and other patients from harm by the first dentist.

Occasionally, individual dentists will have personal and professional relationships with the first dentist that are close enough that their individual personal contact with the first dentist will be effective in protecting this and other patients. Sometimes, these personal contacts can be more effective than reporting to a reviewing agency. When this is the case, a dentist may be justified in working toward this end without reporting the matter to the appropriate dental organization, for the goal is enhancing and protecting patients' well-being rather than bringing about punitive action toward a dentist. Feelings of collegiality and friendship, however, may weaken a dentist's judgment on this matter. Dentists who are tempted to forgo reporting a colleague, then, should examine their reasons very carefully before doing so. Failure to act effectively to protect patients from future bad work and possible harm under such circumstances is a serious individual professional wrong, and it is a serious violation of the profession's commitment to the larger community to assure that its expertise is properly applied.

Evidence Sufficient for a Public Judgment and Not Gross or Continual

A third subcategory are those circumstances where (1) the evidence available to the dentist *is* strong enough to justify a statement to the patient that the bad outcome is an instance of bad work but (2) the dentist's judgment is that the bad work probably is *not* an instance of gross or continual faulty treatment. Under these circumstances, if the patient asks, the dentist may not ethically answer that there is not sufficient evidence for him or her to offer a judgment; it simply is not true. Integrity and Professionalism and the commitment to an Interactive Relationship with the patient require the second dentist in these particular circumstances to explain his or her judgment to the patient, along with the supporting evidence.

A dentist, as indicated above, will not often be faced with this decision unless he or she has already conversed with the first dentist about the bad outcome. On those occasions, when this set of circumstances prevails, the second dentist ordinarily maintains his or her judgment that bad work has occurred after communicating with the first dentist because the first dentist has concurred in that judgment or else because, in spite of listening to the first dentist, the second dentist has concluded that bad work has nevertheless occurred. In either of these cases, the degree of evidence required for offering his or her judgment to the patient is so great that the ordinary objection of some dentists to telling the patient—namely, that "you never have enough evidence"—will not apply. If the first dentist concurs with the second dentist's judgment, though, the two dentists can work collaboratively with the patient to deal with the situation and, working together, they can determine what should follow in terms of maintaining the collaborative relationship with the patient to promote the patient's health and well-being. Since it is *not* probable, in this situation, that the patient is at risk of additional bad work or possible harm at the hands of the first dentist, it is important to note that the second dentist's obligation to return the patient to the first dentist, and to support the first dentist's relationship with the patient, remains intact. This may seem ironic, for a patient informed that a bad outcome is probably the result of the first dentist's bad work might seem likely to sue the first dentist or at least leave his or her practice. If there has been a good relationship and good communication with the first dentist, though, that relationship may possibly continue productively.

The second dentist might also—though at some risk because of the cultural environment in the United States in which dentistry practices today—try educating the patient about the difference between bad outcomes and bad work with special attention on the differences between (1) the occasional, minor bad work inevitable in the professional practice of fallible humans and (2) the gross or continual bad work that puts patients at risk (and that is not the focus of this third subcategory). The second dentist might try convincing the patient to allow the same appropriate leniency of judgment—regarding occasional, minor mistakes—that dentists ordinarily make toward one another. The risk, of course, is that the second dentist will be judged by the patient to be less expert, less dependable, and less professional for having said such things. Yet, communicating honestly about these matters is the most truthful and, arguably, the most effective way for the second dentist; these remain the precise truths about professional dental practice needed to support the relationship between a patient who has experienced a minor, isolated instance of bad work and a conscientious professional caregiver who has made a minor, isolated mistake.

A strong initiative in this direction by the dental community as a whole would, furthermore, be a far better approach than expecting individual dentists in difficult circumstances to offer this kind of education. Dentistry as a whole, like the dentist in the circumstances just described, would also run a risk if it challenged head-on the myths of infallible technology and technique and infallible performers—and their corollary that all bad outcomes must be the result of bad work. It is doubtful dentistry can undermine these myths alone, but it could take part in the establishment of a broad coalition of health professions committed to trying to supplant them, as has already been attempted by the Institute of Medicine's "To Err is Human" initiative.

Until these myths are eliminated, they will continue to fuel an environment of mutual suspicion between health care providers and their patients as well as the professions and society. Malpractice costs will continue to increase because juries will continue to believe these myths, despite evidence in the Scandinavian countries that confronting these myths and developing "No Blame" social policies (as contrasted with "no fault" insurance products) greatly decreases costly defensive health care practices, increases direct restoration of harm related to both bad outcomes and bad work, and generates a more open dialogue where practices improve for both individuals and the profession as a whole. All the groundless pressures and consequences these myths produce for dentists, physicians, and others have solutions. If these myths are eliminated, of course, health professionals' expertise may not be held in awe as it has been historically in this society. There may be some consequent loss of social status and perhaps some change in dentists' (and physicians') compensation. This is an interesting and active question for the health professions—whether they are willing to accept these unknown trade-offs.

Setting such cost-benefit thinking aside, the dental profession's norms of Competence and especially Integrity and Professionalism require it to challenge these myths and to work at the collaborative reeducating of the society that accepts them. The profession of dentistry and its practice is based on facts, not myths; these facts include the fallibility of the technologies and techniques its members employ and the fallibility of the members who employ them. The larger community's confidence in the members of this profession should not rest on infallible technologies or infallible performers but on the enduring *ethical* commitment of its members to use its (fallible) expertise for the benefit for every patient served.

Realistic relationships between dentists and patients ought to be founded on these facts rather than on myths. Within such foundational relationships, dentists could inform patients honestly of another dentist's incidental, minor mistake without fear of causing grave loss for the latter. In that environment, it would not be a matter of some relief that the occurrence of this third subcategory is uncommon, because the high standard of evidence needed to tell a patient that another dentist's bad work is involved is currently not often met. In the different environment projected here, dentists might wish to change the social rules about evidence that govern their communications to patients. Then the simple truths about fallible technologies and techniques—and more importantly the simple truths about the relationships of fallible humans working for one another's good—might be more directly communicated and supported.

Evidence Sufficient for a Public Judgment and Gross or Continual

This brings us to the fourth subcategory where (1) the evidence available to the dentist *is* strong enough to justify a statement to the patient—that is, a public statement that the bad outcome is probably an instance of bad work—and (2) the dentist's judgment is that the bad work probably is an instance of gross or continual faulty treatment. Under these circumstances, the dentist must again explain his or her judgment to the patient, along with the supporting evidence. This must be done whether the patient asks or not because of the probable risk to the patient. The dentist must also report the probable instance of gross or continual faulty treatment to the appropriate reviewing agency.

The reasons why these two actions are required under these circumstances have already been explained. The likelihood that the first circumstance will occur is, as has been discussed, not great. The likelihood that it will occur in conjunction with the second circumstance, which is also uncommon, is even lower. But if these two circumstances should ever occur in tandem, the norms of the dental profession require that the two actions indicated be taken.

The First and Second Situations Revisited

Now that we have considered the complex third situation, in which the second dentist judges—on the basis of the clinical evidence and the patient's reports—that bad work probably *is* involved, we can return to the first and second situations. To consider the first situation, recall that the second dentist privately judges that the bad outcome is probably *not* the result of a first dentist's bad work. How should the second dentist deal with a patient who asks directly about the first dentist's role in a bad outcome when the second dentist judges it is *not* an instance of bad work?

In situations of this type, when a patient directly asks about the work of a first dentist, the second dentist may welcome the patient's question, for this is an opportunity to make the point that the first dentist is probably without fault and explain his or her reasons for this conclusion. The rules of evidence needed to make *positive* public judgments of others' actions in our society do not require the same high standard of evidence as is required for *negative* public judgments. The dentist would therefore not be violating standards of evidence to offer his or her positive judgment even though the forum is still a public one, in the sense explained above. This judgment needs no stronger evidence base than what would support any other private judgment. In other words, the positive content of the dentist's judgment does not violate professional integrity or other social rules. But a dentist offering a judgment on only this measure of evidence should indicate the measure of evidence supporting his or her judgment and should not suggest that the evidence is more substantial than it is.

In the second of the three situations, the second dentist is *not able to determine*—from the evidence available—whether or not the bad outcome is the result of the first dentist's bad work. In this situation, if the patient asks, the dentist is obligated to answer truthfully that he or she is unable to determine the matter. The dentist may be tempted to make this uncertainty sound like evidence that the first dentist probably did not do bad work, but doing so would be a violation of the norm of Integrity and Professionalism and of the dentist's commitment to work for as interactive a relationship with the patient as possible. A dentist may fear that the patient will misinterpret his or her uncertainty as evidence that the first dentist certainly did bad work, and the second dentist should counter these mistakes in the patient's judgment, but not by trying to lead the patient to draw incorrect conclusions in the other direction. This may again be a moment in which the second dentist could educate the patient and discuss the myths of infallible technologies and techniques and infallible performers.

What to tell the patient when there is a bad outcome is a complex and well-known ethical issue. This lengthy and critically important analysis, covering three situations and four subcategories within the third one, introduces the major themes underlying the question's complexity. But the "short" answer can be easily stated: The second dentist is obligated to answer the patient's question truthfully and accurately according to his or her best judgment. The answer must also meet the relevant standards of evidence accepted within the larger community for various kinds of questions about other people's conduct. But this general answer points to very different ethical actions, depending on the particular circumstances, as our efforts to divide the question into several parts has hopefully made clear.

The reasoning offered here does support the claim that a dentist rarely has sufficient evidence to justify telling a patient who asks whether another dentist's bad outcome is probably bad work. But it does not support the opinion common within dentistry that there is never sufficient evidence to form or offer such a judgment. More importantly, however, what this reasoning demonstrates is that the second dentist has some very important and often difficult ethical thinking to do before he or she answers a patient's question in this type of scenario. This, however, is not the only conclusion that can be drawn from the explanations offered here. They clearly support the ethical requirement that the dentist truthfully and accurately inform the capable patient about the condition of his or her mouth, including the facts about the bad outcome. There is no exception to this obligation, regardless of what else the dentist may or may not, ought or ought not, say about the situation. There is also no exception to this requirement when, as may often happen, the second dentist fears a patient will draw unwarranted negative conclusions about the first dentist's work from the facts about the bad outcome. The second dentist may, and ordinarily should try to, counter these conclusions in ethically appropriate ways. But the capable patient must always be truthfully and accurately informed about the condition of his or her mouth—including the facts of the bad outcome.

WHEN THE PATIENT DOESN'T ASK

What if the patient does not ask? Is the second dentist still professionally required to inform the patient? And, may the dentist tell the patient who does not ask if it is not required?

The second dentist is always obligated to inform every capable patient accurately and completely about the condition of his or her mouth—including the facts of a bad outcome. This information may not ethically be omitted whether the patient asks or not. But suppose the patient accepts and understands this information but still does not ask the second dentist to offer judgment about the first dentist's role in the bad outcome. Is the second dentist obligated to introduce the subject and offer his or her judgment? May the dentist ethically do so, even if not obligated? Each of the three situations distinguished earlier in the chapter needs examination. When the second dentist judges that a bad outcome probably is the result of the first dentist's bad work, as in the third situation, strong evidence is usually needed to make a negative public judgment about it—that is, to say this to the patient. In the first subcategory, in which this kind of evidence is not available and gross or continual bad work is not involved, the second dentist may not ordinarily justify volunteering his or her negative judgment about the first dentist's role to the patient. Nevertheless, if significant patient benefit would be achieved, this might outweigh this social requirement about evidence; it may justify offering one's judgment even when the evidence does not meet the public standard.

In both the second and fourth subcategories of the third situation, the patient is at risk of future bad work or harm. This is because there is evidence of gross or continual faulty treatment. In both sets of circumstances the patient must certainly be informed of this whether the patient asks about the matter or not for the reasons explained earlier in this chapter.

What about the circumstance of the third subcategory, where the second dentist does have enough evidence to make a public statement about the first dentist's bad work but gross or continual faulty treatment is not involved? As explained above, if the patient asks, the second dentist would have to be truthful and accurate, as has been explained, saying that the bad outcome is probably the result of bad work. Suppose, however, the second dentist knew the evidence was this strong but, after being informed of the facts of the bad outcomes, the patient still did not ask about the first dentist's role. Ought the second dentist volunteer this judgment in this unusual situation?

The basis of any obligation that the second dentist inform a patient who did not ask would be to protect the patient from harm. The authors propose that since the patient is not judged to be at potential risk of future bad work or harm from the first dentist—that is, as long as the bad work is not judged to be gross or continual—the second dentist is not professionally obligated to inform the patient that the bad outcome is probably the result of bad work.

Is the second dentist professionally *allowed* to inform the patient in this situation, even if the patient does not ask? Here the second dentist would have to reflect carefully on why he or she would want to inform the patient. What will it accomplish? Enhancing the patient's relationship with the first dentist would be an excellent goal, but the second dentist's informing the patient of this unusual situation will not likely be the most effective means to this goal. Instead, the prevalence of the myths of infallible technology and infallible practitioners in the current culture makes it likely that the information might lead to a misjudgment by the patient and an undeserved risk of loss for the first dentist, who has, at most, committed a minor, incidental mistake. The discussion about the bad outcome and the possibility of bad work is typically better had between the patient and the first dentist. It will ordinarily be preferable, then, for the second dentist to contact the first dentist rather than directly inform the patient. The most important ethical question is which course of action most serves the benefit of the patient within his or her relationship with the first dentist.

What about the first situation, if the patient does not ask about the second dentist's role in the bad outcome and the second dentist judges a bad outcome is probably not the result of the first dentist's work? Here the second dentist is obliged to tell the patient this fact only if doing so significantly supports and strengthens the relationship between the patient and the first dentist, and it is hard to imagine circumstances in which that relationship would not be better served by a conversation about the bad outcome between the patient and the first dentist.

CONTACTING THE OTHER DENTIST

The two courses of action that were examined in the previous sections—that the second dentist inform the patient of the first dentist's role or that the second dentist say nothing at all about it—are not the only things the second dentist might do. In addition to these options, the second dentist should ordinarily contact the first dentist.

The best place to talk about a bad outcome, precisely for the sake of supporting the first dentist-patient relationship, is within that relationship. Any subsequent treatment decisions that are needed because of the bad outcome are also better made, as interactively as possible, by the patient and the first dentist. In this scenario, the possibility for discussing the first dentist's role regarding bad outcomes will ordinarily be enhanced as well. If the second dentist contacts the first dentist about the bad outcome observed, the second dentist can describe the strength of the evidence, one way or another, that bad work was or was not involved, as well as the second dentist's interactions with the patient. The first dentist will then be in a much better position to talk with the patient about the bad outcome and his or her role in regard to it and to deal with the consequences of this discussion accordingly.

There are good professional-ethical reasons, then, that the second dentist should, in every instance, attempt to contact the first dentist about judgments of bad outcomes caused by the first dentist's work. Such communication is one of the most effective actions the second dentist can usually take to support the first dentist's relationship with the patient and preserve and support the Central Practice Values of the patient's Oral and General Health and Autonomy.

If this path were routine, the second dentist would inform the patient of his or her intention to contact the first dentist in every instance of an identified bad outcome. The second dentist would also inform the patient to either expect the first dentist to be in touch with him or her or to contact the first dentist directly to arrange further examination or treatment of the bad outcome. The dentists' communication must be made and received in a collegial, collaborative spirit to be effective. The benefit to the patient and the enhancement of the dentist-patient relationship must be the clear goals in the eyes of both dentists.

Many factors in the environment of contemporary dental practice in the United States, unfortunately, make this difficult. This path requires dentists to be willing to talk with one another frankly about bad outcomes and possible evidence of bad work that sometimes causes or contributes to bad outcomes. Most dentists hesitate, in today's culture, to tell any dentist but a close friend that they saw a bad outcome, much less observed evidence that it might have been bad work. They see themselves as judging another dentist negatively. Because they do not want to be judged negatively themselves, it might seem best to avoid seeming judgmental.

All dentists already know that many bad outcomes happen without anyone's bad work and that some occasional bad work, involving no long-term harm to anyone, is inevitable in every dentist's practice. If dentists allowed themselves to acknowledge this to one another, this change in the culture of dentistry could reshape dentists' conversations about these matters. The phone call—where the second dentist informs the first of a bad outcome or the evidence of bad work—would not be an insult putting their future communication and collaboration at risk; it would, instead, be an effort by a colleague to enhance the first dentist's relationship with his or her patient. It would thus be an act of positive collegiality based on mutual understanding of the challenges of dental practice.

But this communication between dentists would not support the relationship between them if the first dentist did not, in turn, contact or talk with the patient, nor would the patient's Oral and General Health or the patient's relationship to the first dentist be effectively supported. That is, the first dentist must also be willing to discuss with his or her patients the possibility of bad outcomes, the possibility of bad work, and the role of occasional mistakes that all professionals experience with patients. The first dentist must also be willing to work with patients to make any needed treatment and relationship decisions that result from this conversation. This brings us to the dentist's obligations to the patient when a bad outcome or bad work is his or her own.

An aura of suspicion admittedly lies between professionals and many of their lay clients in the current culture of the United States. The larger community often fears that professionals, including dentists, are more interested in protecting one another than in respecting the norms of their professions. Professionals understandably fear that their clients will take advantage of bad outcomes, especially bad work, to profit through lawsuits and other legal maneuvers, all of this based on the public's wide acceptance of the infallible technologies myth. Public media typically reinforces this environment of suspicion by creating audiences willing to listen to isolated examples of bad work by a dentist or patients suing over a dentist's incidental shortfall that involved little if any irreparable harm, with each side then believing what it feared is even more widespread than before. The two most important facts, (1) that the vast majority of professionals practice conscientiously according to their profession's norms and other standards of practice and (2) that most people respect and trust the professionals who personally serve them, are widely ignored in such reports, and the environment of suspicion worsens.

In such an environment, establishing the third course of action—collegial communication between dentists about bad outcomes and possible evidence of bad work—as the standard pattern of response to a bad outcome is not easy. Attempting to do so—even if it only begins with private agreements among dentists within referral and/or coverage networks—is likely to be more effective than any other tactic the dental profession might attempt to lessen suspicion and persuade the larger community that dentists are not simply trying to protect one another. This third course of action also positively serves the values and norms of the dental profession in dealing with bad outcomes. This is so whether the second dentist judges the bad outcome is not the result of bad work, cannot resolve that issue, or judges that bad work was probably involved. All three of the situations discussed above, then, are best resolved by taking this third path. Talk avoided is often the talk that is most needed.

WHEN A NEW PATIENT HAS ANOTHER DENTIST'S BAD OUTCOME

In the situations examined in previous sections, patients with a bad outcome would ordinarily be returning to their general dentist after seeing a specialist or having emergency treatment by another dentist, or they are being seen temporarily for specialty or emergency care. But dentists also see patients with bad outcomes when a new patient enters the dentist's practice after moving to a new area, changing marriage status, initiating or changing an insurance policy or managed care contract, the death or retirement of a previous dentist, and so on.

In these cases, the patient's chief relationship is now going to be with the dentist identifying the bad outcome (the "second dentist"), not the dentist associated with the bad outcome (the "first dentist"—that is, the patient's prior dentist). These cases differ from the previous examined cases because the dentist identifying the bad work does not have a strong obligation to support the prior dentist's relationship with the patient; that relationship is simply past and done with. Contacting the prior dentist to strengthen that dentist's relationship with the patient is typically of less worth. (It can, however, be important for other reasons. For example, in the case in chapter 8, Dr. Watkins contacted Kathleen O'Gara's former dentist in the hope that this might lead to her getting the care she needed, even though she was unlikely to return to Dr. Watkins's practice to get it.) The dentist, in cases where the patient is new to this dentist's practice, should ordinarily focus on enhancing his or her own relationship with the patient, for this is the chief dentist-patient relationship for these patients.

The second dentist in this kind of situation may be tempted to overemphasize the bad outcome or to offer judgments about the other dentist's responsibility for the bad outcome that cannot be supported by the available evidence. The claims made and argued for in the previous sections, about judging other dentists' bad outcomes and about statements to the patient, all apply to this situation as well. The second dentist is obliged to fully inform the patient about the condition of his or her mouth, including the bad outcome; he or she is also obligated to answer truthfully and accurately—to the best of his or her judgment (and in accord with accepted standards of evidence)—the patient's questions about the role of the prior dentist in relation to the bad outcome (although the immediately prior dentist may not have been the dentist responsible for it). The second dentist must also report gross or continual faulty treatment to the appropriate reviewing body when this is appropriate, as explained above. The dentist may not ethically lead the patient to a lower opinion of the other dentist than the evidence will bear in any of these matters, and the points made earlier about standards of evidence must also be kept in mind.

But this situation can become complicated if a patient wants to maintain some relationship with the dentist associated with the bad outcome, especially if the bad outcome is related to bad work—for example, in order to correct or seek other forms of compensation for the failed work. The patient will often expect his or her new dentist, then, to assist in these efforts. There are no clear professional-ethical guidelines about how a dentist ought to proceed in such a circumstance. This is particularly so if a dentist privately judges that the bad outcome was probably the result of the other dentist's bad work but does not have sufficient evidence to meet the standard required for a negative statement to the patient.

A collaborative effort by both dentists to attempt resolution of the patient's needs will most certainly and effectively support the professional values and norms discussed in this chapter. The pressures pushing the parties toward a conflictual relationship, though, are very strong—particularly in the current environment where the myths discussed earlier are so prevalent.

STILL MORE COMPLEX RELATIONSHIPS

To this point the discussion of bad outcomes and the possibility of bad work has focused on situations in which both the first and the second dentist are imagined as being in solo practices. But many dentists today practice as partners in group practices or, especially among young dentists recently graduated from dental school, as employees in other dentists' practices or in large, multisite and/or corporate dental offices. So the dentist who has experienced a bad outcome or whose work might possibly be bad work—the first dentist—could be the second dentist's partner, employee, employer, or a fellow employee in the same organization or could be a dentist who is part of a different dental care organization, and the second dentist could be part of a multidentist organization as well. Moreover, under any of these circumstances, the culture and character of the relevant organization(s)—whether they consist of only two dentists or of many—will significantly impact the relationship between the first and the second dentist and may mean that other dentists, especially those in organizational leadership positions, will also be involved. A dental organization's culture may actively support respectful, collegial, patient-centered dentist-to-dentist communication, or it may routinely approach relationships about bad outcomes and bad work adversarially (which can easily end up involving lawyers and the courts), or the response could be something in between.

Lastly, a bad outcome or bad work may be a direct result of a corporate policy or directive that leaves its employed dentists with little other option than to quit, or the dentist discovering the bad outcome or bad work may be employed and unable to act with the independence assumed in the discussions so far in this chapter. The obligations of those who employ dentists will be covered in chapter 10. Another possibility is that a dentist might encounter a bad outcome or bad work from an employed dentist and discover that that dentist cannot independently respond to inquiries or efforts to rectify the situation. But it is beyond the scope of this book to do more than point out that still more complex relationships and ethical issues like these can arise.

WHEN THE BAD OUTCOME OR BAD WORK IS A DENTIST'S OWN

If the dentist responsible for a bad outcome responds properly, even when his or her bad work is involved, things turn out better for the patient, and collaboration between professionals becomes most productive. Working collaboratively with the other dentist(s) involved in order to reach a shared understanding of what happened and why is part of this proper response. The norm of Integrity and Professionalism, like dentistry's other professional norms, commits dentists to base their decisions on shared understandings of the facts and the value of dental interventions. The Central Practice Values and the ideal of achieving an Interactive Relationship with the patient are also relevant. What is less clear, at first look, is what the dentist associated with the bad outcome is professionally obligated to do for and say to the patient involved. (These issues are even more complicated if the dentist is not the sole owner of the practice. For many dentists are partners in group practices and many others practice, as already mentioned, as employees or independent consultants in other dentists' practices. We will begin with the issues faced by a dentist who is the sole owner of his or her practice and discuss more complex practice settings after that.) Let us first consider the dentist who judges a bad outcome to be the result of his or her own bad work but sees it as an occasional, minor mistake, not an instance of gross or continual faulty treatment.

When a dentist and capable patient mutually choose some treatment, the dentist is committed, by that agreed choice, to completing that treatment within the accepted standards of the dental profession. If his or her performance falls short of this standard, the dentist still needs to fulfill his or her part of the mutual choice. In addition to any contractual obligation and any more general ethical requirements, the professional norm of Competence is clearly relevant here. There is ordinarily also a professional requirement to carry out the commitment to the agreed-on treatment because failure to do so usually violates the dentist's obligations to respect and support the patient's Autonomy and to work for as interactive a relationship as possible. The only exception to this professional requirement to respect the patient's Autonomy by carrying out the commitment are situations where fulfilling the treatment commitment would violate the dentist's commitment to serve the higher-ranking Central Practice Values of the patient's General and Oral Health. Usually, however, the dentist responsible for bad work is professionally obligated to do the work he or she committed to do. Or, if intervening events have made the work originally committed to inappropriate for the patient's well-being and purposes, different work that fulfills the patient's needs is required. Of course, finding another dentist to do one or the other, within the original financial agreement, may also be an option.

The dentist may fulfill this obligation by simply redoing the work that resulted in the bad outcome or doing the work needing to take its place at no charge, if that is the patient's choice. The dentist may also cover the costs of retreatment—or appropriate alternate treatment—by another practitioner. There are often fiscal and other business reasons for dentists to do this work personally. From the professional-ethical point of view, though, the only requirement is that the work (or appropriate alternate work) be done competently.

Every dentist must answer patients' questions about bad work truthfully and accurately, according to his or her best judgment and in accord with relevant standards of evidence. A dentist who is examining his or her own bad outcomes will ordinarily, though, have much better access to evidence about what happened than any other dentist. This dentist, then, will most likely be able to meet whatever the relevant accepted standard of evidence is for a public judgment—that is, a statement to the patient—about the bad work. Therefore, the obligation to respond truthfully and accurately to patients' questions about one's own bad work will typically arise more often than it does in the case of a second dentist responding to questions about another dentist's bad work.

What if the patient doesn't ask? The dentist who performed the original work is obligated, as argued, to redo the work, do alternate work, or make other arrangements for the fulfillment of his or her contractual and professional commitments regarding the work. The dentist is also obligated to provide the patient with accurate information about the condition of his or her mouth. The dentist's conscientious fulfillment of these obligations will often prompt the patient to question the cause. But if no such question is asked when the dentist judges the bad outcome was likely related to his or her own bad work, is a dentist obligated to acknowledge his or her responsibility anyway?

The answer depends on what will benefit the relationship between dentist and patient. Self-criticism is not easy. If it is carefully and intelligently done, though, it can often strengthen a relationship—sometimes very much. Suppose the dentist sincerely judges that raising the subject—when the patient has not asked about it—will actually hinder their relationship or at least not help it. We propose that there is no professional obligation to raise the matter if the patient does not ask, provided all the other requirements and communication discussed here are completed. Permitting a dentist not to raise the subject under these circumstances does not, though, justify attempts to mislead the patient into thinking the opposite of what the dentist judges to be the case.

What if a dentist believed his or her bad work was an instance of gross or continual faulty treatment? What if a dentist believed that patients were at risk of continued bad work or possible harm in this dentist's practice? Before taking measures to correct the situation, such a dentist must obviously, and immediately, seek the assistance of appropriate organizational units, friends, and other respected colleagues to first determine if such is the case. The obligations about what to do—regarding the work itself and regarding what to say to patients—would be no different from those just described. If a dentist truly is putting his or her patients at risk, that dentist would then be professionally obligated to refrain from practice—or from certain kinds of practice if the defects are localized—until the situation has been corrected. This obligation is obviously supported in the strongest manner by almost every category of professional norms.

When a dentist's bad work results in gross or continual faulty treatment, though, he or she is ordinarily unaware of the seriousness of the problem and is often slow to believe other dentists and review groups that propose there is a problem. How ought a dentist respond to such a proposal from another dentist? Clearly, the dentist must take very seriously another dentist's proposal that gross or continual bad work is being done. Then assistance should be sought from colleagues he or she respects to examine this proposal carefully; they can then work collaboratively to take appropriate action to correct the problem. This is one of the most painful sacrifices a person can make—to take seriously a dental colleague's challenge to one's ability to practice competently and then to respond carefully. But the well-being of his or her own patients and that of the whole profession's patients are at stake.

Moreover, the dental profession is clearly obligated to supervise the practice of its members. Therefore, it needs to identify and correct members who, for whatever reasons, have demonstrated a significant potential to do bad work and put patients at serious risk of harm and to adversely impact the dental profession in its role in society. The dentist is not only required to take the proposal seriously and respond appropriately because it is his or her own work of which the quality is being challenged. The dentist also has this obligation as a member of the profession because every dentist has an obligation to support the profession's fulfillment of its supervisory role.

Suppose a dentist, after considering the matter carefully, does not judge a bad outcome to be the result of bad work on his or her part. What obligations does the dentist have then? The dentist must, of course, accurately inform the patient about the condition of his or her mouth, including the facts about the bad outcome. But the dentist is only obligated to explain his or her judgment about his or her responsibility for the bad outcome if the patient asks about it. In such situations, the dentist will ordinarily want to raise the issue to explain why the bad outcome is not the result of his or her bad work. The dentist, of course, should not conclude too readily that the bad outcome was not the result of bad work; as a professional, a dentist is obligated to carefully consider all the evidence before drawing a conclusion.

A patient in this situation presumably still needs treatment; the work must be redone or replaced with a clinically appropriate alternative that is acceptable to the patient. The dentist who proceeds successfully in these matters is responding in a professionally competent way, presuming the relationship with the patient remains as interactive as possible because the dentist does exactly what he or she was professionally committed to do from a professional-ethical standpoint. We therefore propose that, when an unplanned, unwanted, or bad outcome occurs that is not the result of a dentist's bad work, then the dentist has no professional obligation to do the needed additional work (or have it done by another dentist) at no charge or at reduced fees.

Other ethical standards, though, are more ambiguous about what the dentist owes the patient. One possible position on this issue is that the agreement between dentist and patient is an agreement for an *outcome*, not simply an agreement for a particular set of interventions by the dentist. If this is how the matter should be viewed, then the dentist would not have fulfilled the agreement, because the outcome was not reached. Few dentists would agree, however, that their relationship with a patient involves an agreement for outcomes. They know that only diagnoses and interventions, not outcomes, are within their control. Patients who accept the myth of infallible technologies and infallible performers, though, may well presume that proper performance of the proper intervention yields the proper outcome in every instance. This view mistakenly presumes, then, that when the patient and dentist agree about an intervention they are agreeing about an outcome as well and therefore that all bad outcomes must be the result of bad work.

Dentists must make their actual agreements with patients very clear, particularly in matters where they are aware of possible bad outcomes. If they do not, they risk serious misunderstandings or worse. That is, dentists are professionally required to explain potential bad outcomes before treatment. This is part of the informed consent process that is the legal minimum and is obviously required if a dentist is striving for an Interactive Relationship and a shared treatment decision. Clarifying with the patient each party's respective responsibilities in the event of a bad outcome would clearly be a prudent part of this process as well.

Equal sharing of the burden of retreatment is another position worth considering. If a bad outcome is no one's fault (presuming the patient is not at fault either), then the burden of redoing the work might reasonably be shared equally since both are equally innocent of the unplanned, unwanted, or bad outcome. The presumption of this proposal is that the patient has already paid for the initial work and the dentist carried the burden of doing it, so the two parties are now equal in the face of nature's or fate's impersonal outcome. But theoretically sound though this proposal may be, the fact that dental care involves a commercial as well as a professional relationship may lead the patient to view matters differently. Therefore, many dentists will make a business decision to redo the work at no charge or at cost in order to retain patients. There is nothing professionally or ethically wrong with doing this. But there are risks. Unless the patient is carefully informed, the patient may consider this course of action to be either acknowledgment by the dentist that bad work was in fact involved—thus reinforcing the myth of infallible technologies and infallible performers—or as evidence that the dentist is professionally obligated to make sacrifices of this sort for patients' well-being. The authors consider neither of these conclusions to be valid. A dentist who makes such a business decision should pay serious attention, then, to what the patient is led to learn from it. The best course is to discuss such eventualities in advance. In any case, any of these possibilities that the dentist considers reasonable should be discussed and resolved between patient and dentist, and then all agreements about the situation should be duly recorded in the patient's record and honored.

Finally, a dentist may genuinely be in doubt and unable judge his or her role in relation to a bad outcome. There may simply not be enough evidence available to answer the question. This dentist's obligations in regard to informing the patient who asks are similar to those of the dentist who sincerely concluded that his or her bad outcome was not caused by bad work. This dentist would similarly, we are proposing, have no strict obligation to redo the work at his or her own expense. This dentist's situation, though, is even more ambiguous than the previous dentist's because the available evidence also does not support the judgment that the dentist's bad work was *not* involved.

In practice, the dentist in this situation is probably even more readily drawn to the business solution of simply doing the work without charge or at cost. This is because his or her responsibility has not been ruled out. The cautions already mentioned, then, bear repeating. The dentist should be as clear as possible about what conclusions the patient should draw from the dentist's actions; those actions, although otherwise professionally and ethically defensible, can inadvertently reinforce the myths that have made dental practice so much more complex in contemporary culture.

As mentioned at the start of this section, many dentists are not the sole owners of the practices in which they work. Every dentist whose efforts have produced an unplanned, unwanted, or bad outcome will need to personally address most of the questions discussed above, regardless of their practice setting. But dentists in group practices and dentists who are employees or independent consultants in other dentists' practices will often need to consult others (partners in a group practice, supervisors or owners for employed dentists and consultants) to determine what happens next. Dentists in these situations often will not have the authority to simply make their own arrangements with the patient about whether to redo the needed treatment or replace it with an alternate treatment, about who should do this work for the patient, or about the financial consequences of these decisions. The obligations of those who employ dentists are examined in chapter 10. In addition, insurers, managed care plans, and other bureaucratic institutions may also place limits on how such a sequelae of bad outcomes can be handled, even for dentists who are the sole owners of their practices.

THINKING ABOUT THE CASE

The first obligations of Dr. Alverez to Ms. Stuart are to (1) provide complete and accurate information about the condition of her mouth, including the facts about the bad outcome, and (2) provide whatever emergency treatment the clinical circumstances call for. In the case, Dr. Alverez does explain all the facts she has observed about Ms. Stuart's mouth before removing the bridge and then determines that the bridge and its preparation need to be redone or reengineered. In every version of a bad outcome that can occur, the dentist must fully and accurately inform the patient of the facts about his or her mouth and dentition.

While Dr. Alverez grants some benefit of the doubt to her fellow dentist, she is pretty certain from what she can see that Dr. Singer did not do a good job on the preparations. The length and shape of the preparations are ordinarily completely within the preparing dentist's control unless the carious lesions originally were quite sizable or there are unusual congenital abnormalities; but this does not appear to be the case here. Admittedly, she does not know all the circumstances of Dr. Singer's preparation for the bridge. Perhaps Dr. Singer was being hurried by Ms. Stuart to finish or she was unusually active in the chair or the preparation was hindered in some other way. Perhaps something went amiss with the impressions or in the transfer to the lab, or the lab miscast the bridge. Even so, Dr. Singer should not have permanently seated the inadequate bridge. At most, Dr. Singer might have seated the bridge temporarily if she judged that that option was better than placing a temporary plastic bridge.

Suppose, on the other hand, that Ms. Stuart was actually a very pushy, controlling patient and now she is telling only half the story. Suppose Dr. Singer started to place the bridge, saw that it was inadequate, and told Ms. Stuart the work needed to be reengineered or redone. What if Ms. Stuart then wanted the work to be completed at that visit and demanded Dr. Singer to place the bridge as best she could? Even in that case, Dr. Singer should not have cemented the inadequate bridge in place permanently, regardless of the patient's wishes.

What should Dr. Alverez say? She has no evidence that Ms. Stuart did anything to cause the problem; she cannot ethically take advantage, then, of Ms. Stuart's uncertainty about having done some sort of damage while brushing and flossing. Dr. Alverez also cannot ethically say or try to lead Ms. Stuart to believe that the bad outcome had nothing to do with Dr. Singer's work. That contradicts her own judgment that Dr. Singer probably made an error, possibly several errors.

A point not mentioned previously is Dr. Alverez's need to carefully distinguish between differences in dentists' judgments about treatments that are grounded in differing philosophies of dental practice. Differing treatments can all be within the range of professionally acceptable treatment. But Dr. Alverez is judging that Dr. Stuart's work is outside of that range and therefore is an instance of bad work. As long as Dr. Singer's work met the dental profession's standards of minimally acceptable practice, Dr. Alverez could not ethically judge Dr. Singer's work to be bad work solely because the two practitioners might have different philosophies. The facts here, however, point to a genuine issue of bad work rather than only a difference in dental philosophies.

The question of how the bridge came to be inadequate, which may or may not have been Dr. Singer's doing, needs to be separated from the question of whether Dr. Singer should have cemented the inadequate bridge. Dr. Alverez has differing levels of evidence for answering these two questions, so what she may ethically say to Ms. Stuart about them is different. (Both of these questions presume that Dr. Singer should have recognized the bridge's inadequacies. If Dr. Alverez subsequently learned that Dr. Singer did not recognize its inadequacies, that would raise another, even more serious, issue.)

If Ms. Stuart asks about Dr. Singer's responsibility for the bad outcome, Dr. Alverez needs to separate—at least in her mind—these two questions. Regarding the bad preparations and the inadequate bridge, the evidence available to Dr. Alverez about who is responsible for the bridge being inadequate does not pass the relevant standard for a negative public statement. This situation therefore falls under the first subcategory discussed above. That is, only a significant benefit to the patient would justify Dr. Alverez making an exception to the ordinary standard of evidence for negative public judgments and, thus, justify telling Ms. Stuart about her private judgment that bad work was probably involved in the bridge itself as well as in its preparation. Dr. Alverez will likely need to say she does not have enough evidence to say exactly how things went wrong—that is, how the bridge came to be inadequate or why the preparations are done as they are. At minimum, she would need to talk to Dr. Singer for more information about these matters because a number of different explanations—including the role of the lab and the possibility that carious lesions at the preparation site were in fact considered—are possible.

Regarding Dr. Singer's placing the bridge, however, Dr. Alverez clearly has evidence that passes the standard needed for a public statement to the effect that the bridge is inadequate, that such an inadequate bridge should not have been permanently placed, and that Dr. Singer did place it. Dr. Alverez falls into the third subcategory regarding statements to Ms. Stuart about this. If Ms. Stuart asks a direct question about it, then Dr. Alverez may not ethically remain silent about her judgment that Dr. Singer should not have cemented the inadequate bridge, with the precaution that Dr. Singer might be planning to reengineer or redo the treatment at some future date even though she did not communicate or leave any other indication of this. Therefore, Dr. Alverez must answer Ms. Stuart's question about Dr. Singer's responsibility for the bad work by finding some way to say clearly, "I think Dr. Singer should not have permanently cemented this bridge unless there is something I do not know and Dr. Singer was using a more permanent cement to assure the bridge is secure until the time when an arrangement can be made to redo the treatment needed."

Three-unit bridges can go wrong, even for the best of dentists. There is no basis to consider the bad outcome and work here a probable instance of gross or continual faulty treatment (assuming Dr. Alverez has not seen a lot of faulty bridgework or worse from Dr. Singer's hands lately). There is, therefore, no justification for Dr. Alverez to contact the local dental society's review committee. There is also nothing to suggest that the bad outcome raises a question about whether Ms. Stuart should continue as Dr. Singer's patient; so Dr. Alverez also may not, ethically, try to lower Ms. Stuart's opinion of Dr. Singer simply to attract her to Dr. Alverez's practice.

What emergency treatment should Dr. Alverez provide? This depends in part on how seriously the gum tissue is irritated. Simply replacing the bridge without taking other measures has risks; the gingiva are already involved and causing pain, and Dr. Singer is not due back for another ten days. There may be good reasons to leave the bridge off for several days to let the gingiva in the area rest and recuperate. It might be necessary to make a well-fitting temporary bridge. If the gingiva were not too inflamed, Dr. Alverez could then temporarily cement the bridge and send Ms. Stuart to Dr. Singer for an appointment as soon as Dr. Singer returns. Dr. Alverez's precise plan would depend on further clinical details not provided in the case. But Dr. Alverez cannot ethically decline to provide or arrange for emergency care since the gingiva are inflamed, the bridge is loose, Ms. Stuart is complaining of pain at the site, and Dr. Singer is not due to return for ten days. Dr. Alverez would, however, be fully justified in charging her usual fees for whatever services she renders.

If Dr. Singer were not impossible to reach, then contacting her fairly quickly to consult with her about Ms. Stuart's emergency care and follow-up needs would be prudent. Dr. Singer could then make contact with Ms. Stuart to attend to them, and this would also open up fuller communication between Dr. Singer and Ms. Stuart for the sake of their relationship and Ms. Stuart's long-term Oral and General Health. Because Dr. Singer is unavailable, though, Dr. Alverez should proceed on her own best judgment about emergency treatment now and then inform Dr. Singer after her return about what she (Dr. Alverez) has learned and what she has done about it. Dr. Alverez should also inform Ms. Stuart that she will contact Dr. Singer when she returns to fill her in on what happened and Dr. Alvarez should advise Ms. Stuart to see Dr. Singer soon after her return. It is less clear whether Dr. Alverez should contact the dentist covering for Dr. Singer. If these two dentists were partners, the coverage relationship would be close, and Dr. Alverez would have good reason to call. If the coverage relationship is more remote, as the separate telephone number suggests (and perhaps is given simply as a convenience for patients without any strong sense of collaboration), then calling the covering dentist would make sense only if Dr. Alverez intended to refer Ms. Stuart to that dentist for follow-up care after providing the emergency care Ms. Stuart needs right now.

In addition, regarding a conversation with Dr. Singer, the information that the case provides leaves it unclear whether Dr. Alverez might learn enough from Dr. Singer that Dr. Alverez could determine whether Dr. Singer's bad work was gross bad work (and so requires a report to the relevant peer review committee). Dr. Alverez would need detailed information about the reasons for and the circumstances of Dr. Singer's placement of the bridge in the first place. For example, did Dr. Singer extract the tooth, and, if so, why? Was the tooth already missing when Ms. Stuart entered Dr. Singer's practice, and, if so, was there anything unusual about the abutments, chief clinical concerns, and so on? For the reasons indicated in the chapter, getting detailed answers to questions like these would be essential to such a decision. The case, as presented, leaves these matters unresolved.

Finally, what about malpractice action against Dr. Singer? This book is a study of dentists' professional obligations, not of dental law, so any detailed commentary on the legal aspects of this case would be out of place. As a general comment, however, when bad work is not continual or gravely serious (that is, gross) dental malpractice actions are usually caused by simple lack of mutual, respectful communication between dentist and patient or between the staff and patient. Too often a dentist or staff member will appear to be remote and inaccessible to the patient; they come across as unconcerned and focused only on technical matters rather than communicating that they are concerned and compassionate.

It is not clear if Ms. Stuart has this impression of Dr. Singer or her staff. Her willingness to believe that she herself may be responsible for the problem, though technically naïve, suggests that she views the dental relationship as a joint venture, requiring both parties to collaborate for a common goal. When this is a patient's view and when the dentist is in fact concerned and compassionate and shares this collaborative view, then bad outcomes, and even bad work, can often be dealt with within the relationship instead of breaking it apart. This is the most effective preventative to malpractice actions.

Suppose, however, that Ms. Stuart was of a different temperament than this. Suppose the case had indicated that Ms. Stuart declared her intention to sue Dr. Singer immediately upon learning Dr. Alverez's judgment that Dr. Singer should not have cemented the bridge. Suppose Ms. Stuart proceeded to ask Dr. Alverez if she would testify about what she has found in Ms. Stuart's mouth. How should Dr. Alverez respond?

Dr. Alverez may not wish to get further involved in the case; she certainly may say this. Her statement will be more meaningful, though, if she can articulate her reasons for this wish. If Ms. Stuart were to have indicated this, Dr. Alverez could acknowledge Ms. Stuart's need to follow her own conscience in the matter, but she should not try to manipulate Ms. Stuart one way or the other. Instead, her most valuable and professionally responsible contribution at this point would be educational. Ms. Stuart would gain genuine understanding of her situation if she learned the difference between occasional, minor bad work and gross or continual bad work.

While Ms. Stuart suffered some discomfort and there is some risk of harm from the bad work, she has not suffered greatly nor has she been harmed in any lasting way. There is, furthermore, no reason based on what Dr. Alverez has learned so far for her to fear that Dr. Singer will do similar bad work or harm Ms. Stuart or other patients in the future. Dr. Alverez could profitably try to communicate these points to Ms. Stuart. No matter how the patient reacts, Dr. Alverez is in the role of the second dentist facing a bad outcome and the probability of bad work by the first dentist. Her obligation as a professional is to help both parties draw on the strengths of their existing relationship if possible. Dr. Alverez does this by being thorough and straightforward with factual information so the patient and her regular dentist can then begin discussing the bad outcome, and possible bad work, on even ground. She addresses the immediate problems with appropriate emergency care in a caring and concerned way, even though Ms. Stuart is not her regular patient and she has no other connections to Dr. Singer. In this way, Dr. Alverez makes it more likely that Ms. Stuart does not return to her regular dentist angry about inconsiderate care or lack of concern about her pain. In all these ways, Dr. Alverez not only treats Ms. Stuart's immediate needs in a fully professional manner but serves the patient by affirming and supporting the established, professionally appropriate relationship between the patient and her regular dentist.

Bad outcomes are not the same as bad work. They can be related, but this is uncommon in professional practice even though occasional minor, correctable errors are inevitable in every practice. But the current myth of perfect technologies challenges this reality and makes proper responses to bad outcomes and bad work more complex than need be. In today's culture, concepts like spin, fact checks, and fake news are only a sampling of age-old issues dealing with bad news and good intentions, and they can become more complicated because patients and dentists can find themselves in social and legal climates that place additional moral stress on all parties. Still, in professional relationships, the ethically proper approach starts with the requirement that capable patients receive sufficiently accurate information about their oral condition that they can make appropriate interactive decisions about it. This is the way to demonstrate professionalism in these difficult situations and the way to preserve and support patients' trust. It is also how dentists can help themselves, and one another, to prevent malpractice actions. For in this way, fallible human beings can use fallible human technologies and techniques to serve patients' well-being most effectively and ethically and thereby fulfill the dental profession's commitments to the larger community.

Managing an Ethical Dental Practice

CASE: HAPPY SMILES

Dr. Bob Milford graduates from dental school in 2004 and starts a practice in Montclair. The dentist-per-capita ratio in Montclair is very low at the time, and a local bank happily provides a start-up loan that also offers enough working capital to help service a substantial student debt. His practice takes on all comers and he signs manageable provider contracts with any insurance companies that patients might have. He also writes off accounts when needed for charity purposes. His practice grows steadily and his life grows comfortable. But Montclair's industrial base begins to weaken by 2010, and neither he nor the bank sees much hope for a quick recovery of Montclair's economy. So in 2012 he uses the gains from his eight-year practice, another bank loan, and a relatively minor windfall from the settlement of his parents' estate to buy a good-sized practice from a retiring dentist in Ridgeview, a comfortable suburb of the state's largest city, 130 miles north of Montclair. At the same time, he puts the declining Montclair practice into the hands of the associate he hired three years earlier. He retains ownership of the practice and pays the associate a salary for managing it, plus 35 percent of the profits with provisions for an annual bonus if costs are kept in line. He also drops the provider contracts with any insurance companies that are no longer financially profitable; the associate is not restricted, though, from renegotiating any provider contracts on his own. The profits from the Montclair practice will hopefully help cover Dr. Milford during the transition to Ridgeview.

Dr. Milford arranges to leave the Montclair practice six months before the Ridgeview dentist actually retires, and he takes a wonderful six-week European vacation with his wife and three children. He then spends the rest of those six months attending continuing education programs and workshops all over the country to develop more skills in aesthetic dentistry, pain control and anxiety reduction techniques, and dental marketing. He is well aware of the data from dental economists that predicts a general downturn in the dental market. So Dr. Milford develops, with the help of a highly skilled business consultant he has come to know, a plan that may help his practice not just weather the downturn but turn it into an opportunity.

Upon taking over the Ridgeview practice, Dr. Milford first changes its name to "Happy Smiles, Inc." He then hires the business consultant to contact all the patients of the previous dentist and to create carefully designed and highly polished billboard and radio ads, along with e-mail, Facebook, and Twitter campaigns aimed at reaching every resident in Ridgeview and six surrounding communities. This highly sophisticated campaign announces the establishment of a new dental practice that will bring advanced dental technology to the patients of Ridgeview and that makes "happy smiles" the focus of the practice rather than "the pain, discomfort, and anxiety that the general public associate with dentistry." The messages also include an introductory examination offer for new patients or the next check-up for patients of the previous dentist. The published price of an exam is intentionally well below that of the fees charged by the area's other dentists.

These messages also ask audiences if they know about "all that can now be done with the new dental treatments and materials." Dental and general health, which "are what professional dentistry is all about" are benefiting greatly, the ads says, and the appearance of the smile can be greatly improved as well. Dr. Milford's office offers "the most advanced technology," according to the ads, and people can get "the appearance they want" to help them in their social networks. People are advised to look closely at their teeth and think carefully about what their appearance tells others about them. If they want to change their image to be more attractive and better received, "improving the appearance of your smile, what everyone first notices about you, might be the most direct way to take action," the promotional materials state.

In order to help potential clients decide, audiences are directed to his *Happy Smiles* website. There, various dental defects in appearance are matched with possible treatments and their intended results along with a statement that reads, "our technology and professionals offer accuracy and predictability you can trust" (with a small-print disclaimer that actual results depend on many factors and the pictures do not guarantee these exact outcomes). The website explains that these are not the only possible treatment options and that actual recommendations will depend on the results of a thorough examination and on each patient's treatment goals. Dr. Milford's continuing education credentials in these areas are noted and a free "smile consultation" with intraoral video tours and 3-D imaging are offered to both current and new patients at no charge.

Dr. Milford's marketing consultant also obtains detailed knowledge of the practices of Dr. Milford's chief "competitors," especially those of Dr. Joseph Kamamata, who has practiced in Ridgeview for twenty years, and Drs. Ed O'Brien and Silvia Della Galla, who have a joint practice of ten years in a nearby suburb. On the consultant's advice, Dr. Milford offers Dr. Kamamata's office manager a large raise and better medical benefits. He also offers Dr. O'Brien and Dr. Della Galla's best hygienist the same incentives plus a contractual commitment to support her completion of an MBA degree through an online university. Both women give their current employers the chance to match Dr. Milford's offers, but when he remains the highest bidder, they join Dr. Milford's new office.

The fruit of all these efforts is not only a well-run office with highly skilled and expe-rienced dental hygiene care that complements Dr. Milford's growing technical skills but also an immediate jump in new patients above the already steady flow of patients from the previous dentist's practice. Dr. Milford's business consultant has successfully matched the marketing efforts to the upscale lifestyle of the Ridgeview area. Quite a few new patients come specifically for cosmetic dentistry and then leave their former dentists and stay in Dr. Milford's practice because they see the advantages of having their regular den-tal care in the same office as their cosmetic care.

Within two years Dr. Milford needs another dentist in the Ridgeview office. He adver-tises at several dental schools, proposing to pay a new associate (who will focus almost exclusively on basic diagnostic and restorative work) a fixed percentage of gross receipts in three categories: procedures the associate personally performs, dentistry prescribed by the associate and performed by the hygienist, and all cosmetic procedures performed by Dr. Milford as a result of the associate's educating patients about its value.

Some dental students thought the details of this payment structure and the aesthetic education "script" involved unethical financial incentives to treat excessively. Others, however, had heard horror stories of vague, competitive, or demeaning relationships with employer dentists and the "get your numbers up or get out" culture of huge corporate dentistry shops and welcomed the clear-cut arrangement in a two-dentist office. In any case, since there are plenty of dental students burdened with $400,000 debts from under-graduate and dental school loans who have no easy prospects or desires for independent practice, Dr. Milford has plenty of high-quality applicants. Some of them apply in order to avoid the business of managing an office that now needs to deal with increasingly com-plex insurance contracts, laws, and bureaucracies as well as changing public policies about health care in general. Others are part of dual professional marriages and need options for geographic mobility. Still others just want more freedom in their lifestyles. Dr. Milford eventually hires Dr. Sandra Ballman, who is skilled, personable, highly recommended by her dental school, and a living model of what ideal smiles and oral health should be.

Meanwhile, Drs. Kamamata, O'Brien, and Della Galla had become furious with Dr. Milford. With considerable support from other dentists who have lost patients to Dr. Milford's practice, Drs. Kamamata, O'Brien, and Della Galla submit a petition to the Ethics Committee of the local dental society, arguing that Dr. Milford's mailings and website are unethical because they make claims about aesthetic dentistry that, if not false, are certainly materially misleading.

Dr. Milford is also a member of the local dental society. But he has not participated much in organized dentistry, preferring (on the recommendation of his business consul-tant) to become active in local business organizations and in several other nondental but health-related charitable organizations. With his limited spare time, these activities pro-vided new opportunities to further grow the practice and develop his business skills and connections, as well as assist local philanthropic groups. Dr. Milford suspects the three dentists' petition to the Ethics Committee to be nothing other than an act of revenge for his hiring away their employees. "All they had to do," he says to his business associates, "was pay them better themselves. It's just good business, and they weren't willing to do it. None of them took the time to learn the business skills or work through the business ethics and compliance courses that I took. If they don't like the effects of my business style, they should think about getting some education themselves and start hiring their own consultants. I'm not against fair fights in the marketplace. It's this backhanded business of complaining to the Ethics Committee and trying to undermine my professional reputation that I object to. I've been careful to follow the profession's guidelines about ethical advertising, and my business practices are fully consistent with the best business ethics. As far as I'm concerned, good ethics makes for good business.

"You know, the dental economists' data indicate there are plenty of patients out there now for all of us. I'm barely scratching the surface, and if they would get their heads straight and start to work with me and the other health organizations in the area, especially educating the public about the importance of oral health, we'd only get better at reaching them. Even in this area, less than half the population use dentists regularly for nonemergency care. So why am I some kind of ogre for trying to get them into a dentist's chair?

"I think we should all be marketing aggressively and telling the people what we have to offer. That's good business and what good dentistry should be about—educating people so we can help them. If we don't get them in the door, we can't give them the education they need, and if we don't educate them, we can't help them. I think we should all get together and offer the community a free day of care in our offices, for example, and we should work together to raise funds to set up a volunteer clinic for all the poor people on Medicaid and those women and children whose families are destroyed by addiction. They need a place to be treated, too. Good marketing isn't unethical at all; it's good education, good community relations, and what good dentistry ought to be about!

"Painless Parker once said, 'There's nothing wrong with peddling,' and he was right, as long as you educate yourself and do it ethically. We also need to work together to get the feds and public policy people to make these new pay-for-performance initiatives and the health insurance system really work for all the people who need dental care. I can't tell you how glad I am to see organized dentistry finally starting to get out press releases and published ads about why we professionals need to work together."

CHANGES IN THE DENTAL LANDSCAPE

In the United States dentistry has always been part of the free enterprise system, with most dental care being provided by individual dentists running their own small businesses until group practices became more common toward the end of the twentieth century. But the culture of the dental community and the understanding of the content of dentists' professional obligations, both among dentists and within the larger community, were such in those days that the most prominent characteristics of the competitive free enterprise marketplace were not very evident in dental practice. Active marketing of dental services, competitive advertising, and serious competition by price were less common during most of twentieth century and were discouraged in the American Dental Association's *Principles of Ethics and Code of Professional Conduct* (hereafter ADA Code). But now all three of these, and many other characteristics of the free enterprise marketplace, are well known in dentistry. Events, starting in the 1970s, began to challenge the under-standing—reached in the dialogue between society and dental profession in previous years—that dentistry is primarily a profession and therefore very different from a typical participant in the commercial marketplace. Events were also challenging the conviction that the dental community is responsible for holding its members accountable as ethical professionals, which had been a part of this understanding.

What happened to dentistry during this period involved the coming together of a number of fairly independent sets of events, so its causes are multiple and complex. One was the late 1960s and early 1970s radical increase in dental school admissions in antic-ipation of the baby boomers entering the workforce. The number of dentists therefore grew more rapidly than the population's desire for what they considered ideal dental services. It might have been assumed, for example, that more than half of the population would start to use dentists for nonemergency care if more dentists were available and the population was becoming generally better educated. But this did not happen and still hasn't. Evidence and surveys suggest that there are more influencers to human behavior than supply and demand and targeted marketing campaigns aimed at directing people to make more use of dental services. Consequently, for the next thirty to forty years the United States found itself dealing with more dentists than could be kept busy if their primary focus, based on previous understandings about the nature of dental diseases, continued to be focused only on the treatment of caries.

Meanwhile, the dental community had succeeded in persuading the larger commu-nity to take preventive dental care seriously, to some extent in the dental office and through better-promoted self-care advice but more dramatically through fluoridation of many water supplies. The dental community itself also changed as the preventive theme expanded beyond caries and its consequences—tooth extractions, pulp treatments, and prosthetic appliances—to include more emphasis on periodontal disease, cancers, occlu-sal disorders, aesthetics, obesity, diabetes, smoking disorders, and so forth. The preven-tive efforts on caries, most often through the community fluoridation efforts, did help decrease the severity of the consequences of dental caries, so dentists' needs/opportunities to do restorative work with the half of the population who already sought regular care decreased. The increased provision of a broader array of in-office caries and periodontal preventive care, though, made up for only some of the decrease in traditional restorative care. Dentistry found itself, then, with an increased number of providers and a decreased need for the previous understandings about the nature of basic dental restorative treat-ment that had been the mainstay of dental practices for years. Dental emergencies also remained stable in numbers, though this stability also came with a population shift to a growing number of patients who had lower incomes, were more elderly, and had more medically complex issues. In any case, very few dental practices were able to survive prin-cipally on the provision of emergency care.

Added to this mix was the entrance of insurance companies into the dental care pic-ture. Dental diseases did not fit, however, the traditional characteristics of insurable events—namely, low-frequency, unpredictable, catastrophic financial or social losses that are hard to manipulate. Still, beginning in the 1980s, in collaboration with public health care policies and large employers, many insurance companies began to develop products to help address dental health care needs and, before very long, to influence, if not control, dental health care costs as tightly as possible. These efforts were met with mixed results. Whether basic dental health care needs were being better met or costs were being better controlled remained questionable. But, already challenged with the first two factors, US dentistry now began to face a fiscal situation in which powerful third parties were entering into the once traditional dialogue between patient and dentist about how to treat the patient's oral health needs. At the same time, little happened to change the fact that our society would consistently spend fewer dollars for dental care compared to health care in general, both in absolute numbers and in relation to people's needs.

More recently two other factors have further compounded this picture. One is the aging of the US population. Even though some forms of caries are less common causes of oral disease for this group than in previous years, periodontal disease remains a major factor in their oral health. But with the decrease in painful carious lesions, a significant percentage of elderly patients have, over time, become less interested in dental treatment, especially the long-term forms of dental monitoring appropriate to chronic/silent oral conditions. In addition, many in this aging population find themselves with fewer financial resources or are less willing to devote their limited resources to dental care than previously. Thus, the impact of the aging of the US population on dental practice in our society, while complex and difficult to predict, has further complicated the already complex dental landscape.

Meanwhile, a fashion trend to have one's teeth appear whiter than their natural coloring has swept across almost every demographic of the population. Dentists have long been available to assist patients who wished to restore teeth to their natural tone when they became severely discolored. But this fashion trend for whiter-than-natural teeth began providing dentists with patients they might never have seen for routine oral health care. Ideally, these patients, or at least some of them, continue to be seen and benefit from regular visits. But, as chapter 14 will explain, the provision of cosmetic and aesthetic care focused on meeting the patient's cosmetic interests (rather than the traditional aesthetic goals of dentistry) raises important questions about the relevance of dentistry's professional expertise in providing services of this kind and the insertion of market-based values and market-based thinking into the patient-dentist relationship. So the highly increased prominence of patients seeking cosmetic/aesthetic assistance that this fashion trend has prompted (the trend itself often promoted by dentists themselves) must be viewed as an important change in the landscape of dental practice in our society.

Finally, there has been a significant change in the circumstances of graduating dental students, beginning in the early 1980s. When the federal tuition grants of previous years ended, this put a larger tuition burden on students themselves and/or their relatives, who were already becoming more indebted than in previous generations because of increases in the cost of undergraduate education. Then followed sharp increases, for many reasons, in the cost of dental education, and, with that, a decrease in the number of dental schools and class enrollment sizes. Then the cost of dental school increased even further in order to incorporate ever-growing, though sometimes short-lived, new technologies as well as faculty being drawn to higher paying positions in other parts of the market, and schools' inability to compete effectively for additional financial resources from the government, foundations, and private philanthropy. Consequently, many dental students' tuition bills continued to rise and their indebtedness rose even further.

The graduating dentist of an earlier generation ordinarily moved directly into a practice with the help of a bank loan and a population waiting for his (and occasionally her) services. Of course, the loan had to be serviced, but the ability to easily secure the loan was ordinarily there to help a young dentist get started, and servicing the debt could be factored into the practice's cash flow needs. Since the 1980s, however, fewer and fewer graduates have entered directly into their own practice by starting with a bank loan. Especially since the beginning of the twenty-first century, most have been too deeply in debt from the cost of their educations and not yet experienced enough in practice to be considered for such a loan. Open fields for gaining this experience, however, were growing within the armed forces, public health, growing numbers of hospital-based general dental practice residencies, and the increasing popularity of group practices. But few of these opportunities offer salaries high enough to pay off the higher dental education loans efficiently. What has been found to be financially sound, however, is hiring these newly graduated dental students, bringing returns of 15 percent a year or more for entities investing in recent dental school graduates. So dental students have, understandably, become extremely anxious about their prospects. Most know they will likely begin their dental career in someone else's practice. They hope to be fortunate enough to be an associate of someone who is seeking a younger professional peer rather than merely an employee of someone willing to take advantage of their financial need. A world in which dentists are collaborative and not actively competing with one another is a dream world for them, perhaps seeming like something out of the past. This is because dental students are now unavoidably competing from the moment they enter dental school just for the opportunity to practice dentistry in a setting they can feel proud of.

None of these change factors arise from anyone's ill will toward dentistry or anyone's insensitivity to the norms of professional dental practice. The dental profession, like any social institution, is situated among and strongly affected by many other complex social institutions, and many US institutions have played a hand in the changes just discussed, although broad economic policy decisions and other economic factors seem to have played a particularly important role. It is hard, then, to assign blame for these changes, even if there would be value in doing so. What is needed is for the dental community to ask how it ought to respond to these changes in the dental landscape in order to continue practicing dentistry as professionals and in as professionally ethical a manner as possible.

It may sometimes seem that the changes in the landscape of dental practice over the last thirty to forty years have already turned dentists into typical marketplace producers of services and their patients into typical marketplace consumers. This chapter and those that follow it will look at some of ways that the practice of dentistry is at risk in this respect.

But one of the main themes of this book is that this does not have to happen. Dentistry, like the rest of health care in our society, will continue to be provided in the context of the marketplace for the foreseeable future. But just as dentists in previous generations provided their care in the marketplace but conducted themselves as professionals in their dealings with patients and one another, and were viewed as professionals by their patients and the society at large, so can dentists continue to practice as professionals. But because the landscape has changed, doing so will require some careful thinking about how to do this and possibly some changes in how things are being done in order for dentistry to be carried out in a way that is genuinely professional.

It is very important, therefore, to reflect on how dentistry can be done ethically and professionally in the changed economic and social circumstances that face dentists today. Every practicing dentist needs to ask such questions about every aspect of his or her practice, and the discussion here and in the following chapters can only attempt to survey the most important issues. But there is no more prominent set of ethical concerns for today's dentists than these, so they deserve careful attention.

We will begin in this chapter by looking at some of the management decisions that need to be made in every dental practice and that can be made in ways consistent with dentistry's commitments as a profession or in ways that can make a dental practice look little different from a typical marketplace enterprise. The first of these concerns dental advertising because this is a topic that touches every dental practice and dental organization in our society today in one way or another. We will conclude this chapter with reflections on the theme of patients' trust of their dentists, a topic introduced at several points earlier in this book. Within this chapter, and then in the chapters that follow, we will examine other situations on which a dentist who wants to run an ethical dental practice should reflect.

DENTAL ADVERTISING: SOME BACKGROUND

One of the most dramatic shifts in dentistry, in the minds of many dentists, occurred in 1979. This shift involved changes in the ADA Code in regard to prohibiting competitive advertising and the consequent proliferation of competitive advertising since then. But none of the patterns of change described in the previous section came about simply because of the changes in the ADA Code about competitive advertising. While the proliferation of advertising since 1979 certainly points to a much more competitive relationship between dentists, the reasons for the increase in competition are to be found in the social trends just described, not the advertising that expresses it.

Advertising, depending on its definition, formulation, and uses within the broader concept of marketing, actually has the potential to educate the public about dental care and oral health, as well as how to access dental services. It is clearly a mistake, then, to view dental "advertising" or direct-to-public-education as an unmixed evil. The excessive advertising by some individuals, furthermore, is not proof that dentists should never advertise. Many who have advertised since the changes were made in the ADA Code have done so ethically. The criteria for determining when competitive dental advertising is ethical and professionally appropriate, however, have still not yet been fully articulated, even though the ongoing dialogue between the dental community and the community at large about this issue has been going on for almost forty years now. One important depository of this dialogue within dentistry is the Appellate Disciplinary Decisions of the ADA's Council on Ethics, Bylaws, and Judicial Affairs. The background to the changes in the ADA Code was a consent order that the ADA and the Federal Trade Commission (FTC) entered into in 1979, a consent order to avoid continuing costly legal battles that the ADA was clearly not winning. The actions of the FTC at that time were framed around the claim that the limits on advertising in the professions' codes of ethics were a restraint of trade. Though a final Supreme Court decision was never made, the settlements between the FDA and the professional health organizations in the United States made it clear to the ADA, the American Medical Association (AMA), and other large professional health organizations that they would be challenged in the courts should the prohibition of advertising be reintroduced into their codes of professional conduct. The original claims initiating these complex legal proceedings were as likely motivated by political and economic considerations as by a careful reading of the mind of the larger community. So, one can argue that the elimination of the ADA Code's prohibition against advertising was not necessarily an expression of society's wishes.

The fact that the larger community has never had extensive representation on the ADA councils and other dental organizations' committees that have drafted dentistry's codes of ethical conduct, furthermore, raises an important question. For professional codes, by their nature, ought to be the work of both the profession and the larger community working together. While they may be primarily articulated and enacted by professional organizations whose members are experienced and knowledgeable about the internal workings of their service to the community, any reasonable or pragmatic organization would surely seek the community's voice in articulating the norms that will guide its provision of services to that community. However, the only evidence of the larger community's acceptance of these groups' articulation of dentists' professional obligations, as with its acceptance of the FTC's actions in 1979, consists solely in the larger community's lack of vociferous protest.

It is usually the case when dealing with the contents of professional norms that there are other, more subtle forms of evidence of the community's mind. It is probably relevant that direct-to-consumer marketing in the United States by pharmaceutical companies, hospitals, and health systems is now even more plentiful than dental advertising and, although prompting some political and legal battles, it too has not yet been met with significant objections from the US public, though it is questioned outside the United States. The issue that such passivity raises, then, is whether the US public has reflected with any care on the differences between how the professions aspire to relate to those they serve and the competitive relationships of the marketplace. In any case, it is important to ask what the commitments that the dental profession and each of its members make imply about dental advertising.

THE ETHICS OF DENTAL ADVERTISING

The categories of norms that will be used here will be the nine categories of professional norms first identified in chapter 3 and applied to numerous other topics throughout this book. But as shall become clear, the three most important categories with regard to advertising are the obligation to respect patients' Autonomy as one of dentistry's Central Practice Values, the norm of an Ideal Relationship, and the norm of Integrity and Professionalism. This section will focus on the themes of Autonomy and the Ideal Relationship; the norm of Integrity and Professionalism will be considered in the next section.

Four models of the dentist-patient relationship were considered in chapter 4, and reasons were offered for judging the Interactive Model as most accurately representing what the dental community and the community at large currently accepts as the Ideal Relationship between dentist and patient. The Guild Model views the lay patient as wholly incapable of making judgments, not only about his or her appropriate therapy but even about his or her need for therapy and the values and priorities involved in determining how important it is to address that need. This is why the Guild Model has no place for patient decision-making. Even regarding the original choice of a dentist, into whose hands the lay patient then places his or her well-being, the Guild Model must hold that this choice by the patient is blind; for the Guild Model views the patient as having no understanding of the data that would be needed for the rational consideration of alternatives for such a choice.

Consequently, according to the Guild Model, there would be no justification for dentists, or any other health professionals, to advertise. If lay patients cannot understand or properly evaluate any advertised data that would be relevant to their choice of a dentist, physician, or other health care provider, advertising is at best utterly useless. But for the Guild Model advertising is actually worse than useless because it suggests to the lay patient that he or she *can* form properly reasoned judgments about the choice of a health professional. Suggesting this to otherwise unknowing lay persons might then lead them to believe they are capable of properly making other judgments about dental care—for example, about what sort of care is needed or about the quality of the care that is provided. Consequently, advertising runs a serious risk of interfering with the formation of a proper dentist-patient relationship. If the patient comes to believe that he or she is capable of judgments that only the dentist can make, then the patient may become less receptive to the essentially passive role that is the only appropriate role for patients in the Guild Model. The fact that the Guild Model, then, has no place in it for patient autonomy has seemed to some people to support the proposal that we should adopt a pure Commercial Model of the dentist-patient relationship.

The Commercial Model is obviously the approach supported by the Federal Trade Commission, whose mission is promoting and protecting competitive free trade, not trust in professions with their distinctive expertise and ethical commitments. According to the Commercial Model, the relationship between dentist and patient is simply that of producer and consumer negotiating about possible exchanges in the commercial marketplace. The two parties are viewed as being, from the first, self-interested competitors, each trying to obtain from the other the greatest amount of what he or she desires while giving up as little as possible in exchange. The Commercial Model's supporters claim that, by the working of the "invisible hand" of the competitive marketplace, relationships formed on this model yield the greatest quantity and quality of dental care for the least cost in both natural resources and human effort. Therefore, its supporters argue, the "invisible hand" makes this the most efficient model of social relationships as well as one in which the value of every party's autonomy is most respected.

Thus, the Commercial Model implies that advertising by dentists and other health professionals is a good thing because, its supporters believe, advertising increases competition. Increased competition is believed to improve efficiency through the workings of the "invisible hand." Moreover, the pure Commercial Model does not need to worry whether advertising will mislead the lay patient or will adversely affect the relationship between dentist and patient. For the Commercial Model presumes that the patient can determine whether instances of advertising are of value or not, and the dentist-patient relationship is presumed to be an adversarial relationship from the start. So there is, so to speak, no one to be harmed by advertising and nothing to be lost from doing it. In addition, the Commercial Model views the dentist and patient as equal bargainers who have no obligations to one another prior to their contracting, except an obligation prohibiting coercion and thus supporting some measure of truthfulness and keeping one's contracts once they are made. Consequently, if these minimal obligations are met, the two parties cannot act unethically toward one another. But even the obligation to truthfulness is an obligation only to *truth*, not to the *whole* truth. That is, though the bargainers may not lie, they have no obligation to speak clearly or precisely or to say everything they know. They are not responsible for the other party's understanding. If their statements are not "false or misleading in any material respect," to use the phrase promulgated in the ADA's consent agreement with the FTC and replicated in the current ADA Code (5-A), then either party may say anything he or she judges will be useful to enhance the other's desire to engage in an exchange in a manner profitable to the speaker.

Consequently, the Commercial Model permits a broad range of advertising language and techniques and views all efforts at advertising that do not violate the minimum obligations just mentioned as genuine contributions to efficiency. Therefore, as the mandate of the FTC also requires, the Commercial Model would oppose any efforts at regulation of such advertising, whether by statute or by professional code, that would test advertising by any other standard than whether it is "false or misleading in any material respect." The ordinary consumer of dental care, however, views himself or herself as, in part, lacking the information and skills necessary to meet oral health needs. Consequently, the dentist is in fact at a significant advantage in the relationship. But, says the defender of the Commercial Model, life is like that; some of us are in situations of advantage at some times and of disadvantage at others; but no one owes anyone else equality in such matters unless they have voluntarily contracted beforehand to provide it. Therefore, the dentist may take whatever advantage of the consumer's lack of information and skills that does not violate explicit agreements between the dentist and that consumer. The dentist is not obligated to alert the consumer of the effects of his or her ignorance (provided the minimal ethical obligations of the marketplace are not violated). That is, dental care is no different from the rest of life, says the Commercial Model, and so the relationship between dentist and patient—and the role of advertising within this relationship—has no business being different either.

The Interactive Model of the dentist-patient relationship holds that both of the previous approaches are incorrect. The Guild Model fails to support the important Central

Practice Value of the patient's Autonomy and is too ready to assume that patients can understand much that they often cannot. It also forgets that dentists' expertise in rendering professional judgments about diagnosis, prognosis, and therapy does not include any special expertise in the values of a particular patient. Therefore, the Interactive Model holds that dentists must have the fostering and enhancement of the patients' Autonomy as a central goal of their practice. Moreover, since that autonomy can be diminished by the psychological and physiological effects of their ailments, dentists must in fact *assist* patients to make their own value judgments about what shall be done for and to them, based as much as possible on the patients' own values, goals, purposes, and so on. As chapter 4 explained, the patient and the dentist are both to be considered moral equals and active choosers within their relationship, and they should treat each other accordingly.

At the same time, patients ordinarily *do* lack the technical understanding that is necessary to make sound dental-care judgments, and they lack the technical skills that are necessary to act on these judgments. So they cannot function as equal bargainers with their dentist, as claimed by the Commercial Model, in judging the quantity and quality of alternative dental care options. In fact, since potential patients are motivated to seek dental care because of important needs that they cannot meet themselves and are often fearful and/or in pain, patients rarely interact with dentists as equal bargainers in the way that rational market consumers are supposed to. Thus, while the Commercial Model puts its emphasis on *business equality*, what is important in the Interactive Model is the *moral equality* of the patient and the dentist, not their equal ability to be bargainers in the marketplace.

What, then, does the Interactive Model imply about the characteristics of ethical advertising? Certainly the Guild Model's arguments against advertising are much weakened by the Interactive Model's emphasis on patient decision-making and on the patients' ability to understand, with the assistance of the dentist, much of what is relevant to sound dental care decisions. So a blanket prohibition of advertising is certainly unjustified in an Interactive Relationship. Nor does advertising mislead, as the Guild Model proposes, when it suggests that patients be active decision makers; instead, it says something correct and important.

But the Commercial Model's minimal constraint that advertising merely not be false or materially misleading is inadequate when we know that, prior to actual contact with the dental professional, many patients are not yet well informed for the decisions that they have to make, especially the initial decision about who is an appropriate caregiver. Consequently, the Interactive Model seems to support proposals of many state dental societies that, for example, claims of competency in advertising be regulated to guarantee their accuracy and that comparative data be required when comparative claims are made—rather than the typically vague comments about cost or quality.

Before the Interactive Model's implications for ethical advertising can be developed further, however, the target audience of such advertising must be considered. For example, a *hardened consumer* will habitually doubt the validity of advertised comparisons in terms of cost or quality and will habitually discount associations of a particular dentist's work with elements of "the good life." At the other extreme, a *wholly receptive consumer* will simply accept such comparisons and associations. A more *reflective consumer* falls in between. He or she will attend to the evidence offered in support of comparisons and will weigh its merits and will hold associations with "the good life" up to critical reflection before forming any judgment about the advertised dentist's services.

A dentist hoping to advertise his or her services in a manner consistent with the Interactive Model must therefore consider which of these three groups, or the many variations that lie between them, are likely to be recipients of his or her advertising. For advertising "puffery" that would not be taken seriously by the hardened consumer and that would be evaluated and then ignored by the reflective consumer might be accepted as evidence of quality care by the wholly receptive consumer. Since such a dentist's goal is to assist every prospective patient who receives advertisements in making a careful choice of caregiver, the ethical way for a dentist to judge how to advertise requires a focus on asking whether the advertising will fail to assist, or even positively hinder, the wholly receptive consumers within the projected audience.

Marketers of other goods and services who do not have a professional commitment to preserving and supporting certain values for their clients may be able to justify increasing their sales with "puffery," associations of their product with "the good life," and subliminal content to motivate unwarranted trust that some, perhaps even most, recipients of such advertising will accept without noticing or questioning it. The issues of business ethics raised by such practices are complex and beyond the scope of this book. But dentists should not inflate their advertising claims. For they are committed to fostering as interactive a relationship as possible with those they serve and advancing dentistry's Central Practice Values of Life and General Health, Oral Health, and the patient's Autonomy for *every* patient they contact either with information or in service, and this includes those in their audience who are wholly receptive consumers.

As was noted when the norm of the Chief Client was discussed in chapter 3, a dentist's professional obligations are owed not only to patients of record and those who seek out the dentist for emergency care. Whoever receives a dentist's advertising—whether they are likely to become that dentist's or any dentist's patient or not—is owed, by the advertising dentist, as interactive a relationship as possible and the respect and support needed for his or her autonomous decision-making. Since there will almost always be parties in a dentist's advertising audience who will be wholly receptive consumers, the dentist is professionally obligated to advertise only in ways that will assist rather than hinder, much less harm, the decision-making of the wholly receptive consumer.

In summary, we have argued that the changes that have taken place in dentistry since the 1970s were not caused by the removal of the prohibition against advertising. Nor is advertising necessarily a violation of the commitments of dentistry as a profession or of the individual dental professional, providing it is advertising of the right sort. Indeed, when dentists carefully attend to the ideal of an Interactive Relationship and the obligation of dentists to respect patients' Autonomy and the autonomy of every recipient of their advertising, then the educational effects of properly conceived advertising seem to recommend it as a professionally appropriate and often valuable activity.

What is ethically questionable are certain kinds of advertising. False or misleading advertising clearly violates dentists' obligations to respect patients' Autonomy and contradicts the obligation to work for as interactive a relationship with patients as possible. In fact, false and misleading advertising is seen as unethical because it is coercive, even from the far more accepting perspective of the Commercial Model. But that is not the only kind of dental advertising that is ethically questionable. Also deserving of professional-ethical criticism is advertising "puffery," tactics that target their recipients with subliminal and unwarranted associations with the "good life," and framing and naming genuine issues of public health in ways principally designed to serve the profit motives of the advertiser—that is, anything that fails to assist, or runs the risk of hindering, the decision-making of the wholly receptive consumer. For it is this consumer's ability to benefit from dental advertising that must be taken as the standard of ethical dental advertising.

There is, however, an additional category of professional-ethical criticism of dental advertising that does not come to light in an examination focused on the norms of the Ideal Relationship and respect for patients' Autonomy. This concerns advertising that, even if it meets the standards just explained, sends the larger community the wrong message about dentistry and prompts doubts or raises questions in people's minds about the values that principally determine dentists' actions regarding patients and prospective patients. Such advertising, we will argue, violates the norm of Integrity and Professionalism that obligates dentists, within limits, to act consistently with the values they are professionally committed to—even when they are away from the operatory and the office. This norm was first described in chapter 3. Now it is important to consider its implications for dental advertising.

ADVERTISING AND ITS COMPETITIVE MESSAGE

Many dentists whose views of the dental profession were formed when advertising was more limited by the standards in the professional codes believed in those limitations. They have understandably been critical of dental advertising as it has become more common; their reasons for being critical, though, are quite different from those discussed in the previous section. Their concern is that the very act of advertising and marketing by dentists sends a false and damaging message to the public about dentistry as a profession and about dentists' professional commitments.

The question that needs to be asked here, then, is what kind of message dentists' increasingly energetic engagement in advertising and other marketing efforts sends to the public. Is it a message that says something is more important to dentists and the dental profession as a whole than the well-being of patients? To any audience reasonably cynical about the contents of advertising and marketing language—whether the hardened consumer of the last section or only the reflective consumer—the fact that dentists employ any kind of language or imagery that resembles standard advertising "puffery" or subliminal messages to motivate unwarranted trust suggests that dentists and the dental profession as a whole are not interested in communicating with their clients literally and carefully in terms linked to scientific fact and oral health. The message that the public can easily take from aggressive advertising and marketing, and the competition between dental care providers that such advertising represents and implies, is that dentists are willing to place making a sale ahead of meeting the patient's needs. It says the criterion of success for a dental practice is having more patients and/or earning more dollars than other practices. Such advertising and marketing efforts suggest, as does all advertising, that "beating" their competitors in the marketplace—that is, other dentists—is a dentists' primary goal, whether those other dentists are serving their patients' oral health needs well or not. In such an environment, the ethical criteria of effectively meeting patient's oral health needs, relating as interactively as possible to patients, and bringing about the other Central Practice Values of the profession can easily be lost on the audience.

The same points can be made in connection with earning patients' trust. As previously noted, patients' trust—especially their Trust of the Person of the dentist—derives from the dentist's habitually communicating his or her commitment to the primacy of the patient's well-being over other aims and goals. Because it is in the very nature of most advertising to imply that market success is its primary goal, dental advertising can fail to support and can even erode patients' trust unless it is done with very special care.

The point to this ethical challenge to dental advertising and marketing is that such promotion can easily communicate a negative message about dentists to the public even when the content of the ad or mailing is true and conceived with professional-ethical standards in mind. These efforts can easily be read by the public as communicating that serving the patient's well-being is only important to dentistry insofar as it is instrumental to meeting marketplace objectives. Such a message is certainly the opposite of what dentistry as a whole claims when it says it is a profession and that dentists are professionals committed to giving priority to the patient's well-being. In addition, such a message runs a serious risk of undermining dentists' ability to achieve their professional goals by undermining patients' trust that the dentist really is committed to them.

Note, of course, that dentists not only risk misrepresenting dentistry's priorities to the larger community by advertising and marketing activities. Dentists profess their values and communicate to the public about dentistry and its priorities in how they speak about what they do at chairside, by how they conduct their financial transactions with their patients, and in many other ways. A dentist whose manner at chairside can be perceived as salesmanship, to take one example, rather than as an effort at interactive, collaborative decision-making or whose approach to time management or the management of an office sets other values ahead of the patient's General and Oral Health are at least as likely to undermine patients' trust that the dentist is a committed professional as are aggressive marketing practices. Consequently, every dentist needs to regularly examine how he or she pursues the entrepreneurial goals of dental practice; they need to consider what that pursuit communicates to that dentist's patients and also to the larger community about the practice of dentistry and its priorities. Every dentist needs to make sure that his or her own words and conduct, and the policies and practices of his or her office, do not misrepresent dentists' and dentistry's commitments as a profession. They ought not portray the profession as simply another commercial enterprise in the competitive marketplace. Additional ways in which dentists can send the wrong message—that dental care is first and foremost a commercial activity rather than a professional service—will be examined in this chapter and in chapter 13.

MANAGEMENT EFFICIENCY IN THE PROFESSIONAL SETTING

Efficient management can contribute significantly to a dental practice. But management efficiency must be in the services of the professional goals of the practice. One change in the new landscape of dentistry deserves special ethical attention; this is the practice, widely supported by dentistry's management consultants and employed in most large dental practices and a number of smaller ones, of separating the business management elements of running a dental practice from the direct care of patients. In large dental service organizations this separation is effected by employing accountants and specialists in insurance, purchasing, and so forth to handle all of the organization's billing, purchasing, insurance, and other business activities. In small practices these tasks might be outsourced to specialists outside the practice.

The purpose of doing this, when it is viewed in the most positive light, is to enable dentists to focus on chairside dentistry and the care of patients and to put management tasks into the hands of people who are good at them. But there are ethical challenges that arise immediately when the decisions about a dental practice's nonchairside affairs are formally separated from the direct care of patients. For it is not true that what takes place in a dental office can be cleanly divided into clinical and nonclinical matters, as is sometimes claimed explicitly and certainly implied by those who recommend these arrangements.

Business relationships with patients, for example, are still *relationships with patients*, and therefore the dental profession's ethical norm of striving for the most Interactive Relationship possible still applies. The ethics of the business world, however, do not require this level of attention to the patient's values and priorities—or to the kind of communication that is needed to achieve it. By the same token, decisions about supplies, facilities, schedules, personnel, and productivity are always, simultaneously, decisions about the kinds of practice options that the dentist will have available at chairside in order to provide the most appropriate care for each patient. Therefore, the priority of patients' well-being should be the dominant consideration in decisions about these matters; it is the relevant ethical norm. But as mentioned above, in the commercial world the well-being of the consumer—which is what the patient is from the point of view of the marketplace—has no inherent ethical priority for the seller of services.

It must be granted, of course, that the skills needed to handle business and administrative matters effectively are very different skills from those of the chairside dentist. This fact does nothing, though, to offset the many real consequences that business and administrative decisions have on the chairside provision of care and on dentists' relationships with patients. Many chairside dentists would be grateful if dentists could spend less time trying to be skilled at management decisions; they would have more time, then, to become the best chairside dentists they can be. But the ethical point here can be made in a different way by asking "What is the direct goal of management as a social role with its set of recognized skills?" The answer is that management is about *efficiency*; as a social role, then, management is goal neutral. That is, the job of the manager is to achieve *whatever goals* the organization happens to have *as efficiently as possible*—where "efficiency" means maximizing the achievement of those goals while minimizing the amount of resources (human, fiscal, material, etc.) needed to do so.

But providing professional dental care is not, and ethically can never be, goal neutral. The goals of professional dental care are easy to identify in general terms, as the *well-being of patients* and *Interactive Relationships*, or more fully in terms of dentistry's Central Practice Values. What these goals involve concretely is complicated because achieving them involves sophisticated judgments about each individual patient together with the exercise of complex skills of perception, evaluation, judgment, and action on the part of the dentist, along with often-subtle decisions and judgments about priorities and trade-offs on the patient's side of the relationship. But whether dentistry's goals are stated in general terms or in more detail, providing dental care is not a goal-neutral activity.

However, if dental care is not goal neutral and if the consequences of managers' decisions impact what care can be given and affect patient relationships, then those who make management decisions for dental practices *must* have the goals of professional dental care as *their* goals in every efficiency decision they make. The ethics of the dental profession need to be the ethics of those who manage the provision of professional dental care. The point being made here is not that the challenges of managing a dental practice cannot be solved in ethically excellent ways. Rather, it is the ethical point that the goals of those who manage the business aspects of professional dental care, and who thus have efficiency as their focus, must always be the same goals as those of the dentists whose professional practice they manage—namely, to provide the most appropriate oral health care to each patient and to relate to patients in as interactive a way as is realistically possible.

Doing this will take careful planning in the creation of organizational structures and the relationships between chairside caregivers and those tasked with management work. It will require extremely careful hiring of management personnel. It will require effective feedback systems between managers and chairside caregivers to address any misplaced priorities and directives. Without these, the underlying and unspoken (thus rarely systematically addressed) goal neutrality of management activity, along with the natural management goal of business success in our society, will create serious ethical problems.

The same point needs to be made about practices in which dentists who are not owners of the practice are *employees* of the dentist or dentists who are the owners (and all the more so in any dental service organizations in which the owners are dentists who no longer provide chairside care to patients or where the owners are permitted by law to include persons who are not licensed dentists). In all of these settings, whether small or large, the activities of the owner in managing the employed dentist must mirror what has just been discussed about other kinds of management activities in a dental practice. The prime goal of a dental practice or a dental service organization must be the priority of the patient's well-being, the formation of Interactive Relationships between patients and the dentist(s) caring for them, and the furthering of dentistry's Central Practice Values for every patient. This means that the relationship between owner(s) and employed dentist(s) needs to be structured with the fulfillment of this goal in mind above all.

In addition, whenever an organization of any kind employs professionals, this always brings with it a set of obligations that the organization should not overlook and that have greater moral weight than any business goals of the organization. For, as chapter 2 explained, professionals' ethical commitments are the product of an ongoing dialogue between the profession itself and the larger society about how the members of the profession will use their professional expertise in providing professional services to the people of that society. These commitments between the profession, its individual members, and the larger community not only precede the business organization's contract with the professional in time but have greater moral weight than any conditions of employment or work orders that the organization might attempt to impose on the employed professional. Therefore, organizations that would pressure their professionals to violate their professions' minimum ethical standards are clearly acting unethically themselves. Moreover, in a dental practice or a dental service organization, which is primarily created to provide professional services to the public, this obligation of the organization extends to supporting employed dentists in the other, more expansive norms of the dental profession.

Owners have the "power of the purse," but just as managers' goal of efficiency must not prevent chairside dentists from providing appropriate and competent oral health care to every patient and must not interfere with their establishing as interactive a relationship with every patient as the circumstances permit, so owners' bottom-line goals must not interfere with the delivery of fully professional oral health care either.

Owners should also be particularly attentive to the ways in which "the power of the purse" can interfere with the spirit and goal of working together as professional colleagues, as discussed in chapter 8. They should also remember that, by fostering appropriate collegial relationships with the dentists they employ, owners—who are usually more experienced than their employees—can not only support but significantly enrich their younger colleagues' professional growth, both in competence and in the elements of professionalism that will be discussed in chapter 15.

FIRING THE EXTREMELY UNCOOPERATIVE PATIENT

Suppose Jack Jones, an intelligent forty-year-old lawyer in excellent health, is a patient of Dr. Clara Lewis. Mr. Jones has a deteriorating tooth for which Dr. Lewis's ideal treatment of choice is endodontic therapy with a post and crown restoration. In repeated conversations with Mr. Jones, Dr. Lewis has explained why this is the ideal choice for a man of his age and other health characteristics. But Mr. Jones has repeatedly refused endodontic therapy, though not out of any evident pattern of excessive fear, such as was observed in Roger Vianni in the case in chapter 4. Mr. Jones claims, instead (based on misguided information and reasoning and/or an inability to understand otherwise), that he is against having "dead things" in his mouth. If the tooth needs to be "devitalized, killed," he claims, "then it should be removed and replaced by an implant," which he describes as "a proper artifact, not a dead thing."

Dr. Lewis could extract the tooth and provide the requested implant to fill the space. But she would consider it a serious violation of her philosophy of practice to do so under these circumstances, for she believes, as do many dentists, that maintaining the natural teeth is ordinarily the ideal way to secure patients' oral health. If serious financial issues were the reasons for Jack's refusing endodontic therapy, Dr. Lewis would consider other less costly alternatives that might be within the patient's means. Or if there were some other benefit to be gained by the patient—for example, the establishment of a long-term treatment relationship for a patient who previously had none (as was mentioned in the discussion of philosophies of practice in chapter 5)—then Dr. Lewis might choose to violate one element of her philosophy of practice for the sake of another. But in the situation at hand, Dr. Lewis is being asked to violate her philosophy of dental practice for no good reason at all.

Here the patient's lack of cooperation does not involve obnoxious behavior. That is not the issue. But repeated efforts at education do not change Mr. Jones's insistence on getting "this dead thing" out of his mouth. May Dr. Lewis ethically "fire" this sort of patient? That is, may she decline to treat him further in her practice in order to preserve acting on her commitment to her own carefully considered philosophy of dental practice?

First of all, it is essential that Dr. Lewis provide Mr. Jones with whatever emergency treatment he needs. If he is in pain, for example, Dr. Lewis must provide pain relief and other appropriate temporizing treatment—if Mr. Jones will accept it—independently of the extraction he wants. But, with the proviso that emergency treatment must always be provided for, we believe Dr. Lewis would be professionally and ethically justified in sending Mr. Jones away from her practice. Since Mr. Jones will soon need treatment in any case, Dr. Lewis should also provide him with the names of other practitioners whom she respects, perhaps in this example with the names of several oral surgeons and prosthodontists and perhaps an endodontist. By doing this she fulfills her obligation to preserve the Central Practice Values of this patient's Oral and General Health, even as she preserves her commitment to her own professional philosophy.

Suppose a patient's lack of cooperation was of a different sort. Suppose that, after a year of Dr. Lewis's careful instructions about how to care properly for dentition to lessen the risk of severe periodontal involvement, a patient still showed no sign whatsoever of even minimally adequate self-care. Here, again, it is important that Dr. Lewis would have made extensive and thoughtful efforts to educate the patient about appropriate self-care, including perhaps methods of behavioral self-care, as well as education and motivation programs aimed at getting Mr. Jones to be compliant with what was being taught. For it is by doing so that she fulfills her obligation to try to preserve this patient's Oral and General Health. Doing so may involve some sacrifice of comfort and convenience for Dr. Lewis, as has been noted, but that may be necessary to fulfill Dr. Lewis' basic obligation to attend to this patient's Oral and General Health.

But, with the provisos that Dr. Lewis makes such educational and motivational efforts at self-care and that any emergency treatment needed by this patient is offered, we believe Dr. Lewis would not be acting unprofessionally to ask this patient to seek treatment elsewhere, perhaps with the suggestion that she may not be the best person to serve his or her particular needs. In this sort of case, Dr. Lewis' philosophy of dental practice is implicitly involved; she is acting as a dentist who far prefers to practice in an interactive and collaborative relationship with her patients. The burdens on Dr. Lewis in this patient's case, though, are more the burdens of a lot of additional effort, the affective burden of frustration, and the other negative feelings associated with one's careful professional advice simply being ignored. When the dentist has made appropriate sacrifices for the sake of the patient's well-being, even burdens of this sort may be sufficiently heavy to justify severing the relationship provided the patient has reasonable access to the needed care.

It is worth noting, by the way, that dentists dealing with uncooperative patients are often tempted to *threaten* to sever the relationship when they believe it is a relationship that the patient values—that is, as a way of motivating the patient to cooperate. Such threats may sometimes be educationally useful in helping a patient see that this valued relationship is at stake in the matter at hand. But threats are very often difficult to justify ethically, even under the best of circumstances. This is because they are often manipulative, even coercive. In fact, they would ordinarily not be thought effective unless they were coercive. Threats of this nature are almost always, then, in direct conflict with respect for patients' Autonomy and with efforts to develop as interactive a relationship with each patient as possible. Thus, within dental professional morality, and morality in the larger sense, threats should always be viewed as morally suspect; they require very special sets of circumstances to be ethically justified. Therefore, a dentist should not threaten to sever a patient relationship that could not be ethically severed, because a patient persists in being uncooperative. Patients may ethically be fired, if at all, only for ethically sound reasons and not because the patient failed to respond to an ill-conceived threat.

CONFIDENTIALITY AND PATIENT RECORDS

It is widely held that all humans have obligations to protect one another's privacy regarding certain kinds of personal information and in certain situations and relationships. "Privacy" (i.e., privacy about information) refers here to a person (or a group) being the one who determines who else may learn information about that person (or group) that is not of an inherently public nature and also to how such information may be used. Protecting someone's privacy, therefore, chiefly involves not revealing private matters about them to others and not using such information about them unless the person (or group) has so chosen—either explicitly (for example, because they were asked about it) or by reasonable implication (e.g., they have themselves shared the information under similar circumstances). Another aspect of protecting someone's privacy concerns the person (or group) knowing who has obtained knowledge of private matters about them and also being able to correct such knowledge when it is in error. These aspects of privacy are particularly relevant in relationships where formal records are kept, including relationships between patients and health professionals. They pertain also to informal relationships, however, whether close or not. So one might well be obligated to let a person know that one has, in some way, learned otherwise private information about him or her without the individual having deliberately shared it; to invite him or her, then, to correct it if appropriate; and to ask how, if at all, the information may be used or shared with others.

The general ethical reasons for protecting one another's privacy are numerous. Respecting the value of Autonomy or the right of self-determination certainly implies supporting one another's efforts to exercise control over personal information. Consequently, the protection of privacy has a very important place in our culture's standards, both in social policy and among criteria for ethical personal conduct. For some, in fact, privacy is itself viewed as an inherent human right or a core value of human personality and not only a means of exercising autonomy and self-determination.

Protecting others' privacy is also an essential means for maintaining relationships of trust and friendship, and as a means, it gains moral significance from the importance of friendship and other trust-based relationships within human life. Some hold that the "mutuality of shared knowledge of one another" is at the core of our most valued relationships and is not merely a necessary means to them. There are, in other words, many kinds of harms that humans would suffer, both individually and collectively, if privacy were not widely protected. The term "confidentiality" is primarily used when such obligations of using private information arise. This is because someone is deliberately sharing private information with another person and is doing so with the understanding that the receiver will only reveal or use the information in manners determined by the one doing the sharing. This happens most frequently in friendships (in fact, such sharing is often a measure of the degree of friendship) and in relationships between professionals, especially health professionals, and the people they serve. In this respect, professionals often know things about those they serve that only a person's best friends would know and possibly not even his or her best friends. This quasi intimacy is one of the complexities of the dentist-patient relationship, even as it is a necessary component of this relationship in its ideal form as an Interactive Relationship. For this reason, dentists, like all health professionals, have special additional obligations of confidentiality over and above the general obligations of privacy just discussed.

For in order for health professionals to employ their expertise for the benefit of patients, they need to know many facts about patients' lives, bodies, and behavior and about their values, goals, and fears—many things that most people would not reveal to many other people. Therefore, health professionals have and proclaim an especially stringent obligation of confidentiality regarding the facts they learn about patients; this is so patients can feel secure when providing the information practitioners need to care for them. Thus, the starting point of the accepted standard within dentistry, as in all the health professions, is that every fact revealed to the dentist or other members of the care team by a patient is, in principle, subject to the requirement of confidentiality. Therefore, in principle, nothing may be revealed to anyone else without the patient's permission.

This standard has several built-in exceptions, however, which are so widely taken for granted in daily health care practice and are thought to be so widely understood by patients and by the community at large that they are also considered by most health professionals to be part of the accepted standard of professional confidentiality. First, it is widely taken for granted that other health professionals involved in a patient's care may be told the facts they need to know about the patient in order to provide effective care. Second, some individuals who are not providers of health care but who administer its provision (by keeping records, managing financial affairs, managing the institutions in which care is provided, and so on) will also need to know some of the facts patients reveal to health professionals so they can carry out their jobs. This "need to know" status justifies access by such persons to a patient's record. But it is understood that, in the course of learning from that record the particular matters they need to know for their work, such individuals may unavoidably learn other facts about patients that they do not strictly need to know.

Third, it is an accepted limitation of the health professional's obligation of confidentiality—although many patients may not think about it very often—that relevant facts patients reveal may be communicated for educational reasons to other health professionals and student health professionals not involved in the patient's care. In all instances, these three exceptions also ethically require, however, that such additional persons—who might legitimately learn things about a patient that are otherwise matters of confidential communication between patient and professional—have a similar obligation as the original professional for the same reasons. Facts about patients are also revealed, of course, in biomedical research, but current practices regarding informed consent by research subjects require that patients' explicit written permission be sought for research uses of information about patients. So, this practice is not an exception to the basic obligation that information about a patient may not be revealed without permission.

Unfortunately, many settings in which health care is provided have grown very large and complex over the years, and the institutions involved have grown increasingly interconnected. The cumulative effect of these three exceptions, then, is that a great many people learn facts about patients that were originally revealed confidentially to a single provider of health care. A recent estimate holds that in the course of a three- to five-day hospital stay, for example, these exceptions mean that an average of 150 people will have legitimate access to a patient's medical record. In addition, many of those who learn these facts are not health professionals, nor, in any case, do they have a direct relationship with the particular patient. To be sure, these individuals are bound not only by the ordinary obligations of all human beings about confidentiality but also by the extension of the original health professional's obligation mentioned above and by the obligations of any other roles they fill. Yet, they lack the kind of one-to-one relationship with the patient, and some lack any caregiving relationship to patients, that could reinforce their obligation to the patient and raise their awareness that there is a person who could be harmed and who would be betrayed if confidentiality were violated. Consequently, what is intended to be a very stringent obligation, with three very carefully controlled exceptions, often functions more like a sieve, or even a conduit, of sensitive patient information to parties who are far removed from the patient's health care and sometimes to parties wholly untouched by the health professionals' specific obligations to protect confidentiality.

Most dental care is provided in relatively small settings with only a few people having access to patients' private information. But larger dental practices are as likely as the hospitals mentioned above to give large numbers of people access to patients' private information. The obligation of dentists, as professionals, to carefully guard the privacy of their patients' information therefore extends to all those who work with them and are privy to patients' private information.

As is well known, federal law, the Health Insurance Portability and Accountability Act (HIPPA) passed by the US Congress in 1996, not only supports the obligation of dentists and their staff members to protect patients' privacy but provides specific guidelines about the parties with which information may be shared. Of particular importance are its strictures regarding the sharing of patients' private information, including information about diagnosis, treatment recommendations, treatments provided, and the outcomes thereof, with third parties. Dentists and their staff members should familiarize themselves with these regulations even when they may seem to be even more stringent than the requirements of ordinary ethical standards and the published ethical standards of the dental profession.

LEGALLY MANDATED REPORTING

One area in which reporting of otherwise confidential information about patients is legally mandated concerns evidence of child abuse (and in some jurisdictions, elder abuse). In most United States jurisdictions, health care professionals, including dentists and their staff members, are legally bound to report any signs or symptoms in a child that are suggestive of child abuse, even if they personally believe that these indications are not the result of abuse. But legally, the staff of the appropriate state authority must conduct the investigation of the allegation of child abuse; health professionals are simply to report the indications without attempting to test the validity of the inference to child abuse.

Situations can arise in which a dental professional believes that much more harm than good would be done by reporting a particular case as a possible instance of child abuse than by addressing the matter directly with the child's parents or even, if the dentist is certain no abuse is involved, simply letting it go. What is being considered in such a circumstance is an act of conscientious disobedience of the law in a particular case. But the penalties imposed by the law are severe if a health professional can be shown to have deliberately refrained from reporting indications of possible child abuse. As mentioned above, in some jurisdictions there are similar legal mandates for reporting indications of possible elder abuse to relevant legal authorities.

MAINTAINING APPROPRIATE RECORDS

The obligation to protect patients' confidentiality would be much simpler if it were not for another obligation of dental professionals: to maintain appropriate patient records. Proper oral health care obviously depends on keeping appropriate records of patients' chief concerns, presenting conditions, diagnoses, any treatments provided, their outcomes, and projections of patients' future needs. Many dentists today think the need to maintain careful records is primarily legal, as an important bulwark against future lawsuits. But the ethical obligation to maintain appropriate records is specifically for the sake of proper patient care; the obligation, then, would be there even if dentists were never at legal risk in providing care. This is also why dentists are obligated to provide either original or copied records to other dentists (or other relevant health care professionals) who are caring for the same patient and to a new dentist if the patient changes caregivers. Both of these obligations derive from the dentist's professional commitment to the patient's well-being, not from any implied or specific business or contractual arrangement that may also exist between dentist and patient. Patients' failures in matters of the business contract, then, do not cancel or lessen these obligations.

These are points on which the ADA Code is particularly clear: "Dentists shall maintain records in a manner consistent with the protection of the welfare of the patient. Upon request of a patient or another dental practitioner, dentists shall provide any information that will be beneficial for the future treatment of that patient . . . A dentist has the ethical obligation on request of either the patient or the patient's new dentist to furnish, either gratuitously or for nominal cost, such dental records or copies or summaries of them, including dental X-rays or copies of them, as will be beneficial for the future treatment of that patient. This obligation exists whether or not the patient's account is paid in full" (1.B and 1.B1).

As soon as there are records, however, the number of possible breaches of patient confidentiality is greatly multiplied. What one caregiver hears directly from a patient in a private setting becomes accessible by means of the record to many people, caregivers and administrative staff alike, and becomes potentially accessible (unless appropriate precautions are taken) to other patients, maintenance staff, and others who have reason to be in the dental office. There are some ways in which all of this is well known, so the ethics of protecting patient privacy seems altogether obvious. The complexity of respecting confidentiality and the accompanying ethical challenges, however, has been multiplied still further with the advent of electronic record keeping.

The very inefficiencies of paper record keeping have the benefit of lowering the risk of both deliberate and inadvertent violations of patients' confidentiality. Physical control of paper records requires familiar administrative steps, though it is not error proof; sorting or copying paper records in order to take one inappropriately are still activities that take time, effort, and stealth. The many efficiencies now available through electronic record keeping, however, also bring new opportunities for both deliberate and inadvertent violations of patients' privacy, not just for one patient but all patients, and not just disclosed to a few others but to many others on a global scale and almost instantly. The harms that confidentiality seeks to prevent through means of privacy are thus vastly multiplied. This raises important ethical questions about the relative priority of confidentiality and privacy in comparison to the benefits of efficient recording, access, and use of information. But the ethical reasons for protecting the privacy of patients' records have not changed in the face of electronic record keeping. If anything, they have become more urgent.

One specific reason, related to the points just mentioned, is the increased linking together of the many data-management sites used by health care professionals. The extent of inappropriate access to this linking of information (which is typically unknown to the patient) is very great, so the potential for actual harm to a patient from an inappropriate breach of confidentiality is heightened. Pathways exist by which a single breach in confidentiality might send such information to insurers, government programs, and other third-party financial entities, as well as employers, public medical data pools, and numerous other potentially linked groups. A second concern is that many health professionals, including many dentists, have only a passing knowledge of record-keeping technology; they are therefore unaware of the precautions they need to be taking. When the often-inadequate security of electronic records sites meets the efforts of hackers and the rise of identity theft throughout the world, it is clear that dentists and their staff members have very serious obligations to stay current with new technology and do much more when it comes to protecting their patients' privacy than simply being careful about what they say.

Under the influence of federal regulations growing out of the Health Insurance Portability and Accountability Act (HIPPA), many insurers and financial institutions have begun to provide their customers with detailed statements about record keeping, confidentiality, and customer access to their own records. As dentists and dentists' patients become increasingly leery about electronic record keeping, dental offices might do well, in the spirit of an Interactive Relationship with patients in the matter of privacy, to consider doing something similar.

THINKING ABOUT THE CASE

Dr. Milford's Ridgeview practice differs markedly from the way dentistry was practiced thirty or forty years ago in many respects, and there are many ways in which Bob Milford seems to be a different sort of person from the typical dentist of those years. But differences are not automatically deficits, particularly when everyone acknowledges that the surrounding environment has changed radically for dentistry since 1980 or so. So each of the differences between Dr. Milford's practice and older styles of practice would need to be examined before any overall judgment of his Ridgeview practice could be rendered. We can begin with Dr. Milford's advertising and marketing activities.

The mere fact that a dentist is actively marketing his or her practice to prospective patients is not, we have argued, something that is unprofessional or unethical. This includes, for example, changing the name of the practice (i.e., Happy Smiles), sending mailings to potential patients to inform them of the approach the practice takes to dental care and the services offered, and providing a low first-visit charge for a checkup to get patients into the office. The ethical question that needs to be asked, however, is what these marketing activities communicate to prospective patients, especially what message the wholly receptive consumer will take from them. That is what needs to be evaluated most carefully.

Organized dentistry prohibited trade names like "Happy Smiles" until the 1979 consent agreement with the FTC. The objection to them was that they made dentistry appear to be a commercial enterprise like any other marketplace activity rather than an ethical and professional activity aimed first of all at preserving and enhancing patients' well-being. That objection is not a foolish one, as the arguments in the previous sections have demonstrated. A trade name like "Happy Smiles," simply by itself, would not support a claim that the practice's advertising fosters unrealistic expectations for those who need care or involves a claim of superiority or special ability, especially in a world where even the wholly receptive consumer is unlikely to think that a trade name actually describes the quality of an entity's product or service. (Claims of unethical practice fitting these descriptions are made and can be substantiated, but they require more telling evidence about the practice's advertising materials.) Consequently, unless the wording of a particular dental practice is seriously (materially) misleading—for example, calling a dental practice "Dental Health Guaranteed"—a trade name by itself is unlikely to violate a dentist's professional obligations.

But one reason the public is unlikely to believe that a dental practice's trade name says much about that particular practice is that so many dental practices now have taken on trade names or branding practices that connect dental care with various aspects of "the good life" rather than with oral health as such. That is, in combination with various other marketing activities, the use of trade names may cumulatively, if not already, become significantly misleading about dentistry as a profession. The possibility of this cumulative effect of marketing efforts that are arguably ethically acceptable on a one-by-one basis will be discussed in a moment.

What about Dr. Milford's message? Here, the "happy smiles" motto is explained as indicating an emphasis on dental care that significantly limits "the pain, discomfort, and anxiety that many patients experience in the dental office." Many patients do experience pain, discomfort, and anxiety in the dental office, so this part of the claim is legitimate. But this may still be an unsupportable and misleading claim if the actual wording used by Dr. Milford implies that his dental practice can provide this better than other practices. However, since Dr. Milford has taken continuing education in pain control, among other things, the claim that he is adept at this aspect of care may not be inappropriate. But there is a legitimate question of whether there is an implied comparison with other dental practices that would not be supported if investigated empirically.

There may be some dentists who find Dr. Milford's advertising to prospective patients objectionable in its direct marketing of aesthetic dentistry. The increased emphasis on techniques for improving patients' appearance, over and above dental health considerations, has coincided with the downturn in the amount of restorative work available for general dentists to do. It is worth asking, then, whether dentists who actively propose aesthetic options for their patients are violating their professional commitments because they are serving a goal other than health, and they are doing it first and foremost for financial reasons, not for the sake of patients' well-being. The professional-ethical issues connected with aesthetic dentistry are subtle and will be examined in detail in chapter 13.

With regard to Dr. Milford's actual advertising, the case does not provide full details. It is possible that other statements in his advertising materials would be professionally compromising in some way. But the information provided indicates that it contained an explicit statement about the priority of dental health over aesthetic considerations, a disclaimer statement that treatment decisions will depend on the clinical facts of each patient's situation, and an indication that treatment decisions will be made by the dentist and patient together. From the information provided, then, Dr. Milford's advertising still appears to conform to the hierarchy of Central Practice Values and to the ideal of an Interactive Relationship that is respectful of a patient's Autonomy. So the charge that his advertising or other marketing efforts makes false or materially misleading claims appears to be mistaken.

What, then, about the cumulative effect of all of Dr. Milford's marketing efforts taken together? Is it possible that a dentist whose marketing efforts were each ethically acceptable when taken individually could nevertheless violate his or her professional commitments when all of them were considered together? One of the points explained in terms of the norm of Integrity and Professionalism is that dentists have a professional obligation to speak and act consistently with the values and norms they profess; this is over and above the obligation to conform their individual actions in practice to these professional norms. We must ask, then, whether Dr. Milford's overall marketing effort—along with his competing effectively with other dentists for a new office manager and dental hygienist—misrepresents the dental profession and misinforms the public about what dentistry stands for, even if his marketing activities, looked at individually, are professionally acceptable.

The argument that Dr. Milford's critics would raise is that recipients of his promotional materials will conclude—from their being directed to all residents within a geographic region and from the use of persuasive language, like the "Happy Smiles" trade name and other familiar marketing techniques—that dentistry is a commercial, profit-driven enterprise like any other in the marketplace rather than a profession founded on a commitment to the patient's well-being, even to the point of actual sacrifices for the sake of it. Critics might also claim that not challenging such possible conclusions will only further compound and/or reinforce the unwarranted conclusion that dentistry is not a profession but rather a commercial enterprise. Dr. Milford's reply to this argument is clearly that his advertisements are a form of educating and motivating the public to come to a dentist, education and motivation that dentists are, in fact, professionally obligated to undertake for the sake of the public's Oral and General Health. Who is correct here?

To date, despite a vast amount of research in the field of patient education, no one has yet done any careful comparative research into the actual educational impact of professional advertising as such on the public's view of professions, much less specifically explored and examined the impact of dental advertising since 1979 on the public's view of dentistry. From that point of view, the matter remains an open question, one that the dental community would do well to investigate. It is also important to remember that the principal way in which the public's views of the dental profession are shaped is from direct contact with dentists. This is, arguably, more formative of their views about dentistry than their experience with dental advertising. If each individual instance of dental advertising met the standard of not being materially misleading, which is required even by the minimum ethic of the marketplace, and if each advertisement effort conforms to the norms of respect for patient's Autonomy, the ideal of an Interactive Relationship, and the priority of General and Oral Health and the other Central Practice Values, then one could argue that the cumulative impact of dental advertising is less important than the cumulative educational and motivational impact of dentists' communications at chairside. In terms of this kind of argument, if Dr. Milford and the dentists (and dental hygienist and other staff members) in his practice conform to this standard, he would not be professionally in the wrong, even if his overall marketing effort smacks strongly of the commercial marketplace.

Here the contrast with Dr. Prentice, in the introductory case for chapter 2, is instructive. Once again, as was noted there, we do not have enough detail in the case to make a once-and-for-all judgment of Dr. Prentice's manner of running his practice. But Jack

Williamson's reports and impressions, if accurate, strongly suggest that Dr. Prentice does not place either the General and Oral Health or the Autonomy of his patients or the fostering of genuinely Interactive Relationships ahead of financial success in his clinics. His marketing outside the clinic, and inside, especially in the operatories at chairside, is specifically aimed at producing additional business. It does so first by failing to make a careful distinction between treatment decisions based on patients' dental health and function needs and other work that can be done without harm but is not needed for health and function. It does so, second, by not informing the patients of this difference when treatments are proposed.

Consider the two dentists' arrangements for their dentist employees. Dr. Milford's arrangements for his associate in Montclair and those proposed for the associate soon to be hired in Ridgeview do place some financial pressure on them to practice in a fiscally sound and productive manner. But it is doubtful that these arrangements would produce any greater financial pressure for these dentists than a solo practitioner already feels in trying to keep his or her practice financially afloat. Dr. Prentice, on the other hand, has established per-patient quotas and other quotas regarding work ordered and work done, together with a severe penalty—loss of job—for failing to meet them. These arrangements automatically create powerful pressures on Prentice's employed dentists to persuade patients to have more work done than they would ordinarily be judged to need in a practice run in another way. This is, frankly, the reason for Prentice's quotas.

There are, in other words, professionally significant differences between these two dentists. Chairside communication and conduct in Dr. Milford's practices seems, from the limited data available, to be professionally sound. Dr. Prentice, on the other hand, seems to have no concern whatsoever for the potential of his practice arrangements to misinform the public about dentistry. Indeed, his comments to Jack Williamson suggest that he believes the Commercial Model of dentistry, discussed and rejected in chapter 2, is accurate. In fact, Dr. Prentice actually seems to think that his style of practice ought to communicate a commercial view of dentistry to the public; that is—he says—what dentistry should be. The style of practice that Dr. Prentice requires in his clinic, then, may manage to fulfill the market's minimal ethical requirement of informed consent without coercion or fraud, but it is hard to say, on the evidence the case gives us, if the priority of patient's General and Oral Health over other values and the support of his patients' Autonomy and of Interactive Relationships are the chief determinants of practice decisions there. For all of these reasons, then, Dr. Prentice's clinics clearly seem to be misrepresenting the dental profession and misinforming the public about what dentistry stands for and therefore to be also violating the norm of Integrity and Professionalism.

Why, then, the antagonism against Dr. Milford among his peers in the Ridgeview area? Part of that feeling of ill will is understandable because Dr. Milford has hired away valuable employees from two dentists. He is also drawing patients away from other dentists through his marketing efforts and his emphasis on and skills in aesthetic dentistry. Yet if he is not conducting himself in an unethical manner in these matters, if he is simply a more effective entrepreneur but is careful that his employment of the tools of the marketplace do not yield professionally unethical conduct, why do some consider him to be at fault?

Before the advent of the social and economic changes in dentistry, which were discussed at the beginning of this chapter, most dentists likely shared a similar temperament and style. The dental profession, of necessity, attracts prospective members from a fairly narrow range of personality types. Thus, the particular understandings of the norms of dental practice in place then and the relative ease with which good, hard work could earn a dentist an established practice and a fairly comfortable life probably limited that range even further. This is not to say that all dentists of that era liked each other or recognized their own traits in one another. It is simply to say that it is reasonable to think there were significant affinities that would not be as evident now, for the environment of dental practice has changed greatly.

To enter dentistry in the current era, a person needs to be willing to face considerable risks. The opportunities for practicing in less congenial settings, or risk not practicing at all, are more commonly available. The person who would be a dentist must also be comfortable managing huge debts and financial insecurity. It would not be surprising, then, if there were significant differences in personality type and style between those who become dentists in the twenty-first century and those who became dentists in the previous environment. In addition, even among dentists who entered practice in the previous environment, there may well have been differences of style and temperament that had no occasion to be noticed until the environment for dental practice became unavoidably more competitive. Those who were adept at managing competition but who felt no call for it in the previous environment, for example, might now be motivated to call up those skills and apply them with energy. Thus, they would be able to distinguish themselves fairly quickly from peers who felt less affinity for functioning in a highly competitive environment.

It is likely that many or all of these processes have been at work in recent years. But whatever the psychosocial processes and/or political-cultural movements that could be related to bringing about the current environment, it is clear that dentistry now includes men and women of very different temperaments and styles, particularly when it comes to participating actively in the competition that the present environment makes inevitable.

If it is true that those dentists who will be most comfortable in the current age are those who are able to employ the tools of the competitive marketplace, when these can be used in conformity with the standards of dental professionalism, then the question about the cumulative effect of doing so on the public's understanding of dentistry needs to be asked from a broader perspective. That is, even if each dentist who does this can, like Dr. Milford, arguably be exonerated from the charge of acting unprofessionally and misinforming the larger society, it is still important to ask if the outcome is as innocent when most, perhaps even all, dentists do the same. This question will be the focus of chapter 13 and examined in regard to organized dentistry in chapter 14.

Dentists like Dr. Milford actively engage these challenges; they do so whether or not they understand that this is a delicate professional-ethical enterprise for the many reasons this chapter describes. Some dentists are more like Dr. Prentice, who is practicing, at best, at the very edge of professional acceptability and probably beyond it in some respects. And some dentists have likely turned their practices into frankly commercial enterprises for profit, with dental care merely being used as a commodity; "let the buyer beware" is now their motto. Those in the last group must be recognized as having given up on the goal of being professionals along with the commitments that the members of a profession make to the larger society.

It is our conviction that some features of the commercial marketplace can be adapted for use in fully professional, fully ethical dentistry. This is, though, a subtle ethical task— one that requires constant ethical vigilance. Some aspects of this challenge are beyond the power of the dental profession to change alone. This is because they concern the relative importance of oral health and oral health care within the goals of the larger society and the effects of this ranking of goals on people's ability to access the oral health care they need. These aspects of this challenge will be discussed in chapters 11 and 12. In addition, there are a number of other ways dentistry can be sending the wrong message about itself to the larger society that are definitely within dentistry's control; these will be the focus of chapters 13 and 14.

11

Society's Health Care Resources and Access to Oral Health Care

CASE: DISTRIBUTING HEALTH CARE RESOURCES

Two committees are meeting at the same hour many miles from each other. One is the Secretary's Priorities Committee of the federal Department of Health and Human Services. It is assisting the secretary of health and human services to respond to the president's proposed priorities for the federal health care program in the next fiscal year's budget. The total amount of dollars in the draft is fixed. The secretary and her advisers must determine whether they support the particular dollar allocations among a large number of health care concerns in the president's draft. They must also determine if there are concerns the president's staff left out that also should be included, along with the corresponding loss of dollars in other areas. They are charged, then, with *rationing* health care dollars for the American people. They are charged to do this carefully and efficiently and in a way that is consistent with the moral norms of justice.

One member of this committee, Dr. Willard Brenford, DDS, is director of the National Institute for Dental Research. He was formerly the president of the American Dental Association and before that of the American Dental Education Association. He was also a longtime dean of a highly respected American dental school. Appointed to this committee, Dr. Willard is now the strongest advocate for America's oral health needs that the dental community has ever had in the federal government. Today's meeting is a prime opportunity for him to seek funding for improved oral health care, especially among underserved children and their families in America's inner cities and rural communities. But these very real needs are not the only unmet health care needs that the committee must weigh and prioritize.

The other committee meeting is the board of directors of the newly founded Lancaster Health Trust. The trust came into being when the Lancaster Regional Health System was bought by a still larger health system. Buyers of not-for-profit health systems

237

are prohibited by law from acquiring the endowments of the purchased organizations in order to prevent them from buying organizations simply for the cash in their often-sizable endowments. So, Lancaster's endowment has become separately incorporated as a not-for-profit charitable trust, and its board is meeting for the first time to set priorities for its philanthropic work over the next five years. Every dollar the trust contributes to the health of the public—since it is just beginning operations—will be a new dollar, not one taken away from some other health care service or organization. On one hand, this is a chance for the trust's board to take a fresh look at health care needs in the community and respond to needs that have not been well met to date. On the other hand, the resources available to the board are finite and there are far more unmet health care needs in the community than the board could ever possibly meet. So they, too, are charged with *rationing* health care dollars, even though these are new dollars, and they, too, have an obligation to the community to do so carefully and efficiently and in as just a way as they can.

The former director of the Lancaster Health System's dental service, Dr. Bernice Lichtmann, DDS, has been appointed to the new trust's board. She is widely respected in the community for her work in establishing and developing financial support for public health clinics. She has always made sure that basic oral health care was part of the mix of health care services provided to these clinics' patients. Now, with the unusual opportunity of financing new programs with new dollars, she is hoping the board will see the wisdom of investing in basic dental care for many more patients who currently lack access to it.

How ought these two groups think through the challenges they face? What would a just distribution of these health care resources look like? What are the criteria for just distribution in a rationing plan? Among the many kinds of benefits that health produces for people, and among the many kinds of harms that health care corrects or prevents for people, which should receive greater priority and which less? And, in particular, how ought these boards prioritize oral health care among health care services, and among oral health care needs, which should count as basic needs, and how much priority should they receive?

In actual practice, such committees are typically comparing the benefits and costs of very specific proposals: for example, a set number of dollars for a program to support perinatal care programs or early childhood nutrition programs in inner cities and rural areas, a certain number for the purchase of magnetic resonance imaging (MRI) machines for small hospitals too far from large medical centers to conveniently refer patients to them, and a fixed number of dollars to provide visiting nurses' assistance to elderly home-bound diabetics or dental hygienists to visit schools in areas with no dental offices. But suppose these committees were able to step back and ask the questions in the previous paragraph more generally so they could develop broader guidelines about justice and the ethical distribution of the limited health care resources they need to ration. How might they carry out this thought process?

JUSTICE AT THE SOCIETAL LEVEL

Dental care is not only a matter of relationships between individual dentists and individual patients. Those relationships occur in the context of a complex social institution, the dental profession, whose norms are the product of an ongoing dialogue between dentists as a group and the larger community. Whether a dentist's particular actions toward a particular patient are ethical or not cannot be resolved without considering the dentist as a professional—and therefore examining the dental profession and its dialogue with the larger community and the norms of dental practice that are this dialogue's result. Dentistry, even when it consists mostly of one-to-one interactions, is also by its very nature a broadly *social* enterprise as well.

The point of this chapter is that there is another broad social structure, or set of social structures, that is directly involved in dental practice, even in the most direct one-to-one encounter of dentist and patient. This is the set of social structures that distributes a society's resources and governs their exchange so some are used or exchanged by some people, others by other people. Moreover, like the institution of profession and the particular profession of dentistry with its particular norms, the set of structures that governs the distribution and exchange of a society's resources can be ethically sound as it exists in a given society, or it can be ethically defective. Since our own society's structures for the distribution of resources have such great impact on what kinds of dental care are available to the people of our society, these social structures deserve to be examined here and the question explored of whether they are ethically sound in their impact on dental care or whether they ought to be rejected in favor of other, more just structures for distributing dental care resources.

When a society's structures for distributing resources are ethically sound, a common adjective used to describe such a society is "just." When a society's distributive structures are ethically deficient, one proper term is "unjust." Aristotle labeled as *distributive justice* the effort to determine which kinds of distributive structures are ethically sound and which are not, and the label has stuck.

What, then, are the characteristics that make a society's distributive structures just? This is not an easy question to answer. Aristotle's description of justice at the most general level provides a starting point. He observed that justice of every sort, in every aspect of life where talk of justice is appropriate, has to do in general with treating like cases alike and different cases differently in proportion to their relevant similarities and differences. This tells us something important about ethical distributions, but we won't be able to apply it to any practical area of life until we can answer a further question: In the area of human life under consideration, which similarities and differences between people should be considered ethically *relevant*? With regard to the recipients of dental care, then, we need to ask which kinds of similarities and differences should determine differences in how much and what kinds of dental care resources each patient ought to receive. The next six sections will examine this issue, first in general terms and then in connection with the current structures for distributing dental care resources in the United States. The final section will return to the chapter's introductory case to comment on the work of the two committees and to propose an exercise for the reader to think about the just distribution of society's health care resources and ethical rationing.

EQUALITY, BASIC NEEDS, AND JUST DISTRIBUTION

What should the norms of justice be for distributing a society's resources among its people? A number of criteria have been proposed, but there is room in this chapter for only a brief explanation of some of the most important criteria. As each is discussed here, the reader should be asking, is this the criterion (or one of several) that should determine what and how much dental care ought to be available to each dental patient in an ethical, just society, and why or why not?

The values of American culture and those of cultures and peoples in many parts of the world today make it fairly easy to reject one historically important criterion for distributing resources—namely, *social class* and *birth-based social status*. There is a broad consensus that these are not relevant characteristics for determining the distribution of dental care, or any other form of health care, so a society that distributes dental care on the basis of social class or birth-based social status is considered unethical and unjust. It would be a useful exercise for the reader to pause here to ask *why* this is (or is not) a correct conclusion.

A more complicated criterion supported by many thinkers in recent centuries is *equality*. The claim is that there are *no* relevant differences between people when it comes to the distribution of dental care resources or other kinds of resources to which this criterion is applied. These thinkers therefore argue that a society's distributive structures should be arranged so these resources—in this case, its dental care resources—are distributed *equally*. But *equally* in regard to what? That is a question that must be answered before this view of just distributions will be clear enough to be put into practice. For example, does "equality" here mean that every person in the society gets exactly the same resources as the next person? So everyone would get the same number of porcelain-fused-to-metal restorations as the next person, for example? This makes no sense. People's needs for particular forms of dental care vary, and most people would agree that the dental care a person ought to receive should be determined by his or her need for that care. So the interpretation of equality that means "equal stuff for all" does not seem very useful here. Instead, when *equality* is proposed as a criterion of just distributions at the societal level, it is usually understood to refer to responding equally to people's *needs*. On this view, equality in distribution would exist when the people of the society were *equally able* to *fill their needs*. But this way of putting it leaves two important questions unanswered. What should count as *equal ability* to fill one's needs? And are we talking about *every kind of need* (i.e., everything that anyone might describe as something they need), or, when justice is understood in terms of needs, is the focus only on *a certain class of needs*, and if so, then which ones and why? With regard to dental care, for example, *equal ability* to fill one's needs is most often interpreted to refer to equal time, effort, and equal resources that people have to expend to get access to a certain form of dental care that they need. This is how the concept of *equal ability* to fill one's needs will be understood in this book.

Regarding what counts as needs when the question is about a society's distributing its resources justly, a common distinction within health care is useful—namely, the distinction between treatments that are needed or essential, and treatments that are nonessential and therefore optional. Within health care this distinction is widely taken to be quite clear (although cases that are difficult to call do occur). In contemporary literature on health care ethics and health care policy, this distinction is often expressed by calling essential matters "basic." Thus, the expression "basic health care" has come into common usage as the collective term for health care that is essential for humans. This is in contrast with other kinds of health care that are judged nonessential and that respond to the wants and desires that people have in addition to their basic needs.

But obviously this explanation is still incomplete. When are human needs *basic*? We must ask: Essential for what? Basic to what? Needed for what? For dentistry and the health professions generally, this question is answered by reference to what is considered to be *normal and appropriate human functioning*. Thus, the discussion of Oral Health as part of the hierarchy of dentistry's Central Practice Values in chapter 5 specified Oral Health to be "appropriate and pain-free oral functioning." Declaring that a certain kind of functioning—for example, pain-free functioning—is an essential part of human health and is a way in which humans ought to function depends on answering serious philosophical questions about human nature that are well beyond the scope of this book. (But the reader would do well to think carefully about these matters since one goal of such reflection is, in fact, to determine what *health* consists of for humans, and this is obviously relevant to understanding what dentists are ultimately aiming at for their patients.)

But whatever functions are considered to be normal and appropriate for humans, it seems clear that there are some human needs that must be fulfilled for a human to be able to perform any of these functions at all. These are the needs that are essential in a special sense, and the concept of *basic needs* will be used here to refer to this class of human needs. That is, even though there may be considerable disagreement about which human functions are those humans ought to be able to do, it is clear that there are some needs that must be met before a human could perform any of these functions. An obvious example is food (that is, adequate nutrition) because without adequate nutrition a human cannot perform any of the functions that might be considered important for human fulfillment, no matter which account of human fulfillment one accepts. Other examples include adequate clothing and shelter (and asking what "adequate" means here is simply another way of asking more concretely which needs are *basic*) as well as breathable air. Many people's lists also include adequate assistance in maintaining one's health—that is, health care—as well as adequate education, human companionship, and so on. (Discussions of basic needs sometimes prompt the question: "How much of a particular kind of resource will it take (i.e., to meet someone's basic needs)?" The general answer to this question is however much of that resource it actually takes in order to enable the person to perform whatever functions are normal and appropriate for humans to perform. That is, the concept of basic need is very general, but what it means concretely with regard to a particular kind of resource on the part of a particular person or class of people will depend on the function to be preserved and what in fact it takes to preserve that kind of functioning for that person or class of people. Obviously, this can be determined only through empirical investigation of the relevant resources and what functions are made possible or impossible, respectively, for actual individuals by a certain degree of access or lack of access to them.)

Since the things being counted here as basic needs are absolutely necessary for humans to pursue every other kind of value, goal, or purpose that they might pursue, then it is reasonable to argue that—although they may not be more valuable in themselves than many other valued human goals—they are *practically more important* and therefore *should take priority* over all other human values and goals when a society is determining how to distribute its resources. According to this line of reasoning, in other words, if any aspects of oral health care are *basic needs* for humans, then responding to these needs for *every member of the society* ought to be the first goal of a society's system of distribution if it is to be an ethical/just society. (There is much more that could be said about this line of reasoning that says that *equality* and *basic needs* should be the criterion by which a just society distributes its resources. While this position cannot be examined further here, the reader is again urged to give it serious thought and compare it carefully with the other approaches to justice examined in the following sections.) For present purposes, where dentistry's ethics is our principal concern, the fact remains that the dental community and the community at large in dialogue do view certain kinds of pain-free oral functioning as what counts as oral health for humans, and this is therefore a proper goal for members of the dental profession to pursue. For this reason, from the point of view of the dental profession and the larger society in dialogue, the proper criterion for ethically distributing a society's dental care resources is the *need* of patients for such care. From this it would follow that, if our society has enough resources to do this, then it ought to arrange its distributive structures so that whoever has dental care needs in our society can obtain the needed dental care resources to fill them. Moreover, if these oral health needs are indeed basic needs for humans generally, then any society that has sufficient resources to provide for them but fails to do so is in that measure an unjust society.

Of course, not everything that someone calls a need is a basic need in the sense explained above. So, what aspects of dental care are *essential* to oral health? What aspects of dental care are responses to *basic oral health needs*? This question will be discussed later in this chapter.

It is also important to point out that what counts in practice as a patient's oral health need—whether a matter of *basic need* because it is essential to the patient's oral health or nonessential and therefore optional from the point of view of treatment—is determined in particular cases by members of the dental profession because it is they who have the needed expertise and who have been authorized by the larger community to make these determinations on the basis of what the profession and the larger community in dialogue determine counts as oral health. These determinations happen at chairside for each individual patient for the matter at hand, and they also happen at a broader level by the dental profession collectively in dialogue with the larger community as they identify and authorize standards of competent dental practice. This is a very important point because, as chapter 13 will make clear, there is a very important difference between need as determined on the basis of professional expertise and need determined solely on the basis of a market consumer's (or other market participants') desires. Further discussion of the dialogue in which dentistry and the larger community determine what counts as oral health and what counts as oral health needs will be found in chapter 14.

Up to this point, the focus of this chapter has been chiefly oral health needs as the criteria of a just distribution of a society's health care resources. There are, however, a number of other ways of thinking about justice that do not focus on either equality or need as the determinant of what counts as an ethical, just distribution of a society's resources.

CONTRIBUTION AND EFFORT AS POSSIBLE CRITERIA

Some theorists hold that a society's resources, including its dental and other health care resources, ought to be distributed according to the value of each person's *contribution* to that society. The underlying idea here is that the resources that a society has are mostly *produced* resources rather than resources that are already highly useful in their natural form. Therefore, because these resources wouldn't exist without the contributions of the humans who produce them, each producer has a legitimate claim on that proportion of a society's resources that he or she has produced. Thus, the measure of what each person in a society receives through the operations of that society's distributive structures ought to be the value of his or her contributions. In other words, the ethically relevant differences between people in the distribution of a society's resources are the differences in people's *contributions*.

Only in a world where there were no specialization and no division of labor would people actually want to simply hold on to what they personally produce. Dentists need to eat, and farmers can't provide all of their own dental care. Thus, an exchange system develops, but its operation unavoidably involves a "cost" and unavoidably consumes a portion of the available resources in order to run at all. It follows that the value a person receives from his or her exchanges will always be some fraction less than what he or she put in. This is why the criterion for distributive justice in terms of contributions is actually that each person ought to receive resources *in proportion to* the value of his or her contribution.

Moreover, because children do not contribute much when they are growing up, using this criterion of contribution would also require an exchange system between generations. Children would tally up a debt by receiving without contributing for a time and then repay that debt when they are able to contribute significantly. (A similar system would be needed to cover those who are temporarily unproductive due to accident or illness and whose savings are not great enough to cover their needs during this time.) It is easy to forget, however, how indebted to the society a young adult is when he or she first begins to contribute something of value to it and how many years of prorating one's return (downward) it might take to gradually pay off that debt. It is also important to note that, if one uses natural resources or resources produced by others' contributions in one's own productive efforts, then these resources also need to be paid for out of the value of one's contribution before what is left belongs unconditionally to the producer.

Objectors to this view identify three problems with it. The first asks what standard is to be used for *measuring the value* of each person's contribution, so that differences in what people receive will be proportional to differences in the value of what they produce. Some objectors even hold that there is *no standard* of value that is universally accepted or that has some sort of objective status even if it is not universally accepted, nor even a standard that is widely shared within our own society. Therefore, they argue, the comparative judgments of value on which the practical application of this view of justice depends are impossible to make or defend. So it is a useless theory.

When the focus is on dental care, this is a weaker objection than it might be if other kinds of resources were under consideration. For dental care focuses on values such as relief from pain, comfort in functioning, nutrition, appearance, control over one's body, communicating effectively, and so on that are very widely considered important for human life, not just for human lives in this particular society, but generally. The experience of giving and receiving dental care seems to make it clear that there are some values of universal, or at least of very general, significance.

A second objection concerns one troubling implication of the contribution view of social justice—namely, that those members of the human family who are unable to contribute at all, not only in the present like children or those temporarily unproductive but forever because their disabilities are permanent, ought not to receive *any* resources from their society.

Many people cannot accept this conclusion and would consider providing some resources to those unable to contribute (e.g., resources necessary to meet such people's basic needs) to be a matter of justice for any society with enough resources to do so. But this position cannot be incorporated into the contribution view without changing it radically. Consequently, for many theorists, if contribution has a role in relation to distributive justice, it is only as a criterion for justly distributing whatever resources a society "has left" after its structures assure that everyone in the society has been able to meet his or her basic needs.

Should patients receive dental care in proportion to the value of their contributions to the society? Or should they receive at least some dental care (perhaps basic dental care) in proportion to their need for it, with nonessential, nonbasic dental care distributed in proportion to their contributions?

A third objection to the contribution view asks a more radical question: Do people really *deserve* to receive in proportion to the value to the society of what they produce? This objection argues that people's ability to contribute something of value depends greatly on their inherited genetic and biological capabilities, over which no one has any control and for which no one ought to take credit or receive a return. A person's contributions also depend greatly on accidents of upbringing, education, opportunity, and luck, and, if we are honest, we must acknowledge that a great deal of what we take credit for in our daily work and other activities involves skills and ideas that we received from others rather than our being able to take credit for them as if they were our own inventions. One British philosopher, L. T. Hobhouse, argued that if we all deducted from our claims on society the part of the value of our contributions that, in all honesty, we can't personally take credit for, we would have to admit that the differences between those who seem to contribute the most and those who seem to contribute the least are in fact very slight. If we take contribution as the proper criterion of distributive justice but are really honest about what each of us can take personal credit for, he argued, we would see that we should actually distribute society's resources equally because the differences between us, after everything is properly deducted and prorated, are actually negligible.

But many people would say to Hobhouse, "What about how hard I have worked? Certainly, I have had control over that." In addition, what really bothers a lot of people most is someone who is not working hard at all but who is receiving the same resources as (or even more than) people who do work hard (which most of us presume we are doing). The focus of this response to Hobhouse is on *effort* rather than contribution. It suggests yet another view of the proper criterion for social justice—namely, that the relevant differences between people, when it comes to distributing a society's resources, are differences in *effort*. How *hard* a person works rather than the value of his or her actual contribution should be the criterion.

Some have argued in response to the *effort* criterion that how hard a person is able to work is partly controlled by genetic and psychological factors over which the person has little or no control. So only insofar as a person is able to put out effort by his or her own initiative or choice may that person's effort be used as the measure of what he or she should receive in the society. In addition, note that if distribution were simply in terms of effort, then great effort would deserve great return, even if it did not produce anything of value. Consequently, actually using *effort* as the criterion of just distributions would almost certainly mean there would be less to distribute, which is at least paradoxical.

Should a society distribute its dental care resources in proportion to how hard a patient works, with harder-working patients receiving more dental care and less-hard-working patients receiving less dental care, independently of other considerations, including their need for dental care? Once again, it seems incorrect to ignore need as a criterion of justice, where need is understood in terms of whatever is essential for appropriate human functioning.

The authors' view is that a just society first arranges its distributive structures to meet all the basic needs of all its members and then may choose to employ criteria other than need in the distribution of whatever resources are "left over" after that. The reasons for supporting this view are straightforward. The authors hold that, whatever other goals, values, principles, purposes, or ideals a human being might choose to live by, none of these can be effectively pursued unless his or her basic needs are filled (not just basic oral health needs, of course, but all the needs that are essential to appropriate human functioning of every sort). Consequently, meeting people's basic needs should take moral priority in the arrangement of a society's distributive structures.

The section on basic dental care will discuss what specific forms of dental care should be considered essential responses to basic needs. But one more view of distributive justice needs to be discussed first, one that rejects the authors' view and every other proposal examined above.

THE FREE MARKET VIEW OF JUSTICE

The Free Market View of justice seems to have a wide following within contemporary American society. But it is not clear that all of those who claim to support it have thought carefully through the assumptions it makes about human beings or the conclusions it entails for human social life. Unfortunately, like the other approaches, it can be examined only briefly here. This view holds that a just society is simply one in which all social arrangements and all distribution of resources are the product of voluntary exchanges of the society's citizens in a free marketplace.

This little story helps express this approach to justice: Two dentists decide to take a vacation in Las Vegas, and each sets aside $300 for enjoying Las Vegas's games of chance. Suppose that they both enter the same establishment at the same time, each with $300, and assume also that the games are not rigged so a player is simply playing against the odds (which, of course, favor the house, but everyone knows that).

At the end of the day, the first dentist emerges without a single dollar of his original $300. But the other dentist finishes the day with $15,000! Has anything immoral happened in this story, even though there is now a huge discrepancy in the two dentists' final financial position? The correct answer seems to be no, for the games were fair, and every play that either player made was freely chosen. In other words, in this type of case, the ethical distribution is *whatever* distribution results from adequately informed choosers freely choosing to exchange their goods however they choose to exchange them.

If the dentists had been coerced into playing the games or if they were lied to or defrauded in some other way or if anyone had failed to keep commitments to the dentists that he or she had made, then the story would include something unethical, and the final distribution would not be a just one. Some kind of restitution would then be needed for the party who was coerced, defrauded, or suffered someone else's breach of contract, and it might also be right to punish the guilty party in addition to requiring them to make restitution. But so long as no one acted in these unethical ways in the story, it seems that *whatever* distribution results from the participants' freely chosen exchanges is an ethical distribution, regardless of whether it conforms to the criterion of need, contribution, effort, or any other.

Supporters of the Free Market View of distributive justice claim that what makes the distribution ethical in this story is exactly the same as what makes any distribution in any aspect of human social life ethical: the exercise of uncoerced free choice by the participants. Thus, in this view, a just distribution is whatever distribution results from the participants' freely chosen exchanges, without reference to its conformity to criteria like need, contribution, or effort. The supreme moral value for all social matters on this view of justice is *respect for people's freely chosen actions* (provided the person does not freely choose an action that violates someone else's freedom).

Applied to the distribution of dental care resources, the Free Market View of justice holds that dental care resources are justly and ethically distributed when they have been distributed to whoever the providers of dental care choose to provide them to, whether this is on the basis of ability to pay the prices dentists ask for their services, on the basis of need, or on some other basis or some combination of bases. So long as both parties *freely choose* the exchange, then the resulting distribution of resources is ethical and just.

In the Las Vegas story, the two dentists began with the same amount of money, $300. In the real world, however, people's resources vary greatly, and for many people the resources available to pay for dental and other forms of health care are limited or even nonexistent, as are the resources they need to get access to such care (long distances to caregivers, means of transportation, etc.). Consequently, distributing dental care solely on the basis of the Free Market View of justice in our society would mean that many people would be unable to receive the *basic dental care* they need. In fact, many people's dental needs do go unmet because so much of oral health care in our society is distributed solely by means of free market exchanges.

Unlike in the Las Vegas story, however, people's actual starting points in life are not equal in resources or opportunities. So the only way a society's distribution system could provide every individual with resources for needed dental care would be by taking resources from those who start with more resources or who get more opportunities than other people and then giving those resources, in the form of dental care, to those without. But unless the losers in this redistribution freely choose the redistribution, doing this would violate the Free Market View of justice's commitment to respecting freedom of choice over every other value. A society that did such redistributing over the objection of even one of its people would be, according to the Free Market View of justice, an unjust society.

In other words, if some dental care is considered to be a *basic human need* (a question that will be examined in the next section) and meeting people's basic needs is taken to have some sort of moral priority when a society is determining how to distribute its resources (which is how the dental profession and the larger community in dialogue understand oral health care), then societies should not employ the Free Market View of justice when designing the systems that distribute its oral health care resources.

There is another ethically crucial difference between the Las Vegas story and what is at stake when a society is choosing how to distribute its dental care resources. The players in the Las Vegas story did not *need* to gamble; for them it was an optional entertainment. (Admittedly, some people do need to gamble, but this is not considered a normal human need of the sort that *basic health care*, including *basic dental care*, is. In fact, if the desire to gamble becomes a psychological need for someone, this is considered unhealthy, dysfunctional, and something that ought to be addressed with care and treatment if possible.) Because gambling is not a basic human need, permitting people's opportunity to gamble to be distributed on the basis of whatever exchanges happen to take place in the marketplace may well be acceptable. But basic human needs are understood to be much more important than this. They concern essentials; their absence renders humans unable to participate effectively in other areas of human life, even in free market exchanges concerning other matters.

Therefore, a society's responses to its members' basic needs ought not to rest solely on whatever exchanges people happen to make, on free market justice. As we argued in previous sections, an alternative standard of social justice (namely, to meet the basic needs of every member of society) ought to guide the distribution of dental—indeed, all health care—resources. Just what practical mechanisms and particular structures should be used to meet people's *basic dental care* needs, whether by public clinics, universal insurance, vouchers, or whatever, and how the structures that meet them should be shaped so as not to interfere with dentists' maintaining their professional commitments to their patients, to other norms of their profession, and to other people in their lives are important questions. But they are questions beyond the scope of this book. The principal point of this section is that leaving the distribution of dental care to be directed by the Free Market View of justice alone means leaving many of our society's people with their dental care needs unmet, a situation that we have already argued is unsatisfactory from the point of view of social justice.

BASIC DENTAL CARE

The concept of *basic dental care* has been used so far without further clarification. Now it is time to try differentiating those aspects of dental care that are essential because they respond to basic needs from those aspects of dental care that are nonessential or optional.

Two categories of dental care are the easiest to identify as essential or *basic* in the relevant sense. These are treatments that end or limit serious oral pain—since pain, when severe enough, interferes significantly with numerous other human functions—and treatments that restore functions, the loss of which prevents or severely limits normal nutrition and speech and thereby compromises other human functions for which nutrition and speech are essential. Note that many different kinds of dental procedures will play a role in achieving these goals, depending on the clinical details of the patient's condition. That is, determining which forms of dental care are *basic* in the relevant sense is not a matter of putting certain procedures on one list and others on another list. It requires instead that we ask of every procedure under what conditions it preserves or restores essential components of a patient's capacity for normal human functioning.

The categories of treatment just mentioned, relief of severe pain and restoration of functions necessary to nutrition and speech, are most obviously essential when the conditions to be corrected are emergent; for example, the pain is currently debilitating or function is currently severely impaired. However, intervening sooner, when the pain or impairment of function is less, is ordinarily included within the category of essential or nonoptional treatments whenever these less burdensome conditions are likely to lead to conditions that will certainly require emergency treatment, as is most often the case. (Considerations of reasonable cost-effectiveness and risk-benefit analysis also favor intervening sooner, but not for reasons directly related to the ethical urgency of meeting people's basic needs.) Therefore, it is reasonable to propose that essential or *basic dental care* includes not only emergency treatment of these conditions but treatment of similar conditions less far advanced. This is so not only to limit the patient's suffering but also to subject the undesirable conditions to expert control at an earlier point in their development so as to forestall yet worse complications and thereby more severe limitations of important human functions. (In addition, earlier intervention ordinarily results in dental resources being used more efficiently as well and thus permits basic oral health needs to be met for more people.)

Many diagnostic procedures, such as oral diagnosis and radiography, are necessary predecessors of the treatments just discussed. It is important to note, then, that these are reasonably included in the category of basic dental care whenever treatment is needed. The same is true of the kinds of patient education, aftercare, and so on that properly accompany such treatments and without which they could not be effectively performed.

The themes of forestalling worse conditions and using resources efficiently for patients' dental health raise one of the most subtle questions about what should count as basic dental care. Namely, should routine checkups and prophylaxis, the use of sealants on pits and fissures, and general patient education for self-care be considered essential care or optional care? Certainly the emphasis within the dental community has been to view such preventive care as essential to good oral health. This is a major tenet of most contemporary dental practices. Its inclusion within the specifically professional commitment of dentists, though, does not necessarily mean such care should count as essential—as *basic* in the sense of being a precondition of people's ability to perform whatever human functions are identified as essential to human fulfillment. But it certainly would seem profoundly foolish and a gross waste of dental care resources to pay no or only optional attention to preventing the conditions of oral need that most interrupt important human functions and instead wait until they begin to occur to address them. The US health care system has, overall, been slow to recognize the inefficiency of such an approach, and dentistry is widely admired in the larger community for the providence of its emphasis on these aspects of dental care. But these arguments, by themselves, only establish a close and very efficient link between these forms of dental care and what is clearly essential for human functioning. If there were no other link, the case for their inclusion in the category of basic dental care might still be unsure.

But there is another link. It concerns the point made in chapters 4 and 5 that pain and impairment of oral functioning, even mild and occasional pain or impairment, lessen a person's sense of being in control of his or her body. These experiences involve not only a lessening of many people's sense of effective autonomy but they also disrupt a person's sense of the unity of the self, since one part of the self is out of control and working at odds against the rest. To some people, these may seem rather soft and unscientific reasons for emphasizing the elements of preventive dental care, but from the point of view of many who suffer from oral pain and dysfunction, the fear and disruption of normal functioning attendant on them are far more dysfunctional than the modest pain or oral impairment itself. This is also why support of and restoration of the patient's Autonomy is ranked as highly as it is on the hierarchy of Central Practice Values of professional dental practice, immediately after Oral Health and Life and General Health.

If health care resources were so scarce that the several categories of care listed so far could not all be provided to those who need them, patients would certainly choose to forgo this last category of care before they went without emergent treatment of severely painful and impairing conditions or without timely treatment of the lesser emergent conditions that lead to them. In that sense, the elements of preventive dentistry and education are arguably less valuable to the most important aspects of human functioning than the other two categories. For the reasons just stated, though, the authors propose that preventive dental care and education for self-care are closely connected to normal and appropriate human functioning in ways that deserve close attention when systems for the distribution of oral health care resources are being considered.

An even subtler question concerns whether those aspects of dental care focused principally on aesthetic concerns should be placed within the category of essential, or *basic*, health care. Some kinds of dental interventions aimed at improving appearance are clearly nonessential, even granting their psychological importance to the patients who seek them. But it would be a mistake to overgeneralize from these. What counts as a normal appearance (or normal enough) is quite variable. Consequently, even though dentists are professionally committed to being concerned about the aesthetic value of their work, many aspects of dental treatment that address appearance will not count as basic dental care in the sense under consideration here. Nevertheless, there will be circumstances, and not only in the practice of oral and maxillofacial surgeons, in which a patient's need for dental treatment to rectify or preserve appearance will be essential to his or her normal human functioning. When this is the case, such treatment should count as an instance of basic dental care.

If the claim made earlier in this chapter is correct, that a just society arranges its distributive structures to respond equally to the basic needs of all its people—then it follows from the reasons just offered that the categories of dental care discussed in this section as instances of basic dental care should be available to all members of such a society. It also follows that the availability of these forms of dental care should not depend principally on the generosity of, or on major sacrifices by, society's dentists or on the chance workings of the free market.

THE SOCIAL DEVALUING OF ORAL HEALTH CARE

In spite of the essential connection between *basic dental care* and people's ability to perform the most important human functions, access to oral health care services has been selectively disadvantaged in the United States health system for decades. This has been a continuing pattern in spite of increasingly clear connections between oral health and the health of many other bodily systems. In addition, there are the millions of lost hours of work, school attendance, and other valuable activities society-wide that are due to dental pain and dysfunction. This pattern and its adverse results for the people of this country was powerfully demonstrated in *Oral Health in America*, the 2000 report on oral health by the US Department of Health and Human Services for the US Surgeon General, and confirmed again in the 2011 Institute of Medicine (IOM) report, *Advancing Oral Health in America*. The 2000 report acknowledges "dramatic improvements in our society's oral health during the second half of the 20th century." But it also identifies the "profound and consequential disparities in the oral health of our citizens." It proceeds to speak about unmet oral health needs in the United States as "a silent epidemic" of oral diseases that especially impacts our society's most vulnerable citizens—poor children, the elderly, and many members of racial and ethnic minority groups.

While the defects in our society's systems for distributing oral health resources are certainly major contributors to this situation, another major contributor is the social devaluing of oral health and oral health care in the whole society. As one sign of this, when people—as patients (or as parents or other proxies for patients) determine under what circumstances they will use their resources to access oral health care, they reveal how much they value it in comparison with other kinds of health care and with other values generally. It is well known that at least half the US population does not have a regular dentist and visits dentists' offices only in emergencies. In spite of dentistry's long-standing commitment to prevention and years of efforts at education, dentists still see large numbers of patients whose self-care is inadequate and whose "dental literacy" is deficient. Moreover, if oral health care were more highly valued socially, there would be much more and much broader social support for distribution systems that respond more justly to unmet oral health needs.

At the same time, the second-class status of oral health care in our society has been reinforced and perpetuated by the fact that extending life and avoiding death are seen as primary goals of the health professions and oral health care is not generally seen as contributing to those goals. This pattern of social devaluation is supported by the widespread but mistaken notion that oral health is solely about teeth and the oral cavity. As the 2000 Surgeon General's report and the 2011 IOM report both affirm, though, oral health involves "the whole craniofacial complex" and has intimate connections with the health of many other bodily processes and the health of individuals and society in general.

It seems likely that significant changes in access to oral health resources and in the systems by which our society's oral health resources are distributed will come about only if there are major changes in understanding the importance of oral health and the value of oral health care across US society. But changes in the distributive system are what will be necessary for the kind of one-on-one chairside oral health education—which is what is most effective in helping patients value dental interventions and manage the need for such interventions through dietary and personal oral hygiene habits—to reach those who currently visit the dentist solely for emergencies.

Note that these predictions do not support an attitude on the part of dentists to say, "Let the education go and just do the work." Support by dentists throughout the United States for the efforts of organized dentistry and other knowledgeable institutions to advocate for systems of distribution that are far more responsive to our society's unmet oral health needs will continue to be important. But chairside education—not just about the patient's own oral health needs but about the importance of oral health in relation to general health and in its impact on people's lives generally—will remain dentistry's most effective tool to correct the errors that have led to its being socially devalued.

THINKING ABOUT THE CASE

There are important differences between the circumstances of the two committees described in the case that opened this chapter. Political considerations, for example, will inevitably affect the work of the Secretary's Priorities Committee in a way that they may not impact the board of the Lancaster Health Trust. But it is the similarities between the two committees that are most important from the perspective of ethical or just distribution systems and access to oral health care.

The Secretary's Priorities Committee is operating within the context of a fixed number of dollars, an amount set by a higher authority that is not at all likely to be increased, regardless of the needs it leaves unmet. The reason it is fixed is that authorities above the secretary have many other uses for the dollars in the federal budget, and they have already rationed those dollars among those uses. That is, in all thinking about allocating health care resources, we must remember that a society has many uses for its dollars and other resources, and it determines, by many means both thoughtful and otherwise, that only a certain portion of those dollars and resources will be dedicated to meeting health care needs and oral health care needs in particular.

Some people take the view that health care needs are so important that a society ought to commit whatever dollars and resources are necessary to meeting them, taking these dollars and resources as need be from other uses. But in our actual situation in American society, this is not the consensus view, and every actual individual and group who must allocate dollars and other resources must do so in the context of this fact. In practice, the secretary may be able to lobby the president for some additional dollars for a particular program or two on the basis that the need for them is far greater than something in the defense budget or the environmental budget. And such lobbying, which of course goes on all the time, will sometimes be effective. But even so, the priorities committee would do the secretary little service if it therefore declined to prioritize all the health care needs it is aware of in order to then fund as many as possible of them with the limited dollars available. So long as the relevant resources are considered limited, determining priorities among different kinds of need and benefit is an essential part of social policy-making, and providing reasonable explanations for establishing such priorities is part of the thought process involved.

The board of the Lancaster Health Trust may seem to escape the exigencies of rationing because its money is new money and every dollar they provide has already been designated for health care. That is, the board does not have to deal with interests outside of health care competing for its dollars in the way that the Secretary's Priorities Committee does, and none of the dollars the trust provides for health care will be taken away from existing programs. But, of course, when there are so many unmet health care needs in a society, every dollar the trust provides to meet any one of them is a dollar not being provided to meet some others. And the trust's dollars, even though they are new dollars, are not infinite. So this committee will be engaged in rationing dollars among competing needs as surely as will the Secretary's Priorities Committee, even if the absence of strong, overt political pressures may permit the trust's board to deliberate in a calmer atmosphere. (Both committees may have—for example, through their social influence—resources of other, nonfiscal sorts that they can apply to health care needs in the society. The case is focused on the dollars they have to ration, but questions about priorities and the just distribution of resources apply equally to whatever kinds of resources a committee or an individual or a whole society has available for meeting human needs. Therefore, the discussions about justice and basic human needs in this chapter should be taken to be relevant to the distribution of every kind of resource that might contribute to filling a human need.)

It is also worth mentioning that, once the Lancaster Health Trust is up and running and known to be a source of funding for health care needs, numerous competing programs will be at the trust's door hoping for assistance, and not a few of them will be programs that, without its assistance, will come to an end because they have exhausted other sources of support or perhaps will never come into being for the same reason. In sum, whether the money is new money and wholly dedicated to health care or not, those who are charged with allocating health care resources in American society today are charged with *rationing* a limited number of dollars and other resources. This is the case whether we like to think about rationing health care resources or not.

How should these committees prioritize the various unmet health care needs that are placed before them? The short and too simple answer to this question, from the authors' point of view, is that they should rank basic health care needs, including basic oral health care, ahead of other health care needs, and they should fund programs aimed at meeting all these basic needs of every member of the society before other health care needs. Then, if they have any resources that have not been spent, they should prioritize the remaining health care needs and meet them in order of their priority for every member of the society until the money runs out. This answer is too simple, above all, because it presumes the committees have simple answers, both about what kinds of health care should be counted as *basic* in the sense described earlier in the chapter and about how other kinds of health care should be prioritized.

The people who make up US society are far from reaching a consensus on these matters. It is possible that it would even be difficult to get a consensus within the oral health community about what should count as basic oral health care, whether the authors' account in the section on basic dental care is adequate or some other. It is unlikely that the committees in this chapter's case could determine what kinds of health care are *basic* and the priorities among other health care needs, much less provide reasonable explanations for such judgments, without something much closer to a consensus about these matters than is currently available in US society.

One reason for this lack of consensus in our society is a lack of careful conversation about the issues involved. Therefore, in the interests of furthering this conversation, rather than commenting further on how the two committees in the case might deliberate, the authors propose the following exercise for our readers to assist them in thinking more carefully about health care rationing.

Suppose you were a member of one of these committees and were faced with the task that committee is given in this chapter's introductory case. Suppose, to keep the challenge of this exercise less daunting, you knew that it was some other committee's task to provide the fullest support possible to biomedical and dental research and to provide for the highest quality of education for the next generation of health care professionals. That is, you are relieved of the burden of weighing resources for health care research and education against resources for the actual provision of health care. Now, suppose you were given the following eleven categories of health care services.

Each of these categories of health care services produces a distinct kind of health care benefit for the people who receive it, but the eleven kinds of benefit are quite different from one another. Your task, in order to assist the secretary in her decisions or the trust in its allocation of dollars and resources over the next five years, is to *rank these categories* of health care services in order of priority from first to last (or, if that is simply too daunting, to rank them in sets of three or four) and to *formulate reasons for this ranking* so you can explain your priorities to the rest of the committee. Your working assumption in this exercise should be that the available dollars and resources will be spent as follows: first, as much of the dollars and resources as are needed will be spent to provide for everyone who needs the highest ranking of these forms of health care, then as much as are needed to provide for everyone who needs the second highest in rank, then the third highest, the fourth, and so on, until all the money has been spent. Those forms of health care that cannot be funded in this way will not be available to anyone.

If you object strongly to this set of working assumptions, then you should have thoughtful reasons for accepting one of the alternative views of social justice articulated earlier in this chapter, and your task would then be to work out a reasoned method of just rationing of health care resources according to that system of thought. Also, while you may judge this set of categories to be in need of serious editing or judge that more categories need to be added to it, for the purpose of the exercise you should either accept them as adequate enough to proceed with the exercise or else add the categories you think are also needed and then do the exercise. But do not let that activity get in the way of *prioritizing* the categories and *formulating reasons* for this ranking, for careful reflection on these tasks is the point of the exercise.

Here, in alphabetical order, are the eleven categories of health care services to be prioritized:

- **Curing a life-threatening condition** (e.g., ending an infection) with the aim of return to or maintenance of (more or less) normal forms of human functioning and (more or less) normal homeostasis to sustain them.

- **Emergency life-saving care** (to prevent people from dying by accident).

- **Function-maintaining / function-restoring care regarding non-life-threatening conditions** (excluding dental conditions covered by primary care), with the aim of restoring/maintaining (more or less) normal forms of human functioning and (within limits) the special functional capacities of individuals (special talents, etc.) and including ongoing functional support for those with chronic non-life-threatening deficits of normal function (e.g., arthritis).

- **Life-extending care for people with a life-threatening condition but without cure**—that is, providing both extension of life and restoration of or maintenance of (more or less) normal forms of human functioning but without cure.

- **Maintaining/extending only biological life** without maintaining or likelihood of restoring (more or less) normal forms of human functioning.

- **Ongoing treatment of a life-threatening chronic deficit** (e.g., insulin therapy) with the aim of return to or maintenance of (more or less) normal forms of human functioning and (more or less) normal homeostasis to sustain them.

- **Pain relief or limitation** (excluding oral pain covered by primary care) and control of other symptoms that interfere with normal forms of human functioning, including treatment of chronic pain and related symptoms.

- **Preventive medical and dental care** (including routine oral prophylaxis and education for oral self-care), both individual and in the form of public health measures and education for other forms of self-care.

- **Primary dental care**—that is, initial diagnosis, self-contained on-site dental treatment of emergencies and of caries and infection as well as any other treatments essential to pain-free oral functioning, referral to specialists or other subsystems, explanation of these actions and education for self-care.

- **Primary medical care**—that is, initial diagnosis; self-contained on-site medical treatment; referral to specialists, hospitals, or other subsystems for additional care; explanation of these actions and education for self-care.

- **Support in time of dying** (psychosocial support in addition to pain relief and symptom control).

Care of Patients vs. Third-Party Payers and Other Bureaucracies

CASE: JUST TAKE IT OUT, DOC!

Dr. Ed Witten's receptionist, Mary Rawley, arrives a little early to open the office. Already waiting at the door is Jane Nelson, a twenty-six-year-old graduate student. Mary invites her into the waiting room and checks her daily morning text from the answering service. It says, "Call Mrs. Brown, needs to reschedule."

"Are you Mrs. Brown?" asks Mary.

"No, Jane Nelson. I came to see if I could get an appointment. I've had a lot of pain on and off and it started up again last night. I've been looking for a dentist to help me—all I have is one of those state medical insurance cards. I saw your hours posted online and thought I'd just stop here real early rather than call."

"Well, we're both little early birds," says Mary, "and you may be in luck. But I need to make a few quick calls first."

Mrs. Brown had been the first patient, but Mary needs to check her list of patients who want to be called in case of a last-minute opening.

Within a few minutes Dr. Witten arrives. "Good morning! Mrs. Brown?"

"No, Jane Nelson. I don't have an appointment."

"That shouldn't be a problem," says Dr. Witten. "Mary, can we fit her in this morning?"

"She has some pain and is looking for a dentist. Mrs. Brown has had to cancel and none of the patients on the waiting list can come right now."

"Well, you are way ahead of us this morning," says Dr. Witten. "We need a few minutes to wake up our computers and flip some switches in the back room. Then I'll come back to talk with you. Can I bring you a cup of coffee?"

"No, thank you," replies Mrs. Nelson. "I'm OK."

Mary catches up with Dr. Witten as he heads into the back. "Our first patient, Mrs. Brown, left a message saying she needed to reschedule. I've called the patients who are looking for a cancellation, but none of them is available. So we do have room for her."

"Okay, thanks, Mary. I hope nothing serious happened with Mrs. Brown. Check with her when you have a minute. I'll go talk with Mrs. Nelson in the waiting room to see what she needs. Would you finish getting things up and running?"

"Hello, again!" Dr. Witten greets Mrs. Nelson as he returns to the waiting room. "We do have a cancellation, and no one on our waiting list is available right now. Mary says you're in a lot of pain and you've had trouble finding a dentist."

"Yes, Doc, thanks for seeing me. You can't believe the run around I've been getting, just trying to get these two teeth out. You're the fifth dentist I've tried to see in the past two years."

"Two years?" says Dr. Witten.

"Yes," says Mrs. Nelson. "I only have a medical card."

"Okay, we'll talk about that in a minute. What I want to know is how bad your pain is right now."

"It's pretty bad right now. It started up again last night, that's why I found your web page and office hours. They cut the class I registered for online, and then last night their site shut down and I was stuck. I was feeling pretty mad about it, and the last thing I needed was a tooth going bad. I was going to come this way anyway to see my adviser. I hope he can help me fix it. I need that class this semester to graduate on time."

"Sorry about your computer woes and your registration problem. I hope your adviser can get it fixed," says Dr. Witten. "But to help me judge the pain from your teeth, what would you say, on a scale of one to ten, is the worst pain you've ever felt?"

"A kidney stone—three years ago. It's not like that—at least not yet," says Mrs. Nelson. "About seven, I'd say. It's been worse, but it's pretty bad right now and I don't want it getting worse. For the past month I've been pretty miserable, though it only hurts off and on. Sometimes it's more when I lay down."

"Does the pain keep you up at night?"

"Not really. I take some Tylenol and that helps. It's the teeth in the back on the right side."

"Top or bottom?"

"Bottom," she says, pointing to her lower-right molars. "They don't wake me up if I take the Tylenol, but they do make it slow to get to sleep sometimes. During the day it only hurts for ten or fifteen minutes, then goes away. I know I have other cavities. It makes it hard to eat though—hot, cold, sweets . . . anything like that sets them off."

"Let me take a look at them," says Dr. Witten, escorting Mrs. Nelson into an operatory and getting her settled in the chair. He does a quick exam and finds a deep cavity in #30, which might be the culprit for Mrs. Nelson's current pain, but he also sees another in #29 and a few others as well.

"Well, Mrs. Nelson, your pain is probably coming from the teeth you pointed to, the lower-right first molar in the back and the bicuspid right next to it. But you do have other cavities, quite a few of them. We will need to talk a bit more about them. But since we're just fitting you in here and you only wanted to see if you could get an appointment for your pain, should we just deal with what's bothering you most today and talk about the other issues later? Or I could do a complete exam and you could walk out of here with a long-range plan to deal with all of it. We could work together and get you on a path where you could still keep your teeth. The teeth you pointed to probably don't need to come out, although I'll need some X-rays to be sure of that."

"Look, Doc, I don't want a plan," says Mrs. Nelson. "You're the fifth dentist I've tried to see in the past two years. Two years ago I went to the dentist that I grew up with when I was on my mom and dad's dental insurance that covered me for fillings and all kinds of stuff. But I graduated from high school and got married and all that stopped. My old dentist said he and some other dentists set up a clinic for people like me and he told me I should go there."

"What do you mean, 'people like you'?"

"You know what I mean, people that can't afford regular care, people with a medical card. My old dentist didn't say it that way. I liked him because he always tried to be nice. But he said to go to the clinic, so I went to the clinic. That was two years ago. At that time I couldn't sleep at all because of the pain . . . and I wasn't eating. I was really acting like a total jerk with everyone. The clinic said they couldn't see me for two months, but the pain was terrible, so I went to the ER at the hospital. They gave me some pain meds and antibiotics, and it went away. They also told me I should see an oral surgeon, and they gave me the name of some. So I called them, but the people on the phone always said they didn't take medical cards. But the pain had stopped so I didn't bother going back to the clinic. Then, last year, when it was bothering me again, I started calling around to find another dentist and no one would take my card, or if they would they could only see me months later."

"Well, Mrs. Nelson, I can't say much about all that. I know it happens. But you're here now and I'd like to help you, so can we just talk about that now?"

"I'd like that, Doc, but how much is that going to cost? Can we do payments?"

"Yes, we can work out something, but that depends on what you and I decide to do. Your lower-right first molar has a very large cavity in it and it's probably near the pulp, the part that keeps the tooth alive, and it may even be into the pulp. There's also a smaller cavity in the tooth right in front of it. Let me get a model to show what the problem might be."

Dr. Witten goes back to his office and brings back a small education model. "Here's what your tooth #30 might look like in 3-D."

"Isn't that cute. I didn't know teeth had numbers."

"Yes, all the teeth have numbers, though some people count them in different ways. But what you and I need to talk about is the big cavity in your #30—the lower-right molar that is probably what is hurting you—and what can be done about it. The other tooth there, #29, also needs a filling sometime soon. But for #30, from the way you're talking about it and what I can see, I think we can try putting a sedative filling in it or paint a special silver fluoride coating on it. I think either treatment might work and solve your pain problem for a little while. But the tooth may need something more rather soon if the filling or coating doesn't solve the problem. And I would like to take some X-rays before I do that to be sure the cavity hasn't gone into the pulp."

"When you say 'something more,' do you mean like a root canal? I've heard of those, people talk about them. But they hurt, don't they?"

"It's a way of saving a tooth rather than losing it, and no, they don't have to hurt. They're a way to save the tooth and keep it from hurting, that's the point. But I really think temporarily filling the tooth or treating it the way I described will resolve your pain for now. I just have to say that eventually the tooth will likely need a root canal and probably a crown, but I think a filling will be enough for today. Your current medical card wouldn't cover a root canal or crown. It would only cover an extraction, but we can work out a payment plan like you said to cover the filling. Later on, if it needs a root canal and crown, you may be working by then and may even have some kind of dental insurance."

"I think I just want the tooth out," says Mrs. Nelson. "My husband and I are both full-time students, and we really haven't got much money. I don't think I could get my parents to pay for it either, even if it was just for a small down payment. If the medical card covers for extractions, then I think I would rather have it out, so I won't have to worry about the money or payments right now. I know I have other cavities and some are in front. I'd rather spend money on that whenever we get enough together—we're waiting for tax refunds in the spring. I'm only twenty-six, and I don't want to lose my front teeth. My husband and I could only scrape up $100 this morning between us before I left, and that really needs to go for food and gas this week."

After further conversation, with Mrs. Nelson acknowledging that she would prefer to keep her teeth if she thought they could afford it, Mrs. Nelson asks Dr. Witten again if he will take the tooth out. He agrees, explaining that extraction may be within the standard of care for her situation but that he would need to get her history and take some X-rays before he knows it is appropriate to do it. He adds that she should consider what might be causing her to get cavities and briefly mentions proper nutrition, avoiding sipping and snacking, using fluoride toothpaste, and other preventive dentistry measures. He then says she should make a point of seeing a dentist regularly because the tooth next to it and a few others could also be causing problems—or soon will be if nothing more is done. He reminds her again that even if she decided to take one or two teeth out, she would still need a complete exam and treatment for the other concerns if she wants to keep her teeth, including the ones in front.

"I understand all that," says Mrs. Nelson. "Just take the tooth out so it stops hurting and my medical card will pay for that much. I need to stop thinking and fretting about tooth pain every time I eat or do anything else, and I will try to come back whenever we have some money for it. Are you upset with me for asking you to take it out?"

"Mrs. Nelson, I am a dentist and a professional. I've made a commitment to put my patient's health first whenever I can, and I think it's terrible that your medical card only covers extractions in a case like yours. You're young, you have many years ahead of you, and keeping your teeth and taking care of them is the best way to protect your health over the long run. The people who manage the medical card that is paid for by our taxes know this; but they're given only a certain amount of money and not enough to cover anything but extractions in a case like yours. It really bothers me—mostly because I see how it changes our thinking about what could be done."

"I'm sorry to make you feel bad," says Mrs. Nelson, "but this really is the best thing for me to do right now. Maybe you should send them a letter or something."

"I and thousands of other dentists have sent many letters to lots of people, Mrs. Nelson, as have our many dental organizations. But we're not telling them anything they don't already know. There are lots of wheels turning in dentistry and society and the messages get very complex. It makes being a dentist very hard when our world isn't set up to work with people and offer the dental care they really need."

THIRD-PARTY PAYERS AND OTHER DISTANT BUREAUCRACIES

There was a time not too many years ago when almost all dental care was paid for solely and directly by the person receiving it. The conversation about costs and payments was a two-party conversation, as was the conversation that preceded it about the patient's oral health needs and the ways in which the dentist might address them. Dentists and their patients together worked out what the dentist would do for the patient and what it would cost the patient, including payment plans and other ways in which the dentist could help when patients' resources were stretched thin.

Beginning in the 1970s, some employers began including some form of dental insurance in the health insurance benefits package offered to their employees, and over time this became a common pattern. Various government programs then began to appear that included limited coverage for the oral health needs of some groups of participants. The conversation about what the dentist would do for the patient and how much the patient would need to pay for became a three-party conversation, with the third party far away and impersonal. Nevertheless, at least for a while, these "third-party payers" transferred funds collected by employers from the labor of their employees or from taxes paid by the public to dentists (or else to patients to reimburse them). Payments to dentists were made on the basis of "usual and ordinary" charges for each service; in this way, "third-party payers" simply accepted the providers' internal mechanisms for determining their charges to patients. For a while, then, the third-party payers' participation in the dentist-patient conversation was often not very intrusive.

Beginning in the late 1980s, however, health insurance organizations and government health coverage programs increasingly began to pressure health care providers, both institutional and individual, to bring the charges for health care down. They employed a variety of legal, economic, and contractual strategies to achieve this end, and by these means, as this process has continued and in fact increased in intensity in the intervening decades, they have profoundly changed not only the economics but also the social landscape of health care in American society. The principal impact of these changes on oral health care has been a transformation of the dentist-patient conversation about what the dentist will provide and what the patient must pay. More and more dental care is chosen in conformity with terms set by third-party payer organizations committed to pressuring providers to keep costs down.

In addition, this industry—the "managed care" industry—has come to be made up of many different kinds of organizations, not only insurers but also a wide range of support industries whose research and advice significantly affect how the third-party payers manage their businesses. It doesn't matter much whether the third-party payer is a not-for-profit or a for-profit business or whether it is a government agency or a private organization. Each has its own systems and priorities and its own bureaucracy and rules, and all the administrative costs that go with them. To complicate matters still further, many government programs are actually run by—that is, "outsourced to"—private, for-profit or not-for-profit organizations with these organizations' own systems, rules, and bureaucracies. This process, and its additional costs, has transferred the management of the fiscal side of oral health care to bureaucracies that are increasingly distant from the patient who needs the care. More important than this, the policies of these distant bureaucracies also have a significant effect on the treatments that patients actually receive. Their cost-limiting policies—especially policies that will cover the costs of only the least expensive treatments within the standard of care for a presenting condition—have the effect of limiting the kinds of care that patients actually choose, for choosing any other treatment recommended by the dentist for their condition will mean having to pay "out of pocket" to receive it.

In addition to the financial burden of such "out of pocket" payments for many patients, such payments seem to patients to be excessive because they have already paid out money (directly or indirectly, for example, by accepting a benefits package rather than higher salaries) to have dental care coverage in the first place or because, if their dental coverage is part of an entitlement program, they believe they are justly entitled to the dental care they need. For many patients, having to pay out of pocket to receive the treatments that their dentists recommend rather than those the insurers will pay for feels like a form of financial coercion and a violation of their autonomy.

Of course, patients have always brought their financial constraints to their conversations with dentists. It therefore might be argued that the insertion of the third-party payer into the dentist-patient conversation was not essentially anything new. Moreover, it might be argued that the patient has freely chosen the particular insurance contract that he or she brings to the dental office, including its limits on coverage, and the limitations are all in the contract the patient receives. As for the limits built into government oral health programs, they are all matters of public record. Patients who do not understand these limits, the argument goes, have no sound basis for complaints. If they want better coverage, they should do their homework, find better coverage, and pay for it.

In practice, of course, the contracts and policies that limit coverage of dental care are written by and for lawyers and health care administrators, not patients. Unfortunately, it is typically left to the dentist and the dentist's staff to try to translate these policies and identify their implications for their patients. But this again means that the one-on-one relationship between dentist and patient that aims at their collaborating in judging and choosing what ought to be done is not only interfered with but also significantly controlled by the distant third party. The significant costs of all this for the dental office—what it takes to handle the complexity and unpredictability of the processes that determine patients' eligibility: frequent, unilaterally initiated changes in patients' policies; time limits; coinsurance requirements; inadequate or misleading forms; and so forth—are not just financial. There are also significant costs to relationships with patients for both dentists and office staff, and patients experience their contact with the dental office to be more impersonal as a result.

The dentist's professional commitment to the Central Practice Values of the patient's Oral Health and the patient's Life and General Health require the dentist to do what is needed to care for the patient. So, in addition, it frequently falls to the dentist or the dentist's staff members to intercede with the insurer as the patient's advocate and attempt to persuade the insurer's staff members—who must follow the rules and limits established by the actuarial teams—that the proposed treatment is indeed the cheapest acceptable intervention. In any society as dependent on third-party payment systems as ours is, every dentist is surely required to employ some amount of time and energy to advocate in this way for treatment the dentist judges the patient genuinely needs. But the extent of this obligation and the dentist's practical ability to carry it out is limited by the dentist's similar obligation to every other patient he or she serves. Dental professionals are constantly rationing time and energy among their patients: those in operatories and those in waiting rooms, those presently on the telephone and those waiting to receive a call. The emergence of third-party payers, however, has multiplied the time and energy a dentist needs to expend in order to deal with them and has required dentists to develop an additional set of skills unrelated to providing competent care in order to provide aggressive advocacy on behalf of their patients to the bureaucracies of third-party payers.

Moreover, the dentist-patient relationship as well as patient trust in the dentist can be affected adversely in another way if the dentist's best professional judgment is rejected by a distant, nameless dentist or nondentist aid who has not seen the patient. Many patients find it difficult to understand how fully qualified dentists can disagree about what is the best treatment in a given case without either of them being mistaken; nor is it easy to express in any readable formula that, in dentistry, the standard of care often includes a range of treatments for each particular case and matter at hand, not only the very best or ideal one.

Moreover, whenever the third-party payer, speaking through its oral health professional, appears to give higher priority to cost over better care, patients can easily question whether their Oral and General Health really are the guiding values of the dental profession. In addition, explaining such things to patients is especially difficult in societies like ours where a large segment of the public believes that the only adequate treatment is the one best treatment and no other. Moreover, some third-party payers are for-profit corporations and may well be limiting covered treatments to the least expensive precisely for the sake of market success for the corporation rather than, as for government programs and some not-for-profits, from a conscientious effort to ration limited resources equitably across a whole population of oral health patients. In other words, with some insurers, the patient may be quite correct to see the limitation of treatments as an intrusion of marketplace values into the dentist-patient relationship that ought to be focused primarily on the patient's Oral and General Health.

An even subtler form of intrusion occurs when a practice signs a contract with a corporation to allow them to audit all patient charts within their practice, not simply to assure accurate record keeping and claims reporting but to compare fees accepted by the practice from other third-party contracts. If evidence shows that one third-party is paying more than another, that party can invoke favorite nation clauses in their contracts to recover funds from the practice, thus placing an additional unexpected financial burden on a practice and all patients within the practice that are not insured by the insurance company that benefits from this maneuver.

Finally, the fact that the treatment covered by the third-party payer frequently is not the treatment that the dentist—who is actually dealing with the patient—judges to be the best treatment for the patient's presenting condition is viewed by many dental professionals as unethical in itself. For all these reasons, this insertion of a distant third party—or at least the actual ways in which third-party payers currently do impact dental care—into what once was and ideally ought to remain a two-party relationship between dentist and patient is viewed by many dentists and patients as a severe and ethically questionable intrusion into the dentist-patient relationship. Despite the hope that progress, technology, patience, common sense, and a shared commitment to respond to patients' oral health needs will eventually resolve these intrusions, the continuing experience of most dentists is that no clear resolution and no reassertion of the primacy of the dentist-patient relationship in oral health care is in sight.

MORAL DISTRESS

A sizable body of literature has recently emerged about what is called "moral distress" on the part of health professionals. A health professional is said to experience moral distress when he or she (1) believes that a certain course of action is the ethically correct action to be taken in a given situation but (2) is prevented in some way from following that course of action or must in fact do otherwise or cooperate in doing otherwise (3) due to external constraints so that (4) the person experiences this not acting or acting otherwise than his or her values direct as an undermining of personal integrity, a weakening or even a violation of important personal and ethical commitments.

There are a variety of "external constraints" that dentists encounter that can produce moral distress, especially about providing the best dental care they can to a patient. Dentists encounter many patients who choose a treatment that is within the standard of care but is not, in the dentist's best judgment, what will be most effective for the patient's oral health. In such situations a dentist may be saddened at the choice or simply resigned because the patient has exercised his or her autonomy and the dentist has made their relationship as interactive a relationship as possible under the circumstances. But sometimes a dentist may respond to such a situation, perhaps at the end of the day rather than in the rush from patient to patient and operatory to operatory, by feeling that the patient's choice really was the wrong choice for the patient and that this dentist-patient encounter therefore did not stand up to the dentist's own professional standards.

In this chapter's scenario the dentist was not responsible for the patient's choosing something else but rather the dentist's best efforts at respectful education did not yield the choice that the dentist thought best for the patient. The negative feelings about what happens in such a situation are an example of moral distress, for what happened was beyond the dentist's power to change but nevertheless was at odds with the dentist's goals as a professional. Note that the negative feelings being discussed here should not be identified with feelings of guilt, for the dentist was not responsible for what the patient chose and did not fall short in efforts to educate the patient to the best choice. This is why the phrase "*external* constraints" is so important in the description of moral distress.

Another kind of chairside example of moral distress for dentists are the situations in which parents choose treatments for their children that are not genuinely harmful because they are within the standard of care but that the dentist knows are not the best for the child. Here the word "external" seems even more appropriate because the choice of the less desirable treatment is not being made by the patient but by others who have superior power in the situation.

The reason for discussing the topic of moral distress in the present chapter, however, is to give a name and an explanation for the sadness that dentists experience when patients do not receive the treatment that would be best for them because their coverage is limited and they accept the least expensive treatment within the standard of care because their financial and social situation prevents them from choosing any other treatment. On the surface such cases may look no different from the patients' unwise choices because, in spite of the dentist's careful education about what is at stake, the patient receives a treatment different from what the dentist judges is clearly best or ideal under the circumstances. But there are two important differences between such situations and the dentist's moral distress in the present case. For there are two ways in which what stands in the way in this situation is not only beyond the dentist's control but arises from factors completely outside the chairside conversation about treatment and cost. In the first place, the patient's financial and social situation is often not only beyond the dentist's control (a discussion of the possibility of "charity care" on the dentist's part will be offered below) but beyond the patient's as well, so that the dentist's professional commitment to enhancing the Central Practice Value of the patient's Autonomy is challenged as well as that of providing the best or ideal Oral Health care for the patient.

But what is frequently still more distressing is that the third-party payer's coverage policies are so often specifically designed to prevent patients from being able to obtain the type of dental care that would be best for them. The distress many dentists experience in dealing with this fact may prompt them to engage in advocacy for change in these social systems (over and above any efforts at advocacy for specific patients). But the second-class status accorded oral health in our society and reflected in our society's funding of oral health care, together with the high administrative costs of many of these programs, have made it even more difficult for the dental profession's efforts at advocacy for their patients to succeed. For many dentists, this last fact about our society prompts a sense of helplessness that can make their moral distress all the more powerful.

There is one good thing about a dentist's experience of moral distress when a patient accepts the least expensive treatment because it is all that a third-party payer will cover: It demonstrates that the dentist's professional commitments and values are still alive and remain active in his or her feelings and responses to such chairside situations. But moral distress also takes a toll on a person, and there are statistics showing the correlation of moral distress and professional burnout in the health professions. Dentists should be sure they have appropriate outlets for their feelings of moral distress so they can balance them with more positive emotions and activities and, ideally, join other caring dentists in constructive actions of social advocacy and provide what professionally guided charity care they can to those in society whom the larger society's health care system and its bureaucracies have left without care.

CHARITY CARE

Of course, the question can be asked—and some patients do ask it of their dentists, friends, or themselves when they know their dentist believes a different treatment would be better for them—why doesn't the dentist just provide the better treatment at no cost or at a reduced cost that the patient can afford? The patient may assume that, since the dentist's regular charges for most procedures seem high to him or her, the dentist must be doing quite well and therefore should be able to give a needed treatment at no charge now and then. Patients typically have no idea what percentage of the gross receipts of a dental office is necessary to pay overhead nor the periodic accounting processes necessary to keep fees fair and equitable within their particular practice but also in accord with insurance comparable-procedure formulas nor how many patients dentists encounter whose oral health care could be improved by "charity care" nor the already significant amount of volunteer care and other charity work most dentists do.

As was indicated in chapter 6, it is the authors' view that, in a society like ours where many people have very little access to dental care, a dental professional who did no charity care and was unwilling to offer payment plans and other flexible financial arrangements for treatment—that is, who accepted no financial sacrifice for the sake of his or her patients' needs—would probably be acting unprofessionally. Only very special obligations to the professional's family or other comparable responsibilities would justify so little sacrifice for the sake of meeting patients' dental needs when there are so many patients who cannot get their dental needs met without such assistance. But this position must be carefully qualified in two ways.

First and most important, the failures of our society's social systems to respond adequately to its citizens' needs for oral health care are not primarily, much less solely, due to failures of the dental profession. It is therefore not only unreasonable—because dentists' personal sacrifices to respond to patients' unmet oral health care needs could not possibly meet so much unmet need in any case—but also unjust to think that these shortfalls should be corrected by the sole efforts of dentists doing charity care. As chapter 11 has explained, what are needed are social systems specifically designed and funded to meet this need as their goal. But such systems would need to be very carefully designed so as to be compatible with the professional commitments of the dental profession and at the same time integrated into our society's fiscal landscape in which administered markets and corporate capitalism are frequently at odds.

Second, as was explained in chapter 6, our society clearly does not presume that a dental professional must make extreme financial sacrifices to fulfill his or her obligation to respond to unmet oral health needs. A dental professional in our society is not obligated to ask his or her family, for example, to live in poverty in order to meet more patients' unmet dental needs. Of course, a dental professional's family might choose to make additional sacrifices in order to provide more needy people with treatment. But such actions would be a matter of choice and above and beyond the dentist's professional duty. A dentist who provides charity care on the basis of carefully determining how much financial sacrifice his or her practice can reasonably afford over the course of a year or a quarter, as was suggested in the final section of chapter 6, is almost certainly living up to his or her commitments as a professional.

Thus, though it is a source of painful moral distress for many dentists to observe so much unmet need for dental care in our society, the authors propose that the current content of the dialogue between the dental profession and the larger community in the United States does not indicate an ethical obligation on the part of dentists to try to single-handedly eliminate this need. These needs can be met only through significant changes in the systems by which health care resources are allocated in our society and a change in the society's health value system so that a higher priority is placed on oral health and oral health care than is presently the case. As already indicated, dentists can also fulfill their professional obligations to attend to unmet oral health needs through collective advocacy for such changes. The topic of collective advocacy for change will be examined more fully in chapter 14.

ADEQUATE TREATMENT VS. THE BEST TREATMENT

The discussion in the previous sections has been dependent on the meaningfulness of an important concept that is widely used and understood by providers of dental care but less often employed by members of the other health professions and rarely given careful consideration by most members of the public in American society. It is the concept of *adequate treatment*. Three or four generations of US health care professionals today have been trained to view their obligation to each patient to be that of providing that patient with the best possible care. Most health care institutions articulate their missions and describe themselves to the public in similar terms and often use this language to articulate organizational decisions, whether consistently or not. (Can you imagine a hospital system advertising itself as providing "perfectly adequate health care?") In addition, many segments of the public in the United States, especially the most vocal and powerful, have similarly come to expect that, when they or their family members are patients, "the best" is what health care professionals are committed to providing. This conception of health care practice is so dominant among health professions other than dentistry that when the diagnostic process has not yet identified the single best course of treatment for the patient that process is ordinarily considered incomplete.

Within dentistry, however, many presenting conditions allow for a number of clinically acceptable treatment interventions. All of these are considered *adequate* modes of treatment, with some of them preferable from the point of view of considerations such as durability, aesthetics, ease of treatment for the patient, cost to the patient, or the employment of more sophisticated dental skills or more complex technologies, and others less so.

But those that are thought less preferable for these reasons can still be good enough from the point of view of therapeutic benefit and reasonable outcome.

The ethical dentist explains all the available treatments to the patient, including the benefits and deficits of each, and makes a recommendation to the patient about the best treatment for his or her condition, given the patient's other priorities, financial means, and the like. But the ethical dentist does not tell the patient that the other treatments within the standard of care are defective from the point of view of the patient's oral health at the time of treatment. In other words, within dentistry, treatment that is adequate from the point of view of the patient's current oral health is in fact *adequate*, even if some of the available treatments might be superior in one way or another.

Even though this is true, most dental professionals have been trained for the past three or four generations to recommend that patients accept the best treatment available, so much so that more than a few of them consider it professionally inappropriate to provide an adequate but less-than-best treatment when this is the treatment a patient intends to choose. That is, some dentists have adopted a philosophy of practice, as considered in the discussion of Dentists' Preferred Patterns of Practice in chapter 5, that they provide only the best treatments to patients and refer patients who intend to choose an adequate but less-than-best treatment to other dentists. But even though some dentists practice in this way, the concept of *adequate treatment* has endured as a meaningful and valuable concept in the description of what dental care can offer.

As has been mentioned, one of the consequences of the rise of third-party payers within American health care has been a narrowing of covered health care options for many patients—usually on the basis of cost to the insurer—not only dental patients but for patients throughout the American health care system. In addition, for some forms of treatment, health care providers have to consult with case managers within insurance programs or corporate benefits programs to get permission to provide such treatments for covered patients, and these case managers must often inform the caregiver that the recommended treatment is not covered by the patient's insurance because the policy covers only the least expensive appropriate treatment. What is happening here is that the concept of adequate treatment is gradually being operationalized within American health care generally in the way that it has been operationalized within oral health care for years. Not surprisingly, however, because the concept of adequate treatment has had little use and has therefore developed little operational meaning outside dentistry, many physicians, nurses, and other health professionals, and many patients and their family members as well, interpret such decisions by case managers as decisions to refuse professionally acceptable care altogether. In response to these circumstances, health professionals may claim insurers are requiring them to practice unprofessionally, and many members of the public object in similar terms.

But if adequate care is indeed *adequate* for the patient's health needs in the situation, then there is nothing unethical or unprofessional in providing it, provided the patient has been properly and interactively informed and is choosing his or her care accordingly. Similarly, as long as third-party payers' bureaucracies are supporting truly *adequate* treatments for patients' needs, they cannot be properly accused of trying to force health care professionals to practice unethically. Of course, since long-standing habits of practice are being challenged in this, the feelings on the part of health professionals that unethical practice is being required of them may be understandable. But their feelings that they are being asked to practice unethically, except in situations in which a managed care organization refuses to provide genuinely adequate care, are in fact inaccurate.

Dental professionals who are experiencing such feelings should look at the whole situation from an ethical point of view much more carefully. A dentist needs to think carefully about the importance of greater durability, aesthetics, ease of treatment for the patient, and so on in relation to this particular patient's oral health at this time. He or she then needs to consider if another treatment within the standard of care is so inadequate that the dentist would truly be acting unprofessionally to provide it—that is, would be genuinely harming the patient rather than serving the patient from the point of view of the Central Practice Values of the patient's Oral and General Health. This may require a dentist to do a self-assessment to determine whether his or her emphasis on "better" treatments over "merely adequate" treatments is genuinely grounded in actually doing more good for patients rather than in a misguided effort to maintain, for example, an image of having a better practice than his or her competitors. These are subtle distinctions, but patients' trust depends on dentists continually demonstrating that their commitment to their patients' well-being outweighs their commitment to the success of a business. This means being straightforward with their patients—which will often mean educating them on this point—that in many situations what is considered an *adequate* treatment according to the standard of care is actually adequate.

THE ORAL HEALTH SAFETY NET

Beginning in the late 1990s, some government programs aimed at providing an oral health safety net began to appear, first for children and more recently for adults with lower incomes. These programs, their regulations and bureaucratic structures, and the extent to which they offer access for various dental care services vary from state to state. Typically, where such programs exist, practicing dentists have the option of accepting patients who are enrolled in these programs into their practices or not, and their doing so is frequently made in terms of their practice's ability to absorb lower reimbursements for care given, for most of the payments provided in such programs are significantly less than the practice's standard charges for the same services (even though providing the services requires the same amount of expenditure on staff and overhead).

In addition to varying from state to state and paying lower reimbursements for care given, many state programs are extremely complicated for both patients and providers to navigate, making the burden on participating dentists even greater and weakening the ability of such programs to address the problem of providing enough access to oral health care. This problem is further exacerbated in areas of the country that have fewer dentists. In such areas, people whose dental care is covered under such a program may not be able to find a dentist willing to accept them as patients within fifty, one hundred, or even more miles from their homes.

In fact, many dentists all over the country do not accept patients from these programs. These dentists may still, of course, be fulfilling their professional obligation to respond to people's unmet needs for oral health care through other forms of charity care or energetic collective advocacy for a better oral health safety net for our society. Obviously, though, one way a dentist can fulfill this professional obligation would be to accept patients from these programs. If all dentists did this collectively and collaboratively, it would seem the burden would be spread across many hands and made lighter. Setting up such systems organizationally and systematically among dentists, however, risks violation of Federal Trade Commission regulations designed to avoid restraints of trade and maintain competition. As was mentioned above, however, it is not unethical for a dentist to carefully determine reasonable limits to the financial burden that participating in such programs ordinarily requires, provided these decisions are made in good faith.

In some areas of the country, dentists have responded to the gaps in the oral health safety net by establishing special clinics for patients participating in these programs and/ or for patients who have no form of insurance or government coverage. If such clinics are readily accessible to the people who need care; are well staffed; provide competent, timely, and consistent dental care; and work as hard at establishing Interactive Relationships with their patients as the dentists who volunteer or are employed at them would provide in their own offices, they can be a valuable way to respond to people's unmet oral health needs. This can be particularly true if they are located in areas where traditional dental offices are in short supply, they are convenient to public transportation, have hours of operation helpful to low-income workers, and so on. As mentioned in chapter 6, some dentists travel to work in clinics for the underserved in the third world.

But two important cautions are in order regarding such clinics. The first is that the reimbursement rates for such clinics from public oral health programs in the United States and financial support for charitable third world dental clinics are, in both cases, often insufficient to adequately support a professionally appropriate operation. This is especially true with regard to continuity of care and follow-up care for major dental work. In addition, volunteer dentists, who practice only occasionally outside their habitual and familiar office equipment, staff, and computer systems, often unavoidably practice more on the level of a novice than an experienced expert in such settings. Therefore, this way of addressing patients' unmet oral health needs, at home or abroad, not only requires significant fiscal sacrifice on the part of the dentists and/or community volunteers who support it but also requires extra vigilance by the dentists to make sure that their donated professional services do not in some way actually harm their patients or, especially in third world settings, affect the base clinic staff so they practice less effectively or reduce these clinics' ability to operate in professionally appropriate ways.

In such clinics in the United States, many patients end up having long waiting periods, so the goal of timely care, for example, is not reached. In a similar way, it is important that follow-up care, long-term plans of care for patients with multiple needs, and consistency of providers not become lesser priorities than they would be in a traditional office because of inadequate fiscal and human resources. In some instances, in fact, local or outside corporate agents have established clinics in communities that have inadequate access to care (or by claiming, through false or misleading data, that an access to care issue exists when adequate care is already being provided by established practices in the area) primarily for their own corporate "good citizen" marketing purposes, for long-range real estate business purposes, or for other strategic planning purposes rather than for better oral health care, with less-than-professional oral health care as the typical result.

The second caution is subtler but deserves to be noted. For it is possible for a dentist to be willing to support a clinic for underserved or low-income patients rather than accept patients on public aid programs into his or her practice in order, to state it bluntly, to keep such patients out of the dentist's operatories and waiting room. In the case that opened this chapter, Mrs. Nelson mentioned that she was directed to such a clinic "for people like me." The establishment of clinics located where such populations live may significantly enhance the provision of professionally appropriate oral health care for patients on government programs or patients who are underserved or impoverished. But from the perspective of the dental profession's Chief Client—that is, the persons whom dentistry is committed to serving and whom dentistry is chiefly authorized by society to assist—people on government programs or people who are impoverished are no different from people with greater financial resources that need dental care; they, too, are members of our society who have oral health needs. Therefore, great caution is ethically required so that such persons, if they appear in one's office in need of dental care, not be led to believe that "people like them" do not belong there. Obviously the same issues need to be addressed if a dentist "dumps" patients with inadequate or no dental insurance or patients whom the dentist finds distasteful, no matter where the dentist sends them when refusing to treat them.

Most dentists and other members of the oral health community accept as accurate the proposal offered in chapter 11 that our society's policy makers and large segments of the public severely undervalue unmet oral health needs. This is a many years' long pattern of undervaluing oral health care—in spite of the impact of unmet oral health needs on people's personal lives, on their ability to function effectively and productively in the society's institutions, and on their health in general. This is surely an important reason why our society's "oral health safety net" leaves so much of our society's oral health needs unmet. As the authors have said a number of times in this book, dental professionals may not ethically view unmet oral health needs with indifference, and they are obligated to make efforts to respond to them. But they are not the principal parties responsible for so many oral health needs going unmet in our society. Furthermore, society's and the dental profession's attempts to address these complex needs with increased marketing and less costly technologies and technicians but still-insufficient fiscal programs seems to be more and more counterproductive. What is needed instead is a change in society's understanding of the importance of oral health and a corresponding change in how the society's health care resources are managed and distributed.

UNIVERSAL ACCEPTANCE

Although it is easily overlooked, it is also important to note that there is already an initial relationship between a dentist and a person who needs dental care before the person becomes the dentist's patient. Because of this initial relationship, when such a person contacts a dentist for the first time the dentist cannot ethically say, in effect, "You have no business being here." For, by accepting his or her professional role, the dentist announces to the public that he or she is someone on whom they can depend for oral health care. This does not mean that dentists must provide complete diagnoses and treatments to everyone who seeks their services, thus making them patients of record. But it does mean that a dentist who turns a deaf ear to someone who contacts him or her for oral health care is failing to respond professionally to the person in a way that is often overlooked and rarely discussed in the dental ethics literature.

Authors who have written about this initial relationship to persons seeking oral health care have described two of its important characteristics under the notion of Universal Patient Acceptance. One concerns what the ethical dentist owes the person who makes an initial contact in search of dental care. The other concerns the trust relationship that is implied in this initial contact, a trust relationship that a dentist who turns a deaf ear to this person violates and who at the same time sends a message about dentistry as a profession that contradicts the reasons for patients to trust a dentist and dentistry in the first place.

What does the ethical dentist owe a person who makes an initial contact in search of dental care? The short answer is this: First, listen to him or her, and then tell how he or she might access the care he or she needs. To do this, the dentist, or often the dentist's receptionist and other representatives, will need to talk with the person, which typically includes asking the person what he or she is experiencing or what he or she thinks he or she needs that leads the person to believe he or she needs to see a dentist. This information will ordinarily confirm that the person does indeed need to see a dentist, and the next step is to inform the person how he or she might get the care that's needed. But there are many forms that this information might take. Fulfilling one's professional obligations in this initial relationship does not necessarily imply that the dentist must receive the person as a patient into his or her own practice. It does mean that that dentist represents, in person, the profession as a whole to that particular potential patient.

If the dentist or a trained representative judges that the person is in need of emergency dental care, there may be an obligation to provide emergency care in the dentist's own office right away; but such is not always the case, and telling the person how to get the emergency care they need will fulfill the requirements of this initial relationship. (The thoughtful dentist will make sure in advance that his staff have ready access to accurate information to provide to such persons whenever he or she is not going to treat them as patients in his or her own practice.)

Of course, once the dentist is talking to the person, if the dentist chooses not to invite that person to be treated in his or her office and become a patient in his or her practice, it will be hard to say this without offering an explanation, and obviously the ethical dentist will give an explanation that is truthful. It may be the case that the dentist has a full appointment book (except for emergency care) for the foreseeable future. It may be that the practice has already expended its budgeted allotment of charity care for this quarter or year (and that allotment has been calculated to be as generous as the practice can reasonably support). It may be that the office is currently short-staffed and overwhelmed with care of their appointed patients. These are practical time-management considerations, and there are a number of other ethically supportable reasons why a dentist could in good professional conscience refrain from inviting someone needing dental care to receive it at his or her office, either then and there or in an appropriate time frame based on the patient's wants and needs.

There is no denying that explaining such a decision may feel awkward, even though it is true and based on careful judgments about the dentist's and staff's and practice's capacity to assist. It is also very possible that, even with every effort at transparency on the part of the dentist, the person in need of care will still wonder if the explanation is true rather than just an excuse for getting rid of him or her. But not offering any explanation is not likely to be a better choice in this regard since all professional relationships should be open to dialogue. It is only in dialogue that the person needing dental care can find it and only in dialogue that the professional experiences, learns, and grows in professionalism.

But even though it may be awkward, such "acceptance" of a person seeking dental care—that is, talking to that person to determine his or her reasons for thinking dental care is needed, affirming that person as deserving of dental care, and assisting him or her in finding the needed dental care—is clearly ethically superior to communicating to the person that, even though he or she believes he or she has a genuine need for dental care, he or she does not belong in a dentist's office.

The authors who write about this initial relationship call the ethical dentist's response "Universal Acceptance." The word "acceptance" here refers to the dentist *accepting to talk* with the person seeking dental care. The dentist does not decline to talk to the person, does not treat the person as someone who has no business seeking to contact a dentist. To do so would obviously be to disrespect the person, who is seeking care because he or she has had experiences, most often pain, that lead them to believe they need it. By accepting to talk to the person and providing information about how to get his or her needs addressed in a timely and assured manner, the dentist affirms the person's worth as a person and the importance of his or her health; the dentist expresses sympathy (implicitly if not explicitly) for his or her pain or other symptoms and supports (rather than undermines) the person's belief that, in our society, it is dentists who are committed to caring for people's oral health needs.

The word "universal" stresses the ethical reality that, by accepting his or her role as an oral health professional, a dentist says to *everyone* in the society, "I and my profession are here to help you whenever you need dental care." For good reasons, our society and dentistry's professional ethics permit dentists to determine to whom they will provide treatment as patients of record in their practices. But *anyone* who contacts a dentist in search of dental care is one of dentistry's Chief Clients and is owed help in accessing the needed care. The dental professional has an ethical requirement to provide the *acceptance* that consists in talking with such persons and to provide them the information they need in order to obtain care, and since this applies to all such persons, this requirement clearly must be considered *universal*.

The second aspect of this initial relationship is its connection with patients' trust of dentists. Consider an example from outside dentistry first. Suppose you are about to enter a store even though you know it is near closing time. But no "closed" sign is evident, the lights are on, and the door is unlocked, so you enter. A salesperson sees you entering and says in a sharp tone, "We're closed." You would not have entered the store if it was closed, and you appropriately relied on the shopkeeper to provide the usual signs to indicate whether the store was open or closed. But this shopkeeper failed to provide them, which is why many salespeople would in fact say, "I'm sorry, we're closed." For they recognize (though probably not very reflectively) that, in accepting the role of shopkeeper, they have entered into a relationship with those who seek their services. Namely, potential customers trust shopkeepers to provide potential customers with reliable open and closed messages.

That is, the daily functioning of a society depends on people in social roles understanding what it means to be relied on by everyone else in hundreds of ways, small and large, and the importance of acting accordingly. What is often overlooked, until someone who is being relied on in this particular universal way falls short, is that the rest of us not only expect and depend on such a person's (including our own) reliability but that a kind of trust relationship is violated by such shortfalls. The trust component that is violated in these shortfalls is not only what was called Trust That in chapter 2—that is, our being able to correctly predict that such-and-such a thing would happen (e.g., the store would in fact still be open)—but the trust that is violated in such shortfalls is what chapter 2 called Trusting the Person, for some component of our well-being is at stake in such situations. Sometimes it is a very minor component (e.g., fulfilling the hope of buying something you want at the shop), but often it is a component considered genuinely significant, like getting help from an expert source about how to deal with the pain in one's mouth or many other oral conditions that require expert assistance. The Trusting the Person that a patient invests in a dentist who is actually diagnosing and treating the patient's pain is almost certainly going to be more personal than the Trusting the Person involved in the initial relationship when the person needing dental care first contacts a dentist. But the dentist who fails to provide acceptance in an initial relationship is nonetheless violating a Trusting the Person relationship. Moreover, since the person's health and pain are involved, and especially since the dentist has made a professional commitment to care for the oral health needs of the society's citizens, the violation of this Trusting the Person relationship is clearly of far more ethical importance than the shopkeeper's failure to post a "closed" sign.

It is also important to mention that the Trusting the Person relationship in the initial relationship is almost always a trust in the dental profession as a group rather than in the particular dentist contacted as an individual. Thus, the loss of patient trust when a dentist fails to provide acceptance in the initial relationship is a loss of trust in the dental profession as a whole. This is especially true if it is clear to the person that he or she is being sent away because he or she is in a government-run oral health program or are impoverished (i.e., "people like us," as Mrs. Nelson put it in the chapter's opening case). For them the message is that commercial success or bureaucratic regulations can outweigh dentistry's commitment to assist whoever in the society needs dental care in finding out how to obtain it.

THINKING ABOUT THE CASE

Some of the most difficult moral questions that human beings face concern how they ought to act when they conclude that the social institution(s) that form the context of their actions are ethically inadequate in themselves. This is the situation for many dentists in the United States today, and the authors share this view, as was explained in chapter 11. So, when we ask what Dr. Witten ought to do about Mrs. Nelson's situation in this chapter's introductory case, one of the key issues to consider is whether he is obligated to make up, out of his own resources, for the ethical deficiencies of the US health care distribution system by providing charity care for Mrs. Nelson.

Chapter 6 proposed that dentists are professionally committed to accepting some measure of sacrifice for the sake of their patients' well-being; unmet oral health needs, especially intense oral pain, certainly qualify. These sacrifices include some measure of charity care and other sacrifices to assist patients whom the US health care distribution system would otherwise leave without adequate dental care. But the discussion in chapter 6 also stressed that there are limits to this obligation.

Little long-term good would be done if a dentist's efforts to care for those the system has forgotten brought dentists' practices to financial ruin. In addition, we proposed, the current state of the dialogue between dentists and the larger community seems to indicate that these sacrifices need not be so great that a dentist is obligated to risk the fairly good standard of living that dentists in comparable practices typically enjoy in this society. Sacrifices within these limits, then, are what dentists seem professionally obligated to undertake in response to the deficiencies of the US health care distribution system. Requiring any sacrifices beyond this would be asking them to go beyond their professional duty.

On this basis, Dr. Witten is obligated to accept some financial sacrifices for the sake of his patients who would otherwise receive no dental care or less-than-adequate dental care because of their limited financial means. But there are many ways in which Dr. Witten can make this sacrifice.

One possibility would be for him to spread the sacrifice over his whole clientele by charging lower prices to all patients across the board. But this would be a less desirable way of using his sacrifice for patients left out by the distribution system, since many of a dentist's patients will be able to handle ordinary prices and the lower prices may still be unreasonable for some of the highly disadvantaged patients. In fact, given the distribution system currently accepted for dental care in the United States, Dr. Witten may ethically set his prices according to how they are characteristically set in such a free market exchange system; namely, he may aim to maximize his income, within the competitive marketplace, up to the level that the market will bear. But, in terms of responding to unmet dental needs among his patients, it would seem far better for Dr. Witten to reserve his sacrifices for those patients who cannot otherwise obtain adequate care than to adjust his pricing structure for all his patients in some way.

Of course, the injustice of the surrounding social institution does not excuse, much less justify, further individual injustices. Dr. Witten may not price gouge, or charge more for his services than they are worth by taking advantage of patients' ignorance of the relative value of services and the current market price structure. Such conduct is a violation of justice and trust in the relationship between seller and purchaser. But even before that, it would already have violated the dentist's professional obligations to strive for an Interactive Relationship and even the minimal obligation of informed consent, as well as respect for patients' Autonomy.

Dr. Witten could make his sacrifices in the form of free care for some patients and payment plans for others, as was described in the case in chapter 6. Or he could make them by providing treatment to patients like Mrs. Nelson, who participate in public aid programs, where payment is usually well below ordinary charges and is often long delayed as well. Or he could make his sacrifices by establishing a relationship with a nursing home, a facility for the developmentally disabled, or an orphanage or other child care facility, where the reimbursement level will probably be below standard and where a significant amount of the sacrifice will be in the form of the extra effort needed to provide care, and caring attention, to patients with special needs and deficits.

Should Dr. Witten do any of these things specifically for Mrs. Nelson in her moment of dental need? Or should he direct his professional sacrifice in some other way? Part of the answer to this question depends on what other forms of sacrifice for unmet dental needs Dr. Witten has already committed to, something that the case as presented does not discuss. Another part of the answer depends on the precise nature of Mrs. Nelson's need for dental care. Will a functional three-surface amalgam or silver diamine fluoride (SDF) coating be an instance of adequate or even minimally adequate care? Or would both be inadequate and a crown be the only adequate response to her need? There are many cases in which this is not an easy question to answer.

Suppose Mrs. Nelson's large cavity was on the buccal surface of #6 and not sensitive, rather than on the mesial of #30. The attractiveness of someone's smile is not essential to his or her General Health, but it may well have a significant impact on his or her psychological well-being and social effectiveness. If #6 were involved, Dr. Witten would rightly be weighing other treatments besides those mentioned in the case as presented.

Dr. Witten does not offer to provide the treatment he recommends (the trial filling or SDF coating for #30) at no charge, but he does offer Mrs. Nelson a payment plan for the service. Clearly, offering a payment plan, with its genuine, if lesser, loss of revenue, would qualify as an instance of the sacrifice for patients with unmet oral health needs that Dr. Witten is professionally obligated to undertake (provided that fair loan practices are maintained). Nevertheless, if he were already meeting his professional obligation to sacrifice in other ways, Dr. Witten could also justifiably decline to assist Mrs. Nelson in this way because there are also limits to the extent of sacrifice that a dentist is professionally committed to accepting. In fact, if he were already meeting his obligation to sacrifice in other ways, Dr. Witten's offer to repair #30 with a payment plan, and therefore accrue some fiscal loss, would be an act above and beyond his duty as a professional.

As it turns out, Mrs. Nelson declines the trial filling. She requests an extraction because, even with the payment plan, she judges the trial filling to be more than she and her husband can afford. Although Dr. Witten believes that the trial filling is a far better treatment for Mrs. Nelson's situation, he accepts her decision to extract the tooth, knowing that this treatment would still be professionally acceptable. Dr. Witten's agreeing to Mrs. Nelson's choice in this matter may seem generous on his part because to do so he needed to set aside his own recommendation to her. But from a professional-ethical point of view, as chapter 5 explained, so long as a patient's choice of treatment is within the standard of care and therefore does not seriously challenge the Central Practice Values of Life and General Health or Oral Health, the dentist is obligated to secure the next-ranked Central Practice Value for the patient, and that is the patient's Autonomy. That is, if he is going to treat Mrs. Nelson at all—rather than direct her elsewhere to try to get her oral health needs addressed in a timely and reliable manner—agreeing to her choice to have #30 extracted is professionally required, even if it seems generous in another way.

In this instance, with regard to the extraction, since Dr. Witten does offer to do it under the conditions of her medical card, which will probably mean a shortfall in compensation, this is clearly consistent with his obligation to respond to an unmet oral health need and, if necessary, to make some sacrifices to do so. But at the same time, when Mrs. Nelson notices his disappointment with her choice, Dr. Witten explains that his moral distress is about the safety-net programs that so inadequately respond to our society's unmet oral health needs. He knows that an extraction is within the standard of care for her situation, especially if there was going to be proper follow-up to the extraction (i.e., until the space was ideally filled with a prosthesis or an implant) and Mrs. Nelson's other cavities and overall oral health were being adequately cared for. But he also knows that these things will not be happening for some time to come, probably not before she graduates and she and her husband find jobs. He knows that dentists' sacrifices cannot possibly meet such great needs within our society (even by triaging and staging patients within these different levels of care), and he knows that the oral health community's advocacy for better oral health safety nets have so far produced only the first steps of what is needed. He also knows that our society is intensely focused on other aspects of health and health care, rather than giving oral health its due, in spite of the intimate connections between them.

To Dr. Witten's credit, it needs to be pointed out that he met and talked with Mrs. Nelson at a point when all he knew was that she was having oral pain. In other words, he clearly "accepted" her and undertook to help her meet her oral health needs and continued to do so after he knew she had said she only had a medical card for payment. Universal Acceptance does not require a dentist to offer treatment to the person seeking dental care. Perhaps Dr. Witten offered to treat her and did so in part because he knew she had tried unsuccessfully to get treatment a number of times before. Perhaps he knew that referring her to a clinic contracted to treat patients with her medical card would delay Mrs. Nelson's care for months because of the clinic's long waiting list or decision not to schedule adults needing extractions. Perhaps he knew that, if he referred her to another dentist, he would be burdening a colleague who was not a contract provider for her medical card or else a dentist who would also not be paid for more than an extraction, and not fully for that, and thus he would simply be sending Mrs. Nelson back into the same situation again. But the fact that he met with her, talked with her, and affirmed that she had every reason to be seeking a dentist's help and to trust dentists to take her need seriously means that he *accepted* her in the sense explained above. This was already an important professional step that every dentist and dental practice should consider imitating (by the efforts of the dentist personally or of staff and other representatives of the practice).

If every dentist grew more adept at practicing Universal Acceptance in this way, many more hands would be making for lighter work, and some of the factors behind the unmet dental needs of our society might be more openly addressed. But it remains the case that important changes in our society's health care system are clearly needed to adequately respond to oral disease in our society.

Finally, there is the unfortunate message that all of this sends the larger society. As noted in chapter 11, unmet oral health needs not only involve pain and discomfort but lost hours of work, school, and other daily activities. They interrupt people's lives and sometimes do so in very severe ways, and they are invariably experienced as a loss of control of one's body and a person's ability to manage his or her own life. Some unmet oral health needs are clearly basic needs in the sense explained in chapter 11, and all unmet oral health needs negatively impact the lives of those who experience them. But in the United States, people's ability to address these needs depends primarily on their ability to either pay for care or pay for (the often uncertain value of) dental insurance. That is, our society has chosen and continues to choose to count on the marketplace to distribute most of its oral health care resources.

It is hardly surprising, then, that there seem to be two competing messages about oral health care in US society. One of these is the message that oral health care is the work of an expert and dedicated professional community, the dental profession, which is committed not only to providing competent oral health care and practicing according to established ethical standards but to earning the trust of patients by giving genuine priority to their well-being. The other message is that oral health care is viewed by our society to be a commodity just like any other commodity in the marketplace and that it is to be distributed primarily through the commercial mechanisms of the marketplace, mechanisms driven first and foremost by the competitive self-interests of the participants.

In such a setting, dentists and dental organizations and the dental profession as a whole have to work all the harder to communicate their message and assure the larger society that they have not lost sight of their distinctive calling. However, certain aspects of actual dental practice in our society combine patient-centered dentistry with some of the characteristics of the commercial marketplace. Unless these are carefully monitored from the perspective of dental ethics and professionalism, dentistry's ability to make sure its professional message is reaching the larger society may be seriously compromised. Chapter 13 will examine this challenge to dentistry's commitments in detail.

⬡⬡⬡⬡⬡⬡⬡

The Wrong Message
and Why It Matters

CASE: THE MAGIC OF BOTOX

After Dr. Bob Milford hires Dr. Sandra Ballman to join his office (see the case in chapter 10), the Ridgeview practice grows even faster. Milford is now deluged with requests from dental business consultants who wanted to meet with him and help him expand his practice in new ways. Meanwhile, the complaint Drs. Kamamata, O'Brien, and Della Galla sent to the Peer Review Committee of the local dental society had grown more complex, as several other area dentists joined the petition. Milford's aesthetic marketing was drawing patients from their practices and, after their aesthetic work was done, many of the patients stayed to continue their general dentistry there.

Richard "Rich" Paulson, a dental business consultant, manages to get an appointment with Dr. Milford. Paulson's marketing materials are carefully crafted to stress the enhancement of his clients' dental professionalism and the commitment of their practices to patient-centered dentistry as he helps their practices continue to grow. This appeals to Dr. Milford. His interest in growing the practice is being driven, at this point, by the fact that he is spending all his time doing aesthetic work while Dr. Ballman is handling the general dentistry needs of their patients. Dr. Milford realizes he is missing the kinds of relationships with patients that were characteristic of his full general dentistry practice. He is rarely experiencing this anymore as he focuses almost exclusively on satisfying patients' aesthetic goals. What he doesn't know is that Paulson was known within the dental consultant community as Richard "I'll Make You Rich" Paulson.

Mr. Paulson hears Dr. Milford out about his wanting to get back to doing general dentistry again, about probably hiring a third dentist, and about getting Dr. Ballman or a new dentist more training in aesthetic dentistry. Dr. Milford thinks this will be a way to reach his goal. Unfortunately, Dr. Milford's office is too small for this. He is hoping Mr. Paulson can help him sort out the financial challenges related to building an addition or moving to a larger site, as well as the practical financial and professional challenges of interrupting the practice and patient care during such a transition. However, Mr. Paulson isn't actually interested in these things. Mr. Paulson wants to sell Dr. Milford on Paulson's ways to grow profits without making such major disruptions to Dr. Milford's current practice, which is already a success. "You don't need to do all that to grow this practice into an immensely more profitable operation," says Mr. Paulson. "You've already laid the groundwork for that beautifully. You don't want to interrupt what you have here. You want to build on it. And the best way to do that is to start offering Botox treatments along with the aesthetic work you already offer.

"The market for Botox is huge, and you're already in the business of helping your patients look better and feel better about themselves. Botox just adds to that, and the profit margins on it are fantastic! You also won't need to add an operatory or move to a larger building. The operatories you have here will be plenty. All you'll need to do is hire a part-time person licensed to do Botox injections or make it worthwhile for your second dentist to get licensed. You're already paying her for the work she does herself and giving her a bit more when she sends you a patient for cosmetic work. If she were trained in Botox, the profit margins are so large you could give her half and keep half for yourself, and she would still think it was great.

"Or, if you only bring in a part-time dentist because there's too much general dentistry for her to do that and Botox too, then you'll still get, say, half the profit margin and you don't have to pay any benefits to boot. Either way it's a win-win situation for you and your people. And you escape all the hassle and potential lost business of constructing a new building or moving somewhere else. Why would you want to do that again? I understand that you would like to be doing more general dentistry. You spent years perfecting those skills and you want to be using them. But you don't need a construction project to do that. Say you get Dr. Ballman, like you were saying, trained to do aesthetic work too. Well, in the interim you would take a hit because if you pick up the slack in general dentistry while she's doing that, you'd lose the profits from the aesthetic work you're not doing. But if you add Botox to your practice first, then you would break even during her training time, and the big profits would start rolling in as soon as she's back full-time. And, you two would be sharing general and aesthetic work, however you two want to work that out.

"Either way, trust me, Botox is the path you should take to grow this practice's profits. It will only better your reputation for aesthetics, and that's what is bringing in most of your patients. I'm here to help you make that happen."

Dr. Milford has never considered this as a way to grow the practice. Should he buy into Mr. Paulson's proposal or not?

WHERE IS DENTISTRY HEADING?

It is not the case that there is something wrong with running a commercially successful practice; it is, instead, a necessary component of practicing dentistry in our society. But a fiscally successful practice is not the first goal of a dental practice if dentistry and dentists view themselves and want to be viewed and treated by others as professionals. So it is important for every dentist to be asking what kind of message he or she is sending to patients in the chair, to prospective patients in the community, and to the public at large. Is this a message that is first and foremost about professionalism, collaborative decision-making with patients, fully competent care for them, and the other characteristics of ethical dentistry? Or is it a message that mirrors the commercial marketplace's ways of thinking, valuing, and relating? Dental journals, especially the throwaways, are full of notices that could easily be coming from Richard "I'll Make You Rich" Paulson, and many dental meeting sessions have a similar focus.

So where is dentistry heading? Will it still be a profession in a few decades? Will the larger society not be able to see a difference between what happens in dentists' offices and what happens in the commercial marketplace?

Where dentistry is heading in the United States will largely be determined by what kind of messages the larger US society receives about dentistry. As chapter 2 explained, it is the larger society that accords dentists their special professional authority—to make socially determining decisions and to have the last word—about matters of oral health and to be, for the most part, self-regulating. It does this for two reasons. First, the dental profession has been recognized as having *expertise* that enables its members to respond effectively to people's oral health needs and to dependably secure for them the essential components of oral and general health, autonomy in the sense of control over their bodies, and other important values. Second, the profession and its members make and, with very few exceptions, are ordinarily observed to honor a commitment to make the well-being of those they serve their highest priority and the cornerstone of what counts as ethical conduct and professionalism in dental practice. These are the essential characteristics that our society attributes to dentistry as a profession and the characteristics that every dentist is expected to embody and continually grow in in order to be correctly described as a professional.

It is therefore reasonable to assume that, if dentists were no longer thought to have expertise in matters of oral health, if dentists were viewed as ineffective or not dependable in properly addressing people's oral health needs, or if it was concluded that dentists could not be counted on to ordinarily make the well-being of their patients their first priority, then the larger society would understandably withdraw dentists' social authority and status as professionals. It is worth asking, then, if dentists are sending any messages to the larger community that would indicate such things are happening. The Interim Gies Ethics Project Report, published in fall 2016 by the American College of Dentists (ACD), offered significant empirical evidence that dentistry in the United States may well be sending these negative messages to the larger community. This chapter will examine a number of activities that are fairly common in dental practices in the United States that can unfortunately be easily interpreted as sending just such a message, and (along with chapters 14 and 15) it will suggest ways in which the opposite message—that dental expertise and dental ethics and professionalism are alive and well among dentists in the United States—could be made more prominent.

It is important to stress that, if dentists in the United States are frequently sending the wrong message to the larger society (even if they don't realize it), it will not be enough to simply "say" or advertise the correct message more frequently. It will not be enough to merely repeat the profession's commitments and high ideals. What will need to happen, to emphasize the correct message, is for every aspect of dentistry in the United States—every dentist in every practice and every dental organization regardless of its particular focus—to concretely *practice* what they preach. But dentists' and dental organizations' ability to do that will depend on serious efforts on their part (every dentist in every practice and every dental organization) to learn or relearn in concrete detail what dentistry's ethics calls them to do and to be (to which this book hopes to make a contribution) and to actively engage in the kind of continuing—which, to be realistic, means daily—process of self-assessment and self-formation in professionalism that will be described in chapter 15.

But, as the Interim Gies Ethics Project report stresses, self-formation in ethics and professionalism cannot be effectively accomplished in isolation; it requires support and collegial assistance not just *from* other dentists but *with* other dentists. Therefore, the process of making sure that dentistry is sending the right message to the larger community—about its expertise, its relationships to patients, the effectiveness of its responses to their needs, and its commitment to give priority to patients' well-being—must include individual dentists' participation in dental professional groups and organizations. It must also include these organizations engaging in their own self-assessment and professional self-formation *as organizations*. This last theme will be the topic of chapter 14.

But the task of this chapter is to look at some common kinds of activities by which dentists send messages to the larger society that appear to diminish dentists' commitment to the dental profession's ethical standards and that challenge the conviction that it possesses special expertise about oral health.

CONFLICTS OF INTEREST

Many professions' codes of ethics address the issue of *conflicts of interest* with the simple directive that they are to be avoided. But this is not a useful directive because almost every activity that a professional engages in involves interests that can conflict, and the only way to avoid them would be to have never become a professional at all. Every time a dentist—or any other health professional—cares for a patient, for example, he or she is at the same time expending time, attention, and energy that could also be expended on some personal interest of the dentist (or of some other person that the dentist cares about or is responsible for). He or she is also, directly or indirectly, earning a living. Working for an Interactive Relationship with the patient and trying to maximize dentistry's ranked Central Practice Values for the patient does not invariably mean these will coincide with a dentist's other goals in life or other things a dentist values. At the same time, however, and as explained in chapter 6, the ordinary primacy that the ethical dentist gives to the well-being of the patient does not automatically settle every situation in which the patient's interests and the dentist's other interests happen to be at odds. Properly dealing with conflicts of interest often requires, instead, careful comparative weighing of possible harms in the context of an ethically appropriate relationship between the dentist and the person the dentist is serving.

The ethical question about conflicts of interest in dental practice, then, is not simply whether they can be avoided, although some can be avoided without serious harm to the patient, as will be explained. Careful comparative weighing of possible harms to the patient is required because the dentist's interests in the situation may have the potential to interfere with the dentist properly exercising his or her expert judgment about what is harmful/beneficial for the patient. This comparative weighing can be summarized in five questions, which will be explained below.

The conflict of interest situations in dental practice that are the most complex, and that will be the focus here, are those in which there is commercial benefit to the dentist from an arrangement with the patient that either is not directly beneficial to the patient's General or Oral Health or does not involve the dentist's specific expertise in oral health. Many dentists, for example, sell dental goods. These include oral health compounds like dentifrices, fluoride products, sonic or mechanical toothbrushes, and other oral devices. These are products that the patient can purchase outside of a dental office and without a prescription. That is, the patient's access to such products is not dependent on the dentist's expert professional judgment in the same way as is oral diagnosis and treatment. Similar to these are situations in which dentists are selling health care services not directly involving dental care. Examples of these would include weight loss programs, holistic medicine regimes, some smoking cessation programs, or any number of other services. (Some dentists sell cosmetic products not related to patients' oral health—for example, Botox injections. Those situations will be discussed in the next section on aesthetic dentistry.)

These situations are ethically complex because, if the dentist's expertise in oral health is not involved in offering the product (as in the case of a weight loss program, for example), then the dentist-patient relationship in this respect is a commercial relationship rather than a professional one. Or, when the product does have some connection with oral health (as in the case of dentifrices, sonic or mechanical toothbrushes, some smoking cessation programs) the patient cannot tell—unless the dentist specifically discusses it—whether or not the dentist is selling the products simply to make money and, therefore, whether the dentist-patient relationship in this respect is actually a commercial relationship rather than a professional one. For, if the relationship is simply a commercial one, then the patient has no reason to think that the dentist's commitment to give primacy to the patient's well-being is operative. The dentist can very reasonably be thought to be maximizing his or her bottom line and, therefore, to be indifferent to whether the product or service is actually going to benefit the patient by securing dentistry's Central Practice Values for that patient.

In order to determine whether such conflict of interest situations are professionally and ethically acceptable, the dentist should ask—and honestly answer—the following five questions about each such situation:

1. Is there any harm that might result from the dentist's secondary interests, and, if so, how serious is that harm?

2. How likely to occur is the harm identified in question 1?

3. If the dentist chose not to act because of the conflict of interest, what benefits would be lost and what harms would occur and to whom?

4. How likely to occur are the harms and benefits identified in question 3?

5. Which course of action available to the dentist is most likely (taking account of the answers to questions 2 and 4) to yield the least harm or the greatest benefit (taking account of the answers to questions 1 and 3), given the professional nature of the dentist-patient relationship?

Before applying these five questions to dentists selling oral health products, for example, there is another conflict of interest situation that arises daily in every dental operatory and that was already mentioned above—namely, that dentists earn their living by caring for patients, and the more services they perform, the more money they earn. This situation is regularly managed ethically—though not always—but it will be useful to apply these five questions to it to illustrate how they work.

Question 1: We can certainly imagine a dentist being tempted to recommend treatments to a patient not because they are needed but because they are lucrative for the dentist. Many dental patients seriously suspect that this has happened to them, a topic that will be discussed in a later section of this chapter. This possibility means that the answer to question 1—about possible serious harm to patients—is surely yes.

Question 2: If every dentist lived by the commitment to practice according to dentistry's professional standards and to give priority to patients' well-being, the likelihood that a dentist's interest in business success will interfere with a dentist's professional judgment on behalf of his or her patient would be zero. Although there certainly are exceptions, the public still ranks dentists among the most trustworthy of occupations. Therefore, it is reasonable to propose that the answer to this question is that the likelihood of harm in this circumstance is typically low.

Question 3 and question 4: The risk of harm to patients from dentists' commercial and other secondary interests is assumed to be low, and this is important. For the only alternative currently available would be to have no one practicing dentistry at all; the harms and lost benefits of that action, of course, would be very significant. In addition, they would be all but certain.

Question 5: The potential harms and lost benefits of having no dentists would be far greater than the harms inherent in our current system. In addition, the likelihood of harms from dentists failing to put secondary interests in proper perspective, for whatever reasons, has been judged to be low.

It is therefore reasonable—assuming that the proposed answer to question 2 is correct—for the larger community to continue to support dentists' authorization as the profession charged with caring for our society's oral health needs; this is in spite of the fact that earning a living is, and will likely remain, an important secondary interest for dentists in our society. (Patients' suspicions that this assumption is not accurate will be examined in a subsequent section of this chapter titled "Dental Expertise, Differing Diagnoses, and Overtreatment.") When a dentist is selling oral health products, however, the ethical character of this particular relationship becomes much more ambiguous.

Question 1: Should the patient assume that the dentist is as committed to the patient's health in this relationship as the dentist is to matters of professional diagnosis and treatment? Or should the patient just know that this is now a commercial relationship to be managed by the "let the buyer beware" principle? Without further information, the patient really cannot tell. That is, because of its apparently commercial character, harm to the patient is possible, and the probability of this harm needs to be considered.

Question 2: The patient needs more information in order to make a dependable judgment of the role of the dentist's secondary interests in the transaction. In other words, absent more information about the dentist's true reasons for selling the product, the risk of harm could well be significant.

Question 3 and question 4: Because of this lack of information, some patients would prefer to separate the commercial and professional relationships; that is, they lose less by buying the products at an ordinary commercial establishment where they know the rules of the game.

Question 5: Such patients would, in effect, be saying that the advantages of separating the commercial and professional relationships are less risky than combining them in the same setting. In the language used earlier, they are saying it is likely that there is more benefit in forgoing this particular relationship with the dentist than in dealing with its potential harms.

Many dentists who sell such products seem to be aware of the ethical ambiguity of these commercial transactions. They may work to ease the ambiguity by explaining to patients that they sell such products simply as a convenience to their patients, to save them a trip, or to assure them that the product they are purchasing is exactly the right one. But such explanations, however reasonable, don't address the ethical ambiguity of the situation. What would be needed to address it carefully would be the equivalent of the disclosure statement like those offered by speakers at dental conferences in which their conflicting interests are identified.

That is, to lessen the patient's uncertainty about the likelihood that the dentist's special secondary interests might be interfering with his or her professional judgment on behalf of the patient, the dentist would need to provide details about those secondary interests. The dentist would need to say, and of course to say honestly, that he or she is not profiting at all from the sale of this product and is providing it at cost (though "at cost" can legitimately include some charge for handling, storage, billing, etc.). Or if there is a markup on the cost of the product, then the dentist needs to say that—like the drug store on the corner—his office adds a 30 percent markup above cost, or whatever it is. Of course, some dentists who are making a few dollars by charging the usual markup might be embarrassed to disclose that so frankly to their patients. But if so, it would be valuable for them to ask themselves why they would be embarrassed. Is it because they are admitting that they have set aside the professional components of their relationship with the patient for the sake of a few dollars?

In any case, the weighing of benefits and harms according to the five questions must be done in the context of the requirements of the professional relationship between dentist and patient. One thing that requirement implies is that protecting the dentist's privacy (about details of the sale, etc.) is not valuable enough to outweigh the value to the patient of making well-informed judgments about commercial products that the dentist recommends. For, because of the ethical ambiguities just discussed, the patient's judgment can hardly be well informed without such disclosure.

For the dentist's part, of course, the answer to question 5 might be that, rather than having to make such disclosures to patients, the best way to avoid such ethical ambiguities is to refrain from selling products at a markup. Since the patient can buy the same product elsewhere (our example has been assuming this is the case), the harm to the patient of not being able to buy the product from the dentist is ordinarily very small.

This same reasoning applies to situations in which dentists are selling health care services not directly involving dental care. The dentist needs to be asking the five questions carefully and should be able to see that, since nothing in recommending these products depends on the dentist's expertise as a professional, the relationship to the patient in such situations is almost certainly only commercial. But that means that the risk of the dentist's secondary interests interfering with his or her judgments, about what will harm or benefit the patient, is even greater than in the case of selling oral health products. In fact, there is good reason for the patient—and the dentist—to wonder why the dentist believes he or she has any business recommending such products when they are so far removed from the dentist's expertise in oral health.

The importance of these ethical concerns is heightened whenever the dentist explicitly recommends the product or service without having personally studied the evidence supporting its effectiveness. Such recommendations are ethically problematic even if, when the dentist has previously recommended the product or service to patients, they have not been harmed or have not complained. Dental expertise requires that a standard of evidence considerably higher than this be employed in a dentist's explicit recommendations. Moreover, even if the dentist does not explicitly recommend the product or service, the fact that the dentist offers it to the patient for purchase may appear to be an expert recommendation in the eyes of the patient. Thus, not saying anything but merely offering the product or service may well be misleading. If the dentist does not have sufficient evidence to recommend it on the basis of his or her actual professional expertise, the dentist should explain this to the patient in order to avoid misleading him or her in this way. (Obviously, the simplest way to avoid the ethical challenges of these situations is again to refrain from offering products or services in the first place, especially those not directly connected to patients' Oral Health. In other words, asking the third of the five questions seriously is a necessary first step in practicing dentistry ethically.)

It is also important to mention, in connection with using the five questions to ethically assess conflicts of interest situations, that there is strong empirical evidence supporting the position that, no matter how impartial we may think we are able to be, when our own personal interests are part of a transaction, we will tend to overvalue them in comparison with the interests of other parties. At the very minimum, when we ask the five questions about a conflict of interest situation, we should assume that, on close calls, we are underestimating the risk of benefits to ourselves interfering with our ability to make dependable expert judgments about the well-being of other parties.

In addition to the subtlety of the ethical judgments that conflict of interest situations call for, and the need to avoid bias in favor of ourselves in such situations, it is important to ask what kind of message a dentist sends when what happens in the operatory moves beyond professionally guided dentist-patient interactions to include commercial transactions. For many patients, the professional-patient relationship still has a special character that is very different from a commercial relationship, and this is the message that dentistry as a profession has long proclaimed. But if the two relationships are mixed together in practice, and especially if the patient is left uncertain about whether the dentist is aware that they are different, the message to the patient—and to those with whom the patient interacts afterward—can very well be that dentist-patient relationships are in the process of changing from professional to commercial. That message does not bode well for the future of dentistry as a profession.

AESTHETIC DENTISTRY

As chapter 5 explained, Aesthetic Values rank as one of dentistry's Central Practice Values, although they rank below Life and General Health, Oral Health, Autonomy, and the dentist's Preferred Patterns of Practice. So a dentist would certainly be failing professionally who paid no attention to Aesthetic Values in his or her practice. One set of Aesthetic Values are the standards regarding the size of teeth, their shape, color, placement, and so on that are accepted criteria for practice within the dental community in our society. But especially since the turn of the twenty-first century, dentists in the United States and elsewhere have encountered a marked increase in the public's interest in aesthetic dental procedures that are not directly connected to preventing or repairing oral health needs and are unrelated to the dental profession's own accepted aesthetic standards.

There is no single standard of appropriate appearance to which all patients, or even the majority of patients, adhere; this includes the preference for whiter-than-natural teeth that has become fairly widespread in recent years. In relation to patients' own aesthetic judgments, then, the dentist honors Aesthetic Values principally by guiding each patient to judge oral and facial appearance according to the patient's aesthetic standards, provided doing so does not harm the patient's Oral Health. In addition, if a patient's personal aesthetic standards seriously violated community standards of oral appearance, and thus put the patient at significant risk of psychological harm, a dentist's support of aesthetic goals of this sort would almost certainly violate the psychological components of General Health.

But there is a fundamental difference between the provision of professional dental care for the sake of patients' Oral Health (or their Life and General Health) and the way in which the dentist functions in the provision of aesthetic services not directly connected to preventing or repairing Oral Health or General Health needs. For in this setting, it is the consumer, not the dentist, who makes the determining judgment about two important things: (1) judging the *need* for aesthetic services and (2) judging whether the dentist's intervention *succeeded* in filling the perceived need. In the provision of professional dental care, both of these judgments must be made by the dentist because they depend on the dentist's professional expertise. So in aesthetic care, in two very important aspects of their relationship, the dentist is no longer acting as a professional in relation to the patient.

In addition, when what is being offered are services not for the sake of patients' Oral Health (and/or other Central Practice Values of the dental profession), then the dentist is providing the patient with something about which the dentist has *no professional expertise*. Indeed, if it is true that there is no single standard of appropriate appearance for all patients, then no expertise even exists that the dentist or anyone else could acquire. For the patient's *need* for aesthetic services and the patient's determining whether the services offered have been *successful* depend solely on the patient's personal aesthetic values. This is why there are serious ethical concerns about the provision of aesthetic services not offered for the sake of patients' Oral Health (or other Central Practice Values) and why dentists should engage in these kinds of relationships only with great care, as will be explained, and on the basis of careful ethical reflection.

Of course, dentists who are successful in offering patients aesthetic services will ordinarily have become skilled in identifying the kinds of interventions most likely to meet the patient's needs and fulfill their aesthetic wishes. But, even though dentists' technical knowledge of the oral cavity and of the chemical and physical properties of various interventions are obviously involved in developing such skills, in this setting they are not using this knowledge *as dentists*, for they are not using it, and the skills it makes possible, for the sake of patients' Oral Health (or other Central Practice Values).

In other words, in these important respects, the relationship between the dentist and the patient in providing aesthetic services not for the sake of the patients' Oral Health (or other Central Values) is a *marketplace relationship*. (It might be argued that the relationship here is an example of what was described in chapter 4 as the Agent Model of the dentist-patient relationship, for it is the patient's values that determine both need and success, rather than the dentist's Central Practice Values. But it would be very strange if a dentist providing aesthetic services was thought to have no values other than the patient's values directing his or her actions. In fact, the dentist is providing these services in the interest of being paid for them—that is, in order to complete a successful business transaction. Therefore, the relationship here is clearly a marketplace relationship, not an example of the Agent Model.)

But if it is a marketplace relationship—and since the patient is clearly acting as a marketplace consumer, that is, by doing his or her own determining of need and making his or her own judgment about whether the dentist's intervention has been successful, then the relationship must be considered to have the other characteristics of marketplace relationships. As explained in chapter 4, marketplace participants are competitors, each trying to obtain the most of what they value from the other while giving up the least to the other. If both parties succeed in this, this is a matter of good luck. But contributing to the other's well-being, or preventing the other from being harmed, is not a primary goal for either of them. That is, dentistry's commitment to giving primacy to the well-being of the patient has no place in a marketplace relationship.

In addition, if this is a marketplace relationship, then the dentist's advice in these situations, like the patients' statement of need and assessment of success, is just one person's judgment. It is not authoritative and not representative of the expertise of the whole dental profession or of any expertise whatsoever. Instead, it is no different in principle from the purchase advice offered by any knowledgeable salesperson in the marketplace and is, from the perspective of the marketplace consumer, indistinguishable from marketing to produce a sale. It is no wonder then that serious ethical questions arise about dentists providing aesthetic services to patients when these are not being done for the sake of patients' Oral Health and other Central Practice Values of the dental profession!

But many dentists who provide aesthetic services will protest that they are in fact acting for the sake of patients' Oral Health because, if they as dentists provide the aesthetic services patients want, they can protect the patients from the harm to Oral Health that could occur if the services were offered by others who are not dentists. In that respect, even though dentists providing aesthetic services are not preventing or repairing Oral Health needs in the usual sense, it can be said that they are serving their aesthetic customers' Oral Health.

This is a legitimate claim, but it does not negate the importance of what has been said about the professional relationship between the dentist and the patient in these situations—that is, the relationship looks at the same time very much like a marketplace relationship and, even more important, is almost certainly being interpreted by patients as *being* a marketplace relationship because *they* determine the need for the service and they determine if the service succeeded in meeting their need. This is particularly important in an environment in which patients "shop" for dentists (comparing accessibility, price, and other aspects of various dental practices). Furthermore, as chapter 10 stressed, dental advertising—especially dental advertising of aesthetics services—strongly suggests that dentists are not professionals committed to their patients' well-being but rather just competing producers in the aesthetic marketplace. In other words, as the title of this chapter asks, in providing aesthetic dental services, are dentists sending a very incorrect message about dentistry to their patients and to the larger society?

Yet it is true that, given the ways that whitening agents and procedures could harm healthy teeth, and even more so teeth with previously undiagnosed weaknesses or disease, it would be far better if people purchased aesthetic services from dentists rather than from someone else. So when a dentist is doing aesthetic work for a patient, what can the dentist do to maintain a focus on what the dentist is contributing to it *as a professional?* Even though aesthetic work is driven by the *patient's* judgment of need and then by the *patient's* assessment of success, what can the dentist do to maintain a proper professional dentist-patient relationship in the midst of this commercial transaction?

The dentist can emphasize that the first and most important criterion he or she will use when choosing a method for meeting the patient's need and achieving the patient's goals is that the method *not be harmful* to the patient's Oral (or General) Health, for judgments about this require the dentist's professional expertise. They are not matters that depend on patients' views or choices, and they are not matters about which, like patients' judgments about looking good, there is no expertise to be had. Of course the dentist should be careful not to turn this emphasis into a demonstration of the dentist's power in the situation, for the ethical standard of striving for an Interactive Relationship still applies. Moreover, while the patient may not realize it, in so doing the dentist is also assuring that the dentist's efforts are aimed, above all, at securing the Central Practice Values of the dental profession for the patient rather than whatever the parties in a merely commercial transaction happen to value. In both respects, the dentist will be relating to the patient primarily *as a professional* rather than primarily as a market competitor.

In addition, regarding the dentist's relationship to the patient, both the dentist's professional commitment to work for as interactive a relationship as possible and the dentist's commitment to give priority to dentistry's Central Practice Values of Autonomy and (the psychological components of) General Health require that the dentist not be the one who initiates discussion about improving the patient's appearance. For most people, an unsolicited comment about the possibility of improving one's appearance will almost always be interpreted as implying a negative judgment about his or her appearance. For most people, an unsolicited negative judgment about one's appearance is ordinarily felt as a devaluation of him or her as a person. Marketers in the commercial marketplace will often begin with a question such as, "Don't you wonder . . ." or "Do you ever feel . . ." and similar phrases to appear as if they are not initiating a question about the person's appearance. But given the risk of their being taken seriously (for example, by the *wholly receptive consumer* of chapter 10), these phrases would be just as likely to be unethical as an oral health professional's unsolicited question about appearance. Moreover, because oral health professionals do have extensive expertise about the oral cavity, then especially if they are offering aesthetic services, some of their patients (again, remember the *wholly receptive consumer*) may think they have expertise about matters of oral aesthetics that are actually matters of personal taste and not matters of expertise at all.

For all these reasons, the dentist who offers aesthetic services has an obligation as a professional to refrain from initiating the conversation about patients' needs for these services. In addition, for the same reasons, the dentist needs to be very cautious about how he or she answers patients' questions about their appearance. This is both to avoid giving the impression of expertise in matters where there is none and being perceived as authority figures in sensitive matters well beyond the range of dentists' actual expertise.

The core question is again the question of whether dentists are sending the wrong message. The provision of aesthetic services combines commercial components (being driven by *patients'* determinations of need and *patients'* assessment of success) with professional components (establishing as interactive a relationship as possible and determining the best method of fulfilling the patient's need—first of all on the basis of protecting the patient's Oral Health and then striving to protect the psychological components of the patient's General Health if these are at risk). There is a constant risk during the provision of such services, then, that the commercial aspects of the transaction will dominate in the patient's awareness and will cloud the patient's perception that what the dentist is providing is *also* professional expertise and a professional relationship. If this last message is lost, the patient will be that much more prone to interpret his or her next visit to the operatory, even though it is clearly for professional dental care, as just another commercial exchange with the dentist. Dentists need to be constantly vigilant that their provision of aesthetic dental services, then, does not lead patients to forget that dentistry is a profession and that dentists are not just another group of purveyors of commercial goods in the marketplace.

Finally, there are Botox and other cosmetic services that might be offered in a dental office but that do not, in any but the most unusual of cases, depend on or involve the specific expertise of the dental profession. Of course, only a person who is trained and licensed to provide Botox injections should do so. But the point here is that this expertise is not part of the expertise of the dental profession. So it is not, in any proper sense of the phrase, professional Oral Health care. The dentist's (or dental hygienist's) role in providing this service, if a dentist (or hygienist) is the one providing the services, is not connected with maintaining the patient's Oral Health (i.e., all the ethical issues mentioned in the section on Conflicts of Interest are equally relevant here). Nor is it primarily connected (as in the case of aesthetic dental services) with protecting the patient's Oral Health from harm. It is a different kind of service from professional oral health care altogether, and the expertise needed to provide it safely is wholly distinct (except in very rare instances) from the specific expertise of the dental profession.

Along with the ethical requirements just identified in relation to the provision of aesthetic dental care, a dentist in whose office Botox treatments (or other cosmetic procedures not related to professional oral health care) are offered has an additional obligation. This is to explicitly inform his or her patients that this service has no direct relationship to professional dental care and that the medical expertise involved is not part of the dentist's professional expertise. The reason for this is that few patients would know of these distinctions on their own. Both the obligation to establish the most Interactive Relationship that is possible and the obligation to respect the patient's Autonomy require, therefore, that the patient be explicitly informed of this.

Returning to the theme of sending the wrong message, a dentist who is thinking about offering Botox (or other cosmetic procedures not related to professional oral health care) in his or her practice should consider the following. The *wholly receptive consumer* may not wonder why a dentist is offering Botox (or related) treatments, naïvely accepting the implied or perhaps explicit rationale that the dentist is trying to meet as many of his or her patients' needs as possible. The *reflective consumer* and the *hardened consumer*, however, will know—whether they could explain it technically or not—that Botox and similar things are not part of dentistry's ordinary repertoire of oral health services, and they will certainly suspect that they have no direct connection to oral health. That is, they will know that the dentist is offering these services to increase his or her bottom line rather than for the oral health of his or her patients and that the dentist is offering these services not as a dental professional but merely as a purveyor of commercial goods in the marketplace.

So what is the message that they will take away? Perhaps it is "only" that this dentist does not know the difference—or worse than that, does not care about the difference—between being a professional and being a participant in the commercial marketplace. But it may well be the message that dentistry—not just that particular dentist—is losing its way and forgetting what it means to be a profession. For every dentist, whether he or she likes it or not, represents all of dentistry to the larger community when he or she acts with integrity as a member of a profession and also whenever he or she portrays the practice of dentistry as just another activity in the commercial marketplace. The message really does matter, and its impact reaches much further than the individual dentist, all the way to questions about where dentistry will be in the future.

NEW TECHNOLOGIES AND PROCEDURES

Many of the new technologies and procedures that the dental research community has devised in recent years have enabled dentists to provide new treatments or perform procedures for patients that are more effective (e.g., direct and indirect restoration materials, sealants, immediately available digital X-rays, etc.). Some innovations help to complete procedures more accurately or more quickly (better hand pieces and ultrasonic devices, cleaning and carving aids). Some provide greater accuracy for diagnoses and treatment (intra-oral cameras, three-dimensional diagnostic and fabrication devices, multiple types of lasers). Some innovations make treatments less painful or uncomfortable for patients (better local anesthetics and sedation techniques). In other words, many new technologies and procedures have either contributed to improvements in patients' Oral Health or have made patients' experience of needed dental treatments less burdensome. It may therefore seem strange to include a section on new technologies and procedures in a chapter that asks if dentists are sending the wrong message—that is, a message about dentistry as commerce rather than a message about dentistry as a profession—to the larger community.

But not all new technologies and procedures improve patients' health or the delivery of needed treatment, and most new technologies and procedures involve a learning curve for the dentists who use them. That is, the fact that a particular technology or procedure is new does not automatically tell us that a dentist ought to use it in his or her practice. Instead, in addition to being a practical and a financial decision, a dentist's decision to incorporate a new technology or procedure into his or her practice is also a professional-ethical decision.

The most important ethical question a dentist needs to ask about a new technology or procedure is of course whether it will enhance the dentist's ability to provide needed dental care to his or her patients. Besides the kinds of improvement in treating oral health needs already mentioned, the new technology or procedure might enable patients to make better-informed treatment decisions and thus enhance the chances of achieving a shared judgment and shared choice of treatment, which is the goal of an Interactive Relationship. Or it may improve patients' oral health indirectly by enabling the dentist to educate patients more effectively in oral hygiene and self-care. Since the newness of a technology or procedure does not guarantee that it will improve patients' Oral Health and the dentist-patient relationship, however, it is incumbent on the dentist considering the purchase of a new technology, or learning a new procedure, to ask the ethical questions, not only the practical and financial questions.

In fact, it is worth asking why a dentist would purchase a new technology or learn a new procedure if it did not improve the dentist's ability to care for patients. (It is being assumed throughout this section that any new technology or procedure added to

a practice will not make patients' care worse since doing that would be blatantly unethical.) Two answers suggest themselves. One is that the dentist considers mastering the
new technology or procedure to be a challenge that he or she will find personally satisfying, independent of whether it enhances patient care in any particular way. The second
answer is that the dentist believes having the new technology or procedure will make his
or her practice more attractive to potential patients—that is, essentially as a marketing
activity—or it will enable the dentist to offer new services to patients that, while neither
harming them nor contributing to their Oral Health, will enhance the practice's bottom
line. Each of these answers deserves some careful ethical analysis.

If the dentist's goal is merely to achieve the personal satisfaction of successfully mastering
a new technology or procedure that, we are assuming, neither harms patients nor contributes to their Oral Health, it may seem that there is nothing professionally unethical about
doing this. But for this to be the case, the dentist would need to refrain from ever using the
technology or procedure when caring for patients, since there is no professionally viable
reason to do so. Or the dentist would have to be totally honest with his or her patients when
offering to employ the technology or procedure while caring for them, informing patients
clearly that it will not benefit their Oral Health in any way, explaining that the dentist's reason for employing it is for his or her own personal satisfaction, and admitting that employing it will take some of the patient's time and explaining how much the dentist will charge
them for its use (unless no charges are involved). But even then, if a patient says it is okay
to go ahead, there is still an ethical problem because it is possible that some patients would
agree in the hope that this will render the dentist more attentive to them.

Obviously such a scenario is truly bizarre and unlikely to take place. But it is worth
considering because it is a reminder that personal satisfaction in successfully mastering a
new technology or procedure is not a patient-centered reason for accepting a new technology or procedure. Moreover, a dentist who conformed to the ethical requirements of
the scenario just described would still be challenging the dental profession's commitment
to the primacy of the well-being of the patient (and, it could also be argued, is also
violating the Central Practice Value of Efficiency in the Use of Professional Resources).
In addition, such a dentist would be sending the wrong message about dentistry to the
patient and anyone the patient told of his or her experience. This "wrong message" is
not specifically about dentistry being excessively commercial, but it would support two
important aspects of the commercial message about dentistry—namely, that dentists are
first and foremost interested in themselves rather than their patients and that the values
that guide dentists' actions are—like those of every participant in the commercial marketplace—their own rather than the Central Practice Values of professional dentistry.

If the dentist adopts a new technology or procedure into his or her practice as a marketing activity or, while neither harming patients nor contributing to their Oral Health,
to enhance the practice's bottom line, the falseness of the message the dentist is sending
is quite clear. Of course, a scenario like the one described above—in which the dentist is
fully honest about the uselessness of the new technology or procedure from the point of
view of proper dental care and honest about his or her reasons for adopting it and offering
it to the patient—would not happen in this case. Actors in the commercial marketplace,

as was explained in chapter 2 and elsewhere in this book, have no obligation to tell the whole truth, and a dentist whose reasons for adopting a new technology or procedure are purely commercial would surely not reveal this fact or the fact that it will make no contribution to the patient's Oral Health.

This kind of situation obviously involves gross violations of dentistry's ethical norms and seriously violates a dentist's commitment to Integrity and Professionalism. If patients or the larger society believed that such things happen with any frequency, this would certainly do serious damage to dentistry's reputation as a profession. So we can certainly hope that it rarely occurs. Pointing out its errors, though, is a useful reminder that every dentist considering the adoption of a new technology or procedure needs to carefully evaluate his or her interest in doing so; he or she must be sure its direct or indirect contribution to patients' Oral Health, or to establishing an Interactive Relationship with the patient, really is the primary reason for doing it. As mentioned in the section on Conflicts of Interest, it is very easy to be biased in favor of what we like—whether it is personal challenges or a better bottom line—and to be drawn to believe that the technology or procedure we are considering is beneficial for patients in ways that it isn't.

Those who sell the new technologies and procedures, furthermore, are highly skilled in supporting these biases and attributing patient benefits to products that don't deserve them. So, in order to reinforce the goal of adopting new technologies or procedures primarily in order to serve patients better, it may be very useful, in doing our ethical thinking, to also ask if, when we introduce our patients to our new technologies or procedures, we will be sending them and those they talk to the wrong message about dentistry as commerce or the right message about dentistry as a profession.

There are two other ethical issues that need mention in relation to those new technologies and procedures that are beneficial to patients. Both of them concern the learning curve that is necessary for almost all such additions to a dental practice. One obviously important category of professional norms concerns Competence, as chapter 3 pointed out. For every professional is obligated both to acquire and to maintain the expertise needed to undertake his or her professional tasks. But almost anyone who acquires something new wants to use it as soon as possible, and this motivation is reinforced if using it will produce revenue that will eventually cover its cost. Therefore, careful ethical judgments are needed to make sure that a new technology or procedure is not employed in patient care in the office until the dentist is definitely able to use it safely without supervision.

In addition, some new technologies and procedures can be employed safely only if the practitioner has also mastered the relevant science behind how it works in order to properly calibrate, titrate, or in other ways adjust it to conform to the specific needs of the patient and its clinical purpose. Attending to this aspect of the learning curve is a serious ethical requirement for the use of a new technology or procedure. If the dentist has not yet learned to use a technology or procedure safely, the dentist, as a professional, is ethically required to refrain from using it in patient care or to arrange to use it under appropriate (i.e., expert) supervision.

Finally, there is the complex ethical issue of patient participation in the use of a technology or procedure when the dentist is not yet fully competent in its use. In some cases, the use of a technology or procedure can be learned to the point of fully competent independent practice outside of the office in training environments in which a dentist's own patients are not involved. But for many new technologies and procedures, advancing to the level of competent practice—that is, use that is not only safe but also dependably beneficial for the patient—requires practice on actual patients. Therefore, beyond the ethical question posed in the previous paragraph about safety until the dentist's use of the item is competent, there is an ethical requirement that the patient be adequately informed about the fact that, at this point in the dentist's learning curve, the use of the technology or procedure is safe but not yet dependably beneficial, and the patient must then give permission to the dentist to employ it under these circumstances. (Similarly, if a dentist who could not yet use a technology or procedure safely was to practice with it in patient care under appropriate supervision, then in such situations both the dentist and the supervisor are obligated to make sure the patient is fully informed and is voluntarily participating in the learning event.)

If patients or the larger society learned that dentists "practiced" on patients—that is, employed technologies or procedures that are not dependably beneficial (in this dentist's hands at this point in the learning curve) as if they were dependably beneficial—without the patients' permission in order to gain competence in the use of a new technology or procedure, again the message that the public would be receiving would be damaging to their understanding of dentistry as a profession. Even if the false message in such a case might not directly associate dentistry with a commercial enterprise, it would still undermine trust of dentists and challenge the assumption of the profession's commitment to give primacy to the well-being of its patients, as well as a number of other ethical norms of the profession.

SELF-REGULATION AND PEER REVIEW

The preceding two sections have discussed situations in which the professional message about dentistry is unavoidably mixed together with a message that says what happens in a dental office is the same as what happens in a marketplace transaction. In both kinds of situations, sending the right message depends on the dentist finding ways to explicitly emphasize the professional aspects of what is going on with the patient and deemphasizing or even deliberately weeding out commercial messages that are not essential to serving the patient appropriately (e.g., "fluff" in advertising, "cool" technologies that don't actually improve patient care or patient understanding, and recommendations that are not based on the dentist's expert judgments of the evidence).

Dentistry currently has the opportunity to be, for the most part, self-regulating. In its commitment to the larger community it ought to be working to prevent prioritizing commercial ways of thinking and acting. The peer review processes are, ideally, the primary formal mechanisms by which dentistry can carry out this function. It ought to be possible for the profession's efforts at self-regulation—both formal and informal—and its peer review processes, then, to focus chiefly on collegial assistance of a dentist who needs it in order to improve their competence in some matter or help them practice more ethically. This ought to be possible, but in fact it happens only occasionally. Every dentist knows that raising a question about a particular dentist's competence or professional conduct is far more likely to become an adversarial matter than one of mutual collegial assistance.

Is there a connection, then, between this problem and the theme of sending the public the wrong message about dentistry and its fulfillment of its commitments as a profession? There certainly is. Fortunately for dentistry's public reputation, what are generally less-than-effective efforts at professional self-regulation have, so far, not become a major concern of the larger society. This may be because the worst violators of the profession's standards of competence and ethical practice ordinarily end up in court and the law processes their cases, and it is these cases that the media pay the most attention to. But the profession typically deserves little credit for this.

Admittedly, few existing peer review committees lack work to do, and they take their work seriously. Few who are called before a peer review committee come there, though, expecting collegial assistance in rectifying errors in competent or ethical practice. Most consider the peer review process to be essentially accusatory—about wrongs done—and punitive in outcome, and in some cases, there are good reasons for this to be so.

The more important issue, though, is about dentistry's opportunity for and commitment to being self-regulating—and how the majority of dentists view this task. Some, perhaps most, might wish that it were focused on the collegial assistance of dentists who need it. But their practical experience—whether personal or vicarious—tells them that raising a question about another dentist's competence or ethical conduct is most likely to become an adversarial matter. This ordinarily makes them slow, if not wholly unwilling, to raise the issue. Multiply this reaction across the whole dental profession in our society, and it becomes a self-fulfilling description of the actual state of self-regulation. Minor, correctable shortfalls that are most effectively corrected collegially are routinely not addressed. This leads to the impression that the only shortfalls in competence or conduct worth addressing to a peer review committee are serious ones. This implies, of course, that any shortfall actually addressed to a peer review committee *is* of a serious nature, making dentists increasingly unwilling to have their own shortfalls reported and still more unwilling to report others' shortfalls, and so on.

Chapter 9 argued for a distinction between bad work and the bad outcomes that every dentist, no matter how skilled or how careful, will experience. In an ideal professional world, dentists who observe a bad outcome in another dentist's work would contact the other dentist out of collegial concern for that dentist (as well as, of course, out of concern for the patient's well-being, if that would be advanced or protected by such a call). That dentist would appreciate the call, possibly even inviting the calling dentist to offer counsel on how to avoid such issues in the future. Both would end the call grateful for the other's response and for their mutual commitment to practice as competently and ethically as they can. That is the ideal that professionalism calls for in dentist-to-dentist relationships.

This kind of informal collegial assistance does occasionally take place, but the dentists who do practice it together have usually become friends first or else are in the same practice and view this kind of relationship as necessary for the success of their partnership. It rarely happens among strangers. This is because the calling dentist must believe that the dentist receiving the call holds dentistry's commitment to self-regulation as something that every dentist should be working for as collegially as possible. The common adversarial attitude that was described above toward raising such questions makes most dentists unwilling to believe that such calls will be received as they are intended. So such calls don't happen very often, and the adversarial pattern is reinforced still further.

It is no wonder that, when a report does go to a peer review committee, there is little likelihood that the party reported on will view the report as an effort at collegial correction. Consequently, even when the peer review committees might have collegial correction as their goal, their ability to interact with the dentist reported on in a collegial way may have already been rendered impossible.

All of this is, of course, even more exacerbated by the litigious character of contemporary US society and the risks involved for dentists accused in patients' malpractice suits. A dentist who would ideally prefer to address another dentist's shortfall collegially might well hold back anyway to avoid possible legal involvement.

There are two ways, then, that this negative pattern connects with the theme of sending the wrong message. If this pattern is in fact significantly hampering the dental profession's fulfillment of its commitment to self-regulate—so that significant numbers of correctable shortfalls in competence and/or professional-ethical conduct are going uncorrected—and possibly some numbers of uncorrectable shortfalls are also going unreported, then the larger community may begin to wonder if the message that the dental profession can be trusted with self-regulation is true. As mentioned above, however, the members of the larger society do not easily observe this shortfall from professionalism on the part of the dental profession (which is certainly not alone among professions in this respect). This last point may be "good news" (at least for now), but it is no solution to the problem.

What is much more visible is the attitude of "potential adversary" that so many dentists seem to have toward other dentists. Dentists, of course, socialize together and build friendships and other important social relationships, many of which bear fruit in shared efforts at community service. But in most communities there are large numbers of dentists who are strangers to one another, and in regard to them, the attitude of "potential adversary" seems to be all too common for the reasons just explained. Since dentists are, from the point of view of the health care marketplace, competing with each other—which is going to be obvious to most members of the public—then their adversarial attitude toward dentists not already known to them (or known only in adversarial situations) will reinforce a message that the dentists in the community are no different from other competitors in the marketplace.

It is clear that a massive recommitment to professional collegiality would be required for this negative pattern to be corrected. But it is hard to see how the dental profession can become effective at self-regulating, either informally (where it is most likely to be effective) or formally (through peer review committees) without a serious effort at such a recommitment. The dental profession collectively—and especially through its professional organizations—needs to readdress this problem with self-regulation and the negative message about its commitment to professionalism that it may be sending to the larger society. Like the ethical concerns expressed in this discussion, this conclusion is also supported by the empirical studies of these issues in the 2016 Interim Gies Ethics Project Report of the American College of Dentists.

Each individual dentist can contribute to this collective process; each can personally turn the message he or she is sending into something more positive. Is it possible that his or her attitude toward other dentists—who are not friends or close associates—is in fact adversarial or at least untrusting? Are his or her comments to patients or others, perhaps without his or her being aware of it, communicating the view that those dentists are competitors and nothing more? Are they, therefore, considered persons whose actions toward other dentists are not to be trusted? Even though they do compete in the marketplace for patients, other dentists are members of the same profession; they try to live, in fact, by the same commitments. Communicating that message to the larger society would be very helpful.

DENTAL EXPERTISE, DIFFERING DIAGNOSES, AND OVERTREATMENT

The previous sections have raised ethical concerns about individual dentists and the whole dental community sending the larger community a message that the practice of dentistry is more like commercial activity in the marketplace than the work of professionals primarily committed to caring for the well-being of their patients. But another essential characteristic of a profession is its expertise; it is a group's expertise, its ability to respond effectively to important human needs—along with its ethical commitments—that accords it the special authority in a society that marks it as a profession. Surely, the reader might say, there is no doubt that the dental profession has such expertise. Why, then, is there a section on dental expertise in a chapter about dentists sending the wrong messages to the larger society?

Again, the 2016 Interim Gies Ethics Project Report of the American College of Dentists is relevant. Its studies of dentistry as it is practiced in the United States included patient focus groups. What these studies strongly point to (though it was an interim report, so the research was not yet complete) is something that any nondentist likely already knows from conversations with friends or neighbors—namely, that many patients hear different stories from different dentists about the same presenting conditions in their mouths. Not surprisingly, this leads patients to distrust dentists because the dentists seem to tell them—as patients interpret it—whatever is most beneficial to the dentist's own practice. Given this disparity, what is most natural for patients to assume? Obviously it is that what these dentists say is whatever contributes the most to their bottom lines.

This is why such experiences send a message to these dentists' patients that dentistry is first of all a commercial enterprise wherein what the dental salesperson says has no direct relevance to the patient's well-being. It is also not surprising that many patients who have had such experiences assume that they were overtreated by one or more of the dentists they have visited.

Of course, there may be other, even professionally appropriate, explanations of these dentists' reasons for having differing views about what to recommend. But this topic is included in this chapter for another and much more troubling reason: If dental expertise exists, then two dentists listening to the same patient's concerns, examining the same mouth, studying its X-rays, and then telling the patient what is going on ought to offer similar *descriptions* of what they observe and how this affects the patient's oral health needs (their diagnoses). Furthermore, unless they have differing judgments of what the patient's needs are, their explanations of the dental *treatment options that are within the standard of care* for those needs ought to be similar, if not the same. For the standard of care for a patient's diagnosed need and what are reasonable treatment options does not vary from dentist to dentist, and the physical makeup of a patient's mouth does not ordinarily vary over short periods of time.

Admittedly, some amount of variation in what patients "hear" can be explained by differences in patients' attention and level of understanding—although the ethical question then becomes whether the dentists were working for as interactive a relationship as possible, or even just for informed consent. But the number of patients who have had this experience is too great for this to be the only explanation. It is also too great to be explained by actual variations in patients' dentition between the two (or more) dentists' examinations.

Is it possible that many dentists are not providing their patients with complete diagnoses but rather only with a description of the work they want to do at the time? Is it possible that many dentists are describing the treatment they want to perform rather than all the treatments that are within the standard of care for the patient's presenting oral health need? Both of these things are possible, and unfortunately many patients have concluded that one or both of these things has happened to them and have assumed that values other than the primacy of their Oral and General Health—not to mention their Autonomy in making a well-informed decision about their treatment—have motivated the dentist. Perhaps more extensive research will make it clearer which of these patterns of practice, or some other factor, explains such patients' experiences.

However these patients' experiences are explained, they raise a different kind of concern about the message the larger society receives about dentistry. If enough dentists are contributing to experiences of this kind for patients—where different dentists say different things about the same mouths—the message it sends the larger society is that there is no such thing as a body of dental expertise that all properly trained and licensed dentists employ in their practices. This puts dentistry at risk of leading the larger society to doubt that there is such a thing as dental expertise.

There have long been people who have claimed there is no such thing as expertise so valuable to a society that those who are expert in it should be accorded special social authority in its use. There have also been people who have held that the social power and financial rewards that such authority brings with it are so great that it is a mistake for a democratic, equality-seeking society to grant anyone this kind of authority. Dentistry and our societies' other professions have nevertheless been supported and accorded the authority and status of professions. This is, first of all, because their expertise has been believed to be both genuine and effective in responding to important human needs. But if dentistry's message to the larger community raises questions about whether it has such expertise, the consequences for those who practice dentistry and for the society that benefits from that practice could be very serious.

The remedy, of course, is obvious. Every dentist must be focused, above all, on communicating thoroughly and effectively with the patient about the condition of his or her mouth, about the needs that are present, and about the prognoses if these are treated according to the various options within the standard of care or if not treated at all. In addition to attending to the patient's concerns, every dentist must clearly separate his or her diagnostic judgment and the observations of the patient's condition on which it is based and the description of acceptable options for treatment that it supports from any personal preference for any of the recommended treatment options available. Obviously, for the same reasons, dentists must never overtreat.

It would be a serious mistake for dentistry—or any dentist—to run the risk of communicating to the public that dentistry's expertise, which certainly is genuine and effective, does not exist.

THINKING ABOUT THE CASE

Richard "I'll Make You Rich" Paulson clearly knows what he wants to sell and, like a good salesman, finds a way to make it appear that his product—setting up Botox services in dental practices—will enable Dr. Milford to accomplish his goals. But it is hard to imagine that Dr. Milford would simply take Mr. Paulson at his word and immediately start working to set up Botox services in his practice. For one thing, Dr. Milford has been described as a careful man who gets a lot of information together before he makes a major move. More importantly, Dr. Milford has been described as someone who, while very savvy commercially, is concerned that his use of commercial techniques to enhance his practice is done ethically, and nothing has been said about Dr. Milford to suggest that he does not view his patients' well-being as the primary determinant of how he treats patients and how he runs his practice.

One would expect, given this picture of Dr. Milford, that in his dealings with patients, both in aesthetic work and in general dentistry, he carefully describes what his diagnosis reveals and explains all the treatments that are within the standard of care and the benefits and risks of each, as well as the consequences of not treating at all. If he has mechanical toothbrushes or dentifrices for sale at cost or for the same price as the local drugstore, it is not just for the convenience of his patients but because he has researched them to be sure they are as good as or better than other brands, and he explains this when he sells them. His judgments about adding new technologies are similarly made on the basis of their value in enhancing patients' Oral Health or education or patients' experience during treatments.

We would also expect that he tries to respond to instances of other dentists' bad outcomes by contacting them whenever he can and works as collegially with dentists as he is able. Even though a petition was brought against him by other Ridgeview dentists, he would be the kind of person who does not bad-mouth these dentists to patients or colleagues. His practice has two dentist employees, one of whom also manages the Montclair practice, and as an owner he has offered contractual arrangements that pay them fairly and enable them to practice as autonomous professionals at chairside, in full control of their time and work and their relationships with patients.

Given this picture of Dr. Milford, the most that Rich Paulson could realistically hope for from the dentist after giving him the pitch for Botox services would be a polite "I'll think about it." But there is value in imagining a longer conversation between this commercially savvy but ethically committed professional and a salesman who views dentistry as a commercial enterprise.

"That's very interesting, Rich, but I have a real problem with bringing Botox into my practice."

"I don't see why, Doc. You're already so focused on aesthetics. It's the natural next step, still addressing people's facial appearance but offering a more comprehensive approach to improving it and giving your patients the look they want. I've read your ads and that's your main pitch. You bring them in to improve their facial appearance and keep them to fix their teeth. What sort of problem do you have with this? We'd certainly set it up so the person doing the Botox treatments here was fully licensed, whether it's your other dentist or someone you bring in part-time to do it."

"My problem with it, Rich, is that it has nothing to do with Oral Health. Dentistry is first and foremost about caring for people's oral health needs, prospectively by prevention and education and therapeutically when there are deficiencies that need to be corrected. Botox has nothing to do with that."

"I'm afraid I don't follow you, Doc. Aesthetic services are your bread and butter, and your aesthetic patients don't come to you for Oral Health, they come for better looks. They may stay for the sake of Oral Health, I'll grant that, but that's not why they come in the door."

"I'm happy to help them achieve the oral appearance they want, Rich. But one reason I am in the aesthetic dentistry business is because people's teeth and other oral features can be seriously harmed if what is done to improve their smiles is done by someone who doesn't know their dentistry. Back when I was in Montclair, I had patients come in whose enamel had been ruined in the patients' efforts to get whiter-than-natural teeth. And I'll admit it, after a couple of those cases, I used to try to persuade patients to leave their teeth alone, to forget whitening them and leave them their natural color unless they were badly stained and we could get them back to natural coloring. But then I saw more and more patients, especially young patients with otherwise very healthy teeth, using products that I didn't trust. So I decided when I made the move here to Ridgeview to invest in getting properly trained to do aesthetic work so I could make sure it was done in a way that wouldn't harm teeth. And I'll tell you, especially after coming here and having a couple of patients who wanted aesthetic work done but who had previously unnoticed problems with the teeth they wanted to treat, I'm even happier that I've followed this path because if they hadn't come to me, who knows what someone else might have done to them!"

"OK, Doc, I understand. You do aesthetic dentistry to prevent the kinds of aesthetic work that can damage teeth. That's fine! But Botox doesn't damage teeth, so there's no reason to refuse to add it to your practice. You sell other products, don't you, like mechanical toothbrushes? They don't damage teeth, but you sell them."

"I'm sorry, Rich, but you don't understand. A dental practice is about Oral Health first and foremost. If we help people's appearance, that's a bonus. But we're here first and foremost for their Oral Health. If I were to bring Botox into this practice, I'd only be doing it to make money, not as something that's part of what dentistry is about."

"But what's wrong with making money, Doc? You make money on your aesthetic work, you make money on your general dentistry, you make money when your hygienist cleans someone's teeth. That's what a business is about. Botox is no different from any of that."

"I don't think money is a value for its own sake, Rich. Of course I want to make money. I have a family I want to support, and I want to retire someday. And when I started out I had debts to pay off. But I am a professional first, not an entrepreneur. I am trying to help people achieve something that is a real value—health. That's a real value. It's not just about money, which is only a means to other things and nothing more. I don't want the people I serve or the others out there in the community to look at dentistry and think it is just another business in the marketplace aimed at earning as much money as possible. That's not what dentistry is and that's not who I am as a professional. And for me, Botox just doesn't fit into that picture, but thanks for stopping by."

Dr. Milford is being portrayed here as a dentist who thinks carefully about the professional-ethical characteristics of every aspect of his practice. Dr. Milford is not necessarily a dental hero. He has not practiced long enough to be the kind of dentist who embodies chapter 1's definition of dental professionalism as "the internalized and habitual ways of thinking and acting that characterize the life and practice of the most admirable members of the dental profession." But he is being described as someone who clearly understands and has thought carefully about dentistry's ethical norms and is striving to be in accord with them in every aspect of his practice. Most likely such a person would have turned many of these norms into habits and therefore does not have to stop and think hard about how to practice ethically unless a case is particularly complex or a decision is a major one, like determining whether to add an operatory, move to a larger building, hire a third dentist for the Ridgeview practice, or change responsibilities within the office so he can spend more time practicing general dentistry.

But one of the main points of this chapter is that Dr. Milford—even if he isn't yet one of the "most admired members of the dental profession"—is nevertheless the kind of dentist who, while making solid use of the marketing tools of the marketplace, is still sending the right kind of message about dentistry to the public—and one reason such a person would do that so dependably is because he is someone who regularly asks himself what kind of message he is sending.

Every dentist needs to be asking this question on a regular basis. The topics covered in this chapter have been chosen because each of them, depending on how a dentist deals with them and speaks about them, can tell the larger community that dentistry's claim to be a profession is well supported by its practice—or, alternately, that dentistry and dentists are looking more and more like typical, self-interested participants in the competitive commercial marketplace. This is clearly a very important question for every dentist to be asking because, in the long run, dentistry cannot have it both ways.

14

The Obligations of Dentistry's Professional Organizations

CASE: PROFESSIONAL ORGANIZATION OR COMMERCIAL ENTERPRISE

You have recently become editor of the prestigious (and fictitious) *American Journal of Dental Prosthetics*, the official publication of the (also fictitious) American College of Fixed and Removable Prosthodontics (ACFRP) and a leading journal within the American dental community. You were appointed editor in chief of *AJDP* because of years of hard work, careful teaching, and significant research. You now face an important decision about advertising in the journal. Your managing editor and your chief associate editor, who have been with the journal for years, are seated before you. They are deeply divided about an expensive, full-color, four-page ad that the Peterswill Corporation wishes to place in *AJDP* for its new product, Capwright.

Peterswill has been a leading producer of dentifrices and other oral hygiene products for years. Its advertising has been a mainstay of *AJDP*, and the Peterswill Foundation, heir to most of the fortune of the company's founder, Peter Roundsmith, has long been a major supporter of ACFRP programs. But the Peterswill Corporation has gone through some difficult years recently. Sales of its mouthwash declined significantly after federally mandated changes were made in Peterswill's advertising claims, and the firm's share of the dentifrice market also slipped badly, chiefly because of the corporation's complacent attitude toward fluoride research. Now a new senior management group is in place, trying to turn things around by expanding Peterswill's markets. Their new senior researcher, hired away from a competitor, has developed Capwright. The firm's management believes that Peterswill's ability to survive now rides on the success of this product.

Capwright is a bonding adhesive and cementation seating compound for fixed prostheses. Its appeal lies in its claim of being durable years longer than any current cementation or restorative product on the market. It also claims and presents data that it adheres to all dental, metal, glass, and composite surfaces, both in the preparation of and in the seating of the prosthesis itself. It appears to be capable of filling any gaps that might occur between the two surfaces without weakening the bond, thus making up for errors in a dentist's preparation of the tooth or in the impressions that the dentist takes for the prosthesis and some other possible errors in the transfer models and fabrication processes.

The ad copy from Peterswill's advertising agency doesn't make this point quite so explicitly, of course; it stresses Capwright's "potential to expand the general practitioner's ability to place caps and bridges while giving even the most expert prosthodontist new confidence that his or her appliances will seat perfectly." But any dentist who reads the ad will understand what is being inferred.

The chief associate editor speaks first: "The first thing you have to ask yourself, Doctor, is what it means to say that we are professionals. We claim to be committed to quality treatment and to placing our patients' oral health ahead of our own desire for money and a flourishing practice. There isn't any doubt that quality treatment and the best care for our patients means that teeth must be properly prepared for prostheses. Impressions, imaging, castings, and all fabrication procedures must be done with precision."

"What do we teach our students in the dental schools?" the associate editor continues. "Certainly not to just come close and then fill in any gaps that are left with a good cement. We teach them that an exact fit is expected from preparation to prosthesis. We teach them the skills to carry this out in routine cases, and we expect them to refer more difficult cases to specialists because that is what the standard of care requires.

"If that is true, then how can this journal publish an ad like this, which says to general practitioners and specialists alike, 'Don't worry about your sloppy work. We'll cover your mistakes!' This journal has a reputation to protect. That's one thing, and I think it is important. But something more important than that is at stake. We are a profession. We hold a public trust, not just as individuals but collectively through organizations like the college. If Capwright is a superior bonding agent, or if it is better at handling the microscopic imperfections that occur in even the highest quality prosthetic preparations and castings, let them say that and provide the long-term clinical research to prove it. We would be guilty of a serious violation of our professional ethics and we would be sending a terrible message about our profession if we were to publish an ad that encourages dentists to tolerate substandard preparations because they can cover up the results with Capwright!"

The managing editor responds: "Of course I respect the values that the associate editor refers to, but there are four additional facts that you need to take account of in your decision, Doctor. First of all, there is the financial issue. We rarely get a chance to run a full-color four-pager, much less to have a chance to contract for one each month for the next two years. Besides, Peterswill has been one of our major advertisers. There is good reason to think that the firm's new management would pull their other advertising from the journal if we refused to run the copy for Capwright.

"You know as well as I do that if the only funding we had was the grant from ACFRP, this would be a quarterly journal of forty or fifty pages, not a monthly that has room enough to serve our community in dozens of important ways on top of the first-rate research we publish. We can't ignore our advertisers and still serve the members of the college and the larger dental community. They are depending on us. That's the second point. In addition to our own bottom-line considerations, we have an obligation to continue serving our readership because they need us and count on us for all that this journal does for them.

"In addition, this product has been field tested by reputable laboratories. It has FDA marketing approval for what it is claiming. So far as the FDA and we know, it won't harm anyone's teeth any more than products in current use and it won't compromise patients' health. The associate editor says he would be willing to advertise a product that claims to fill in microscopic imperfections. Well, we all know that there are many general dentists out there who prepare prostheses with more than microscopic imperfections in the fit, and some patients eventually pay the price in sensitivity, pain, and/or lost function. Why not encourage the general practitioner to use a product like this that will raise the quality of the general dentist's prosthetic work? It is the GPs who are the most pressed right now, with the economics of dentistry changing so much. Don't we owe them some consideration?

"Besides that, this journal isn't published just for the members of the college. The journal says it serves the whole dental community. That's its mission. In the name of the college it's trying to educate dentists generally about good prosthetic care. Here is a way that the care that ordinary dentists actually give their patients can be significantly improved. The standard of care in the dental schools is not the standard of care out in the offices, and it is *that* standard of care that we have a chance to improve here.

"Finally, I want to ask whether the editors of this journal are the ones who ought to tell practicing dentists what is and what is not appropriate care. Dentists are professionals— the associate editor has already stressed that point. But that means they are the ones that have been entrusted with making decisions about the proper care of their patients. Each of them must make that decision about each particular patient. We cannot make those decisions for all of them. Our job is to inform them of the clinical techniques available to them, and you know as well as I do that our advertising is as important a vehicle for doing that job as our articles on current research. This product has FDA marketing approval and is the result of extensive research in Peterswill's own labs and at several universities. So I submit that we would be going beyond our mandate, and doing a disservice to the dental community as well, if we refused to publish this ad, not to mention tightening the financial noose around the journal's neck instead of taking the opportunity to let it take a deep breath for the first time in years."

You are the editor in chief, Doctor. What should you do?

THE PROFESSION AS A WHOLE AND DENTAL ORGANIZATIONS

To this point, this book has principally emphasized the obligations of chairside dentists because of the commitments they have made in becoming professionals and because of the nature of the profession they have joined. But each profession as a whole also has obligations, and so do its professional organizations. This chapter will examine the obligations of the dental profession as a whole in our society and especially of its professional organizations, for these play important roles in the ongoing dialogue between the profession as a whole and the larger society.

First, however, the general idea that organizations and even a profession as a whole organization can have obligations deserves some examination. The cultural bias mentioned in chapter 4 that views all judgments and choices as the actions only of individual humans, rather than seeing some of them as the actions of groups of people acting as a unit, can easily get in the way of our thinking about obligations in regard to groups of people. But groups of people working together collect data, process it, examine alternative courses of action, make judgments about how to act, and then actually do things. When individual humans do these things, under the proper circumstances, we have no trouble thinking of them as actors and as having obligations. There is no good reason, in the authors' view, why we shouldn't understand organizations to be actors that have obligations in the same way, and in fact, many people who look at how various organizations act are quite ready to say they acted wrongly or, sometimes, admirably. That is, organizations are often viewed as having obligations.

What may be less obvious is that groups that are not formal organizations and do not have established roles and offices (i.e., what might be called "informal groups") can have obligations. Among these, for example, would be groups of friends, larger groups like the people at a political rally, and also the whole people of a nation. Such groups can have characteristics in common that, when exercised collectively, give the group the ability to collect data, compare alternatives, and select actions that are rightly considered to have been performed by the group. The dental profession as whole (within a given society) is such a group, and under proper circumstances it is rightly—by analogy with individual actors and formal organizations—considered to act as a single actor and to be responsible for what it does. That is to say, it can have obligations.

It is beyond the scope of this book to delve further into the arguments that philosophers and other social theorists have made for (and against) the idea that groups can perform actions and have obligations. It is, however, a premise of this chapter that the dental profession in our society and its professional organizations have obligations. Therefore, it is important to reflect on what these obligations are.

Of course, groups of humans function as actors—gathering data, evaluating alternatives, selecting among them, and acting—only by virtue of and by means of the actions of the individuals who make up the group, and these individuals therefore have whatever obligations come with the roles they play. But this fact does not mean that a listing of all the individual actions involved will be enough to completely describe what is going on in such a situation, without anything missing. Part of what is meant by saying that a group acts and has obligations is that, even after all the actions of the individuals involved have been thoroughly described, there will still be more to say about what the *group* as a whole does and ought to do.

But because such a group acts only by virtue of and by means of the actions of individuals, it follows that the group cannot fulfill its obligations unless the relevant individuals, playing various roles within it, act as they need to so the organization acts as it ought to. This means that every member of the dental profession has, by reason of membership in this group, an additional professional obligation to do what is necessary so that the profession as a whole acts as it ought. Similarly, and especially, since it is dental organizations that most often represent the dental profession as a whole in our society, every professional dental organization and every member of these organizations has an obligation to act in ways that support dentistry as a whole and each of its professional organizations acting as they ought.

Exactly what an individual dentist ought to do to fulfill these obligations will depend on many factors in the dentist's professional and personal life. Some of the obligations of the dental profession as a whole, for example, are such that individual dentists work most effectively to fulfill them by their actions and what they communicate about the dental profession day in and day out at chairside and, as the previous chapter stressed, by what message this sends to the larger community about what dentistry is committed to and stands for as a profession. For whether a dentist is reflective about it or not, he or she is continually and unavoidably acting in the name of the profession as a whole. Every act of a dental professional organization, whether the members or leaders of the organization are reflective about it or not, similarly communicates a message (either positive or negative) about the dental profession as a whole and what it is committed to and stands for. This fact means that individual dentists (and nondentist staff) who are active in dentistry's professional organizations have obligations to make sure the organization is acting ethically—not only by the minimal standards of organizations in the marketplace but by the norms of professional dentistry—and that its message to the larger community about the dental profession is a positive one.

As every dentist knows, the extra burden of being active in organized dentistry cannot be made to fit into every professional life in the same way. Most dentists find some times in their professional lives more suited to playing an active role in dentistry's professional organizations and other times—for example, when their children are younger and their practices are not well established—less suited for the demands of such activity. But because of the importance of the actions of professional organizations in the public's view of the profession, no dentist may ethically look on the activities of dentistry's professional organizations simply as matters that "someone else" is responsible for. At some appropriate point, every dentist ought to be active in shaping the actions and policies and contributing to the activities of organized dentistry in other ways. This is an important element in the collective life of dentistry as a whole and is a major contributor to the larger society's continued conviction that dentistry is a profession. That is, every dentist bears a share of the responsibility for the character of the dental profession as a whole. Every dentist must take seriously the obligation to shape that character from within dentistry's professional organizations as well as representing the whole dental profession in how he or she practices at chairside.

What obligations does the dental profession as a whole have and what obligations do dentistry's professional organizations have? The nine categories of professional obligation introduced in chapter 3 and employed in the discussion of chairside dentists' obligations throughout this book can be used to offer answers to these questions.

CHIEF CLIENT, CENTRAL VALUES, AND COMPETENCE

One of the most important roles of the dental profession in our society is its contribution to the society's understanding of what counts as oral health and what indicates its absence, especially with a view to professional intervention. As will be explained, the profession's obligations in carrying out this role require consideration of three different categories of professional norms—namely, Chief Client, Central Practice Values, and Competence.

The most general meanings of the concepts of health and disease are probably fairly consistent across cultures and eras. But as these meanings are specified more concretely and grounded on more and more concrete understandings of desirable human functioning, the distinctive values of a given society's culture and even of the accepted modes of practice of each particular health care profession become incorporated into them. Thus, what counts as Oral Health in a particular society like our own is not something timeless, though it seems connected to or is a specification of something of lasting and general human value. Instead, its functional content has been determined in large part by cultural conceptions of acceptable versus unacceptable levels of pain/comfort and function/dysfunction. These, in turn, are significantly affected by the interventions that are performed by those considered expert in the society in addressing and modifying people's oral pain/comfort and function/dysfunction.

Those who play this role are the society's dental professionals both when acting as individuals and through the actions of dentistry's professional organizations, for the interventions that dentists judge appropriate to perform at chairside or that dental organizations recommend for chairside use do not include all possible interventions that might be performed in, on, or for people's mouths. The dental community considers only certain types of possible interventions constructive for Oral Health, so the dental community, to a significant degree, determines what counts as appropriate and pain-free oral functioning (i.e., Oral Health) and what counts as oral dysfunction.

At the same time, however, which classes of interventions are considered proper is also partly determined by the larger society's values regarding oral pain/comfort and oral function/dysfunction. Thus, these two groups—the society's dental professionals and the community at large that carries and shapes its culture—work together in subtle, ongoing ways to shape the concept of Oral Health and its absence, and these concepts, in turn, guide the practice of the former and the expectations of the latter.

To take an absurd example, suppose a patient came to a dentist and requested assistance to strengthen his or her teeth and bite so that the patient could routinely crack especially hard nut shells as squirrels do. Today's dentists might reasonably refuse the request as being dangerous to the patient's Oral Health and may even view the patient as a crackpot, and they would easily be supported in this judgment by the larger community. But suppose that the vast majority of people in the society began to routinely make this request of dentists and they did so for nutritional or environmental reasons that had become significant social goals in the society. Long before such a scenario became commonplace, the dental community would have begun to address the issue. It either would have started looking for alternative solutions for those with such a need or begun working to challenge the rationale that made what is considered very risky from the point of view of society's previously accepted understandings of oral health appear to be a reasonable health request. If these efforts failed over a period of time—how long is difficult to say— eventually the society's views of oral function and dysfunction would have changed, and very likely, the dental community would come to the point of devising modes of assisting the society's people in performing this function in as safe a manner as possible from the point of view of other oral functions and people's General Health.

The point here is certainly not to recommend this strange scenario. It is simply to illustrate the fact that the dental profession does not unilaterally determine the content of Oral Health in a society. Nevertheless, its contribution to this process is far greater than that of any other definable group in society and is even equal to that of the larger community as a whole as long as the community continues to recognize and affirm the dental profession's relevant expertise.

Because it has this important social role, the dental profession also has an obligation to contribute carefully and conscientiously to the shaping of these important concepts. The dental profession makes its contributions to this process in three ways, which correspond to three of the categories of professional norms identified in chapter 3: the profession's Chief Clients, the Central Practice Values of the dental profession, and Competence.

Dentistry's Chief Clients are the class of persons whom dentistry rightly serves, and there are also classes of persons whom it does not serve—for example, the "nut cracker" patient of the previous example. Those whom it rightly serves are served because their conditions and needs are considered appropriate for dentists to address. Those whom it judges it should not serve fall outside the classes of persons whose needs are appropriate for dentists to address. In identifying certain classes of persons as those rightly served by dentists—that is, dentistry's Chief Clients—the dental profession and the larger society in dialogue partly define the society's understanding of Oral Health.

Regarding Central Practice Values, as has been stressed often in these pages, there are certain values that dentistry is rightly committed to achieving for its patients, and there are other values that dentistry has no particular commitment to serve. In determining what dentistry's Central Practice Values are and especially how these values are to be understood concretely as the specific goals of dental practice at a given time in a given society and how they are to be pursued in a given, ranked order or hierarchy, the dental profession contributes in a second way to the society's understanding of Oral Health, even as the society also contributes to this process.

Finally, there are interventions that members of the dental profession rightly perform under certain clinical circumstances and other interventions that no dentist could appropriately perform under those circumstances. At work here is the professional norm of Competence. The guidance that the profession's determinations of what counts as Competent practice offers at chairside is minute and it may appear to be solely based on scientific and technological fact. But these determinations are partly controlled by an understanding of what counts as Oral Health in the larger society, which is then embedded in the profession's criteria of Competence. As the dental community employs these criteria of competent practice in teaching new dentists and also judges practicing dentists by these criteria of Competent practice, moreover, this process in turn shapes the culture's understanding of Oral Health in its clinically important details.

Therefore, the dental profession, as it engages in dialogue with the larger community about the contents of the profession's norms of Chief Client, Central Practice Values, and Competence, has an obligation to attend carefully to the ways in which this dialogue shapes its own and the larger community's understanding of Oral Health. But the larger community also has an obligation to participate thoughtfully in this dialogue. The concepts and professional norms this dialogue yields will of course be employed more self-consciously by members of the dental profession. Moreover, the larger community typically accords first place in this dialogue to the dental profession by reason of its expertise. Since the dental profession has a special obligation to guide this dialogue carefully and to thoughtfully shape the contents of these important concepts for the whole community, each of dentistry's professional organizations and each dentist also has an obligation, insofar as it plays a role in this dialogue, to contribute conscientiously to the fulfillment of the dental profession's obligations in this regard.

MORE ON COMPETENCE

The most obvious obligation of the dental profession as a whole concerns competence in dental practice. That is, it concerns the profession's supervision of the application of dental expertise by dentists at chairside so it is used (and not misused) in caring for individual patients and also, in the case of public health measures, in caring for the community at large.

This obligation is fulfilled in a number of ways. First, the profession maintains standards of practice through dental schools, continuing education programs, and professional organizations. Many individual dentists contribute to the profession's fulfillment of this obligation by serving as dental school faculty, mentoring young dentists formally or informally, supporting continuing education programs of many sorts, and providing financial support for all of these activities.

Second, the profession supports continuing research and quality control regarding procedures, materials, and many other aspects of clinical practice. It also supports the systems of licensure and, especially through professional organizations, has an active voice in legislative and other public forums dealing with competent dental practice. These are the settings where the ongoing dialogue between the dental profession and the larger community regarding standards of practice, society's understanding of oral health, and the contents of the dental profession's ethical norms is most visible.

Third, as discussed in chapters 8 and 9, the profession supports the efforts of individual dentists to provide to one another—and, where necessary, through referrals to appropriate review bodies—appropriate communication about bad outcomes and bad work, whether minor and occasional or serious or continual. The pressures on individual dentists against doing their part for the fulfillment of this aspect of the dental profession's obligations were discussed in chapters 9 and 12. But without a committed effort on the part of individual practitioners to contribute to the work of the profession in this way, the dental profession will not be able to fulfill this aspect of its obligation. It was for this reason that the idea was stressed in chapter 9 that every patient of any dentist is, in this respect, a patient of every other dentist, for every dentist is acting in the name of the Competence ascribed to the whole dental profession in this matter. Every dentist has an obligation to assure every patient of the profession that dental expertise will be appropriately used to the patient's benefit rather than misused.

A fourth and more subtle way in which the dental profession fulfills its obligations of Competence through the actions and judgments of its individual members and through its professional organizations concerns the theme of different philosophies of dental practice. The point was made in chapter 5 that, within the range of acceptable dental practice, there are a variety of philosophies of dental practice that a dentist may legitimately incorporate into his or her Preferred Patterns of Practice. Dentists are not automatons, and neither are patients. Both groups benefit, and the Oral and General Health of patients and their Autonomy are better served, when the profession supports different Preferred Patterns of Practice and different philosophies of dental practice, provided the profession's norms of Competence are observed.

In all four of these areas, individual dentists and dentistry's professional organizations have obligations to continue to assist the profession as a whole and, where necessary, to help it improve in its efforts to fulfill its obligations under the norm of Competence.

MORE ON THE CENTRAL PRACTICE VALUES

Another obvious component of the obligations of the dental profession as a whole concerns its efforts to achieve the Central Practice Values of Oral and General Health and support and enhance patients' Autonomy in oral health care outside the dental office.

With regard to Oral and General Health, the profession fulfills this obligation above all through the activities of every individual dentist and the members of his or her professional and nonprofessional staff who educate individual patients for self-care. It also fulfills this obligation through the educational efforts of its professional organizations and through other public health initiatives like support for the fluoridation of water supplies. The American Dental Association's program for evaluating and approving over-the-counter dental health products is another important example of an organizational effort that contributes to the profession's fulfillment of this aspect of its obligations.

It is worth noting that these efforts, whether of individual dentists or dental organizations, also support patients' Autonomy. For they provide patients with increased control over the challenges to oral health that can affect them, and they enable patients to exercise this control at their own convenience, in their own preferred manner, and in the exercise of their own understanding of what is involved rather than being dependent on another's expertise.

The sixth of dentistry's Central Practice Values, Efficiency in the Use of Professional Resources, has been mentioned only a few times since it was identified in chapter 5. The authors have assumed that such efficiency would be an automatic concern of dentists and patients alike because most dental practices are commercial enterprises and because most patients are concerned about the cost of their dental care. But when this Central Practice Value is considered from the perspective of the whole profession, an ethical concern arises that deserves special attention and that is closely connected to the theme of Availability of Services that will be discussed below.

For the most part, a society looks to the relevant professions to help determine whether its use of resources in one area of human life or another is efficient. The dental profession thus has a role in guiding the larger society to invest its health care resources, and particularly the resources it invests in oral health care, as wisely as possible and, at a deeper level, it must also help guide the society in determining what counts as more or less efficient uses of these resources. For example, the dental professions have been more committed to prevention and education for self-care longer than many of the other health professions in contemporary American society. This is, in part, out of a judgment that this emphasis makes the most efficient use of limited resources for dental care. For this reason the dental profession and the professional organizations that most frequently speak for the profession have a special obligation to guide society wisely in such matters. They must focus their assistance on the maximal health benefit for patients rather than the well-being of individual dentists, dental organizations, or the dental profession as a whole.

IDEAL RELATIONSHIPS BETWEEN CO-PROFESSIONALS AND OTHERS ASSISTING IN CARE

The theme of collaboration among health professionals that was stressed in chapter 8 applies at the level of the whole dental profession as well. America's health professions have a great deal in common (and will likely have more so if the larger community begins to make serious policy decisions regarding the limits of its resources for health care). But this society's health professions have unfortunately spent at least as much effort in political struggles for turf as they have in trying to learn from and support one another or in working to collaborate in achieving the elements of human health that are common among their goals and values.

Health is not neatly divisible into tidy, profession-specific components. Therefore, the dental profession's commitment to patients' Oral and General Health requires that the profession as a collective entity, again through the efforts of both individual dentists and dentistry's professional organizations, work toward increasing levels of cooperation with other health professions and other groups collaborating in the provision of health care. It is difficult to predict what such collaboration might yield, and it is difficult to predict how each health profession's understanding of itself might benefit from the health professions' efforts to work together and learn from one another. Each can surely learn much that is valuable from the others about the institution of profession and about the pursuit of people's health. But to date this learning is almost completely untapped. Therefore, the dental profession has an obligation to begin to make effective use of collaboration with the other health professions and health care occupations to carry out its social role more effectively.

AVAILABILITY OF SERVICES

As chapters 11 and 12 explained, it grows increasingly clear that health care resources are not unlimited, and one unfortunate result of this is the continuance of the pattern of very limited access to oral health services that many people in this society experience. Whether or not this concern will lead our society to an effective national plan for the distribution of health care resources, and whether or not such a plan will be responsive to the kinds of questions about ethical distribution raised in chapters 11 and 12, are questions well beyond the scope of this work. It is also not clear that such a plan would give appropriate prominence to the community's need for oral health care. But these remain important questions that dentists individually, and especially the dental profession collectively, ought to be asking. In particular, these questions and related questions about the typical ways in which today's dental resources are actually distributed ought to be on the agendas of dentistry's professional organizations.

If the dental profession, especially through its professional organizations, does not thoughtfully initiate such conversations, it is very likely that the initiative will be taken, if at all, by others less knowledgeable about what dental interventions can and cannot do and about what is at stake in oral health care. The dental profession is obligated as a whole to work for the availability of dental services for all those who need them, and this requires active and judicious advocacy on the part of the whole dental profession if it is to achieve this goal.

INTEGRITY AND PROFESSIONALISM
AND THE PRIORITY OF THE PATIENT

The obligation of each dentist, under the norm of Integrity and Professionalism, to practice in a manner consistent with the values and commitments of dentistry and to grow in professionalism has been stressed at many points in this book. The theme of personal self-formation and growth in professionalism will be the focus of chapter 15. But this obligation also carries an automatic reference to the dental profession as a whole, for it is the profession's values and commitments, not simply those of the dentist as a particular individual, to which the dentist is obligated to bear witness. But there is another way in which the obligations of Integrity and Professionalism concern the dental profession as a whole: The profession as a whole can also bear witness—or fail to bear witness—to dentistry's principal commitments, in particular those concerned with the theme of the priority of the patient and professional sacrifice discussed in chapter 6.

The obligations of individual dentists to represent the dental profession correctly, specifically in their business affairs, were discussed at length in chapters 10, 12, and 13. It is important that a dentist not communicate to the public that the principal determinant of dentists' treatment decisions and relationships with their patients is for economic gain but rather for the achievement of their patients' well-being, especially as it concerns the Central Practice Values and the ideal of an Interactive Relationship.

For the very same reasons, it is important that the dental profession as a collective entity both act in a manner and communicate to the public in a way that does not misrepresent dentistry's commitments to place patients' well-being and the health of the community ahead of other goals. Statements by dental organizations and their officers, and other dentists identified by the media as spokespersons or representatives for whatever reason, ought therefore to represent the commitments of dentistry accurately rather than presenting a picture of the profession as committed to something else, and the collective actions of dentists and dental organizations should be judged by the same standard.

One important role that dentistry's professional organizations can play in regard to members' growth in professionalism concerns the theme of collegiality that was discussed in regard to bad outcomes in chapter 9 and peer review in chapter 13. The competitive marketplace puts dentists into competition with one another, and our society's litigiousness supports a tendency to see other dentists as potential adversaries in court. But the bonds of shared expertise and shared commitments to dentistry's ethical norms are nevertheless a basis for collegiality among dentists that is often realized through the activities of their professional organizations. In addition, the obligation every dentist has to contribute to dentistry as a whole by responding appropriately to collective obligations can be fulfilled only by dentists working together and communicating and reflecting together on this work. Other groupings of dentists—study groups, shared efforts at charity care, and so forth—are important venues in which the ethical work of the whole profession can be collegially supported. But dentistry's professional organizations play a particularly important role in this precisely because they represent large groups of dentists, and, therefore, how they act is easily read as a mirror of what dentistry as a whole is committed to and stands for. One particular aspect of what dentistry's professional organizations communicate to the larger society about the profession as a whole deserves special attention and will be discussed in the next section.

PROFESSIONAL ORGANIZATIONS OR TRADE ASSOCIATIONS

The operative assumption about many organizations in American society is that they exist principally to serve the interests of their members as those individuals participate competitively in the commercial marketplace. Organizations of this sort will be treated collectively here under the label "trade associations" (although some of them might be formally known by other labels). Trade associations are organizations—that is, groups of individuals with important things in common—formed by self-interested individuals who are in competition with one another but who can each benefit by joining together and pooling certain of their resources in order to fulfill their self-interests. That is, there is no contradiction between how trade associations operate and the ways of thinking, valuing, and competing that are essential to the commercial marketplace in our society. Each member of a trade association aims to benefit himself or herself rather than giving priority to anyone else, which is how, as has been detailed elsewhere in this book, thinking, valuing, and competing in our society's commercial marketplace works. For even intense competitors can have interests in common about which they do not need to compete in order to compete more effectively in relation to other marketplace participants, especially the final consumers of what they sell.

But as has been stressed throughout this book, there are very important differences in the thinking, valuing, and acting between the commercial marketplace and the practice of a profession. Therefore, it is important, under the professional norm of Integrity and Professionalism, to determine if there are ways in which our society's dental professional organizations might be perceived as not being very different from trade associations and, if so, whether these perceptions might be correct.

There are at least three ways dentistry's professional organizations can give the impression that they are little different from trade associations. One of these is the tendency of dentistry's professional organizations to compete with one another for members and to struggle for power and influence within the dental community and in the eyes of the larger society. Trade associations compete in similar ways, but that is to be expected because trade associations are not primarily committed to the well-being of the consumers of whatever products or services their members sell. Both trade associations and professional organizations are better able to serve their members if they can grow their memberships and secure other forms of social influence, but serving its members' interests is not supposed to be the first priority of a dental professional organization.

In fact, dentistry could far more effectively challenge US patients' inadequate access to oral health care services and the second-class status of oral health among our society's health care goals if our society's dental professional organizations were more committed to cooperation than competition. There is also no good reason why one or another of our society's dental professional organizations should view itself as the best protector of dentistry's ethical commitments or the most important resource for dental ethics education. What is needed is collaboration. Enhancing practitioners' and students' ability to practice the profession's ethical standards is far too important an activity for it to be something that professional organizations compete over. Progress in each of these areas will continue to depend on every dental professional organization committing to collaboration marked by the organizational equivalent of selflessness because the primary purpose of a professional organization is not the benefit of the organization nor of its members. The primary purpose of every dental professional organization is the benefit first of all to those whom the profession has committed to serve, dentistry's current patients and all those with unmet oral health needs. This is why competition between dentistry's professional organizations sends a message to the larger society that these organizations are focused on goals other than people's oral health needs.

THE RELATIONSHIP BETWEEN DENTISTS AND THE LARGER COMMUNITY

The second way in which dental professional organizations can give the impression that they are little different from trade associations is in how they, as organizations, relate to the people they serve—that is, dentistry's patients and others in the society with oral health needs.

Many dental organizations engage in or support forms of dental education for patients and the larger society generally, and some of them receive and adjudicate patients' claims of being poorly served or even harmed by chairside dentists. These are valuable services, but they are both services in which the organization makes decisions based on its expertise and delivers these decisions to the nondentist community. That is, there is little evidence that our society's dental professional organizations have seriously considered that the norm of an Ideal Relationship between chairside dentist and patient might be mirrored in the relationship between the organization and the patients and others it serves.

Some dental organizations have made market focus groups, employed nondentist consulting specialists and professional lobbyists, and supported the appointment of nondentist members to some state boards. But as of this writing, dental organizations have rarely sought the input of members of the lay community they serve in their deliberations on any matter in ways that would conform to the Interactive Model. This includes many matters in which technical dental knowledge or practice experience are of little importance. For example, as was noted previously, the deliberations of dental organizations regarding the proper limits of ethical advertising by dentists, though they require information specifically about how nondentists understand and respond to dental advertising, have rarely brought nondentists into the conversation. That is, dental professional organizations have rarely viewed the general lay public as moral equals in the sense of being— as the Interactive Model aspires to—equally invested in the decisions to be made and equally qualified (though for different reasons) to be choosers in the matter. To put this point another way, the evidence suggests that the Guild Model is still the operative model of the relationship between dental professional organizations and the larger community.

The same thing can be said with regard to the work of the ethics committees of the various professional organizations. As has been stressed throughout this book, the ones who determine the professional obligations of the profession are the larger community in dialogue with the dental community. What makes up dentists' and dentistry's professional obligations, it has been argued, is of necessity the fruit of this dialogue if the obligations are to be meaningful at all. Yet, when formal conversations about ethical matters are held by dentistry's professional organizations, one party to that dialogue—the nondentist community—ordinarily goes without formal representation (other than through the occasional consideration of the views of nondentists who are academic specialists in ethics). If the Interactive Model of relationship is indeed the ideal relationship between those with dental expertise and those whom the profession serves, then the dental profession, through its professional organizations, ought to think seriously about applying it conscientiously to the profession's ongoing dialogue with the larger community.

This proposal does not claim to resolve the many difficult questions that will immediately arise about how this obligation, if it is indeed an obligation of the dental profession, ought to be carried out. Clearly, simply working through the most obvious channels within the larger community, such as its legislative or elected officials, is unlikely to answer the need. Nevertheless, however the details are resolved, we propose that a serious initiative to bring representatives of the larger community to whom the profession is committed to serving into active dialogue with the dental profession is in order.

What will be the topics of this dialogue? There may be many. But the most important topic of this dialogue, from the point of view of this book, will be determining the
contents of the professional obligations of dentists and the dental profession. This book
has attempted to identify the contents of these obligations as they currently exist. That
is, it aims to name and frame these obligations as they are currently delineated within the
ongoing dialogue. It aims to help that dialogue become much more explicit *as a dialogue*
and much more self-conscious on both sides.

But discussing the obligations of dentists and of the dental profession as these are currently understood is only half the task. The other half is to inquire whether the content
these obligations currently have matches the content they *ought* to have. This is a question that the dental community and the larger community in dialogue need to continu-
ously ask and keep on asking as the circumstances of social and professional life continue
to change. And, as stressed above, every particular instance of this dialogue needs to have
a formal role for representatives of those whom dentistry is committed to serving, not
only representatives of dentistry.

The larger community is, no doubt, so used to being excluded from dental organizations' processes and activities that it would be surprised to be invited and reminded that it
has an essential role to play. But this fact does not lessen the ethical importance of professional organizations doing so. In fact, it should be clear that such surprise on the part of
the larger community would confirm that those who are the "end users" of dental services
are fully accustomed to being excluded—except in some cases as passive recipients of education or juridical decisions or in other secondary roles—from the activities of dentistry's
professional organizations. This attitude may not itself prompt the larger community
to see likenesses between dental professional organizations and trade associations. But
in any situation in which such likenesses do appear—as in the aspects of contemporary
dentistry in our society examined in chapter 13—this way of viewing dental professional
associations will support rather than challenge that impression.

If dentistry really wants to impress on the larger community that it is a profession, it
will work hard to communicate with the larger community interactively. It is one thing
for individual patients and prospective patients to trust that, for the most part, dentists
hold their patients' Oral Health (and the profession's other Central Practice Values) as
their highest priority. But this does not automatically translate to the profession as a
whole. So dentistry's professional organizations need to energetically engage the larger
community to work with them toward creating a genuine Interactive Relationship in
order to make it clear to the larger community that the goals of the dental professional
organizations and of dentistry as a whole are indeed the well-being of the people dentistry serves.

THINKING ABOUT THE CASE

The third way in which dental professional organizations can give the impression that
they are not very different from trade associations is in their relationships, especially
their financial relationships, to players in the commercial marketplace. The case at the

beginning of this chapter has been crafted to make the problem of association with the commercial marketplace extreme because the issue is whether the product that would secure important advertising revenue could actually support and mask substandard dentistry.

It is reasonable to assume that dental organizations do, in fact, avoid associations with commercial vendors whose products would violate dentistry's commitment to competent practice (in addition to protecting themselves from the legal risk involved). But that does not address the question of the impression the public might well receive if they saw the huge convention display halls filled with dental equipment and supplies, tables of gifts for dentists who are potential purchasers, and the often posh environments in which dental and professional meetings are held or if they were aware of the separate side meetings at these conventions that focus on profit-making or the intense marketing done by business and marketing firms that target their message at dentists or if they learned that the same kinds of language and the same assumptions about dentist-readers' goals are to be found in the ads of most dental professional organizations' journals. All of these scenarios suggest that the thinking, values, and decisions of the commercial marketplace are not only alive and well in the world of dentistry but that they are the dominant ways of thinking, valuing, and acting.

Of course, dental professional organizations *say* their primary goal is the well-being of dentistry's patients and the Oral Health of the community as a whole. But so do many organizations whose actual and obvious goal is to further the interests of their members and to make money for their owners or stockholders. The issue for dentistry's professional organizations is how to meet financial goals while still carefully evaluating every organizational action on the basis of dentistry's ethical norms and professionalism so that their actions do not risk undermining the public's view of dentistry as a profession.

The final decision in the case presented clearly depends on a number of important technical judgments being made in accord with the norm of Competence. These concern exactly what Capwright does and exactly what effect using the product might have on how dentists prep patients' teeth for the fabrication of dental and oral prostheses. But these technical judgments will not themselves resolve the ethical questions in the case.

If the product is in fact beneficial to patient care, the associate editor is correct in proposing that the adoption of this bonding material could change the standard of practice regarding preparations by gradually shifting the point at which general dentists might refer a case to a prosthodontist or allow assistants to aid them at chairside. This is an example of the point stressed previously in this chapter that determinations of competent practice by the dental profession affect what counts as Oral Health in the society and who should be allowed to be the professional experts for this kind of issue. But then the associate editor's suggestion that making such shifts is inappropriate would be incorrect. Instead, the relevant question remains whether patient health will be significantly affected for the worse or, if there is some slight loss of benefit or increase in risk of complications, whether that negative outcome can reasonably be outweighed by a gain in efficiency in the use of dental care resources (i.e., by making certain kinds of care more accessible to patients in general dentists' offices). The case as presented does not offer enough detailed clinical information to decide this matter here. It simply identifies the nature and ethical importance of these questions.

On the other hand, the managing editor is surely incorrect to suggest that decisions about such matters belong solely in the hands of dentists at chairside. The obligation to play a role in guiding the dental profession so it acts ethically—in this case, to properly evaluate a new dental product—is an obligation of chairside dentists. But it is at least equally the obligation of those assigned relevant roles within organized dentistry, with researchers and the technical editors and staff members of research journals having a particularly important responsibility in such matters. The editor in chief of *AJDP* is surely not mandated to make these important technical judgments alone. But he or she is surely mandated to play an important role in them, often enough as the final arbiter, at least from the point of view of publication, of whether the judgments of many different evaluators should be taken to support presenting a new product to the dental community as beneficial to patients or whether he or she should decline to do so.

Thus, this case suggests many difficult questions about competent dentistry and about those who have significant roles to play in confirming (or not) which technologies and products and procedures constitute Competence in the dental community. Some of the questions cannot be resolved here because the case does not provide enough technical data about Capwright. Other questions depend not on details of the case but on views about the proper interplay of various roles within the dental community in fulfilling the dental profession's obligations with regard to Competence and about what counts as Oral Health. While this commentary cannot explore these questions further, they deserve careful reflection both by individual dentists and by the professional organizations within which such special roles are ordinarily assigned.

This case also raises questions about the message that the American College of Fixed and Removable Prosthodontics (ACFRP) and its journal send to the larger community about what the dental profession is committed to and stands for. Of course, very few members of the larger community will even know this organization and this journal exist. But dentistry's norm of Integrity and Professionalism does not say that this is only a commitment for dentists and organizations who happen to be prominent in the public's eye. Every dentist and every dental professional organization has an obligation to ask about everything they do, whether it confirms what dentistry as a profession stands for or raises questions about it.

So again, the question must be asked whether ACFRP—or any other dental professional organization—exists primarily to further the interests and efforts only of the prosthodontists that make up its membership (so that, for example, if using Capwright reduced the number of referrals from general dentists to prosthodontists, publishing the ad would be inappropriate). The managing editor proposes, by contrast, that the association and its journal exist to improve the quality of dental care wherever it is given. Which message about ACFRP will be communicated to its readers if the ad is accepted?

What about the financial security of the journal? Does the managing editor speak against dentistry's commitment to the priority of patients' well-being in proposing that this lucrative ad copy will enable the journal to survive and continue its tradition of service to its readership? May the editor ethically publish advertising copy if he or she judges it to be, if not harmful to patients, at least questionable from the point of view of competent practice? Would publishing the ad in such a case be justifiable if doing so actually preserves the journal from perishing when it provides important services to dentists in their care of patients? Or must questionable advertising copy be rejected in the name of patients' Oral and General Health, even if these might actually suffer in time if the journal's research and other services were less available?

We do not propose that these are easy questions to answer (although they might become easier if the final technical data about Capwright points in one direction rather than another). The point is rather to notice that such organizational questions are, just as much as chairside issues are, important questions of professional ethics in dentistry. Every dentist, not just those in special roles within organized dentistry, ought to reflect on these issues, for the future of dentistry depends on the profession making sure that potential similarities between dental professional organizations and trade associations, together with the ways in which chairside dentists can appear to be participating more in commercial marketplace relationships than in the professional care of patients, are countered with clear messages that dentistry, both at chairside and collectively, is still rightly considered a profession.

15

⬡⬡⬡⬡⬡⬡

Self-Formation and Dentistry's Future: Professionalism or Commercialism

The point was made in chapter 1 that the decisions a dentist or a dental student makes involve not only questions about "oughts" and "shoulds" but also questions like "What kind of dentist am I? What kind of dentist do I want to become? What kind of person am I? What kind of person do I want to become?" Throughout this book, the concept of *professionalism* has been invoked to remind the reader of the importance of these questions. A few suggestions have been made about growing in professionalism. But there are ways to make one's reflections on these questions more and more formative of how one lives and practices as a professional. For the sake of dentistry's future—as well as to try to help every dentist and every dental student keep growing as a dental professional—this final chapter will focus on the process of self-formation in professionalism.

Professionalism was described in chapter 1 as the internalized and habitual ways of thinking and acting that characterize the life and practice of the most admirable members of the profession. This is an aspirational concept, one that identifies a long-range goal. But that does not mean it is something that a dentist should attend to later rather than now. Rather, it is something to be reflected on and actively aspired to from the first days of dental school—or even before—until the last days of one's professional career. But what professionalism as a goal means and what it asks of the dental student is not the same as what it means and asks of the dentist in the first years of practice or of the more mature career dentist now well experienced in caring for patients.

This chapter will try to describe what professionalism as a goal means and what it asks during each of these stages of personal and professional development. It will also try to describe what needs to be learned and practiced and turned into a habit at each stage in order to be ready to move into the next stage. In addition, it will describe some of the most obvious challenges to growing in professionalism that are relevant to each stage in the process.

Many of these challenges connect with the book's numerous contrasts of dentistry's ethical norms and commitment to professionalism with the ways of thinking, valuing, and acting characteristic of the competitive commercial marketplace. These contrasts are important for two reasons related to the theme of growth in professionalism. First, as explained in chapter 10, the dental landscape has changed greatly since the final decades of the twentieth century. Some of these changes, in the science and technology of oral health care, have resulted in significant improvements in dentists' ability to respond to patients' dental needs. But many of these changes have incorporated the attitudes and activities of the commercial marketplace and brought them into much closer contact with the provision of professional dental care than was previously the case. These changes have brought new challenges to dentists at every stage of their growth in professionalism. They require dentists to think more carefully and more often about how to stay true to dentistry's ethical commitments to the larger community. As previous chapters have often noted, these changes have also added greatly to the urgency with which dentists must ask "What kind of message does the influence of the commercial marketplace on my practice send to the larger community?" For dentistry's authority and status as a profession depends on the larger community continuing to see a sharp contrast between dentistry's professionalism and the commercialism of the marketplace.

A second reason for stressing the difference between dentistry's ethical norms and commitment to professionalism with the ways of thinking, valuing, and acting in the competitive commercial marketplace is the fact that this book will likely have some use in educating dental students in ethics and professionalism. That is, it would be a mistake for this book to not look to the future of dentistry as well as its present and recent past.

There is a strong tendency for many people who are growing into a complex social role to focus on learning and habituating the technical skills necessary to practice it effectively and, in matters of ethics and conduct, to regard the practice of the role's established members as simply the way such things are done. But there are a number of patterns of practice in US dentistry today that, even if not strictly violating dentistry's ethical norms, are at serious risk of sending a commercial message about dentistry to the larger society. It is important that dentists entering the profession, those still in their early years of practice, and also those who are well experienced to take serious note of this issue and begin thinking carefully about how to address it. For dentistry's authority and status as a profession depends on the larger community continuing to see a sharp contrast between dentistry's professionalism and the commercialism of the marketplace.

These are challenging times for every one of the professions, and this is especially true for dentistry. Everyone who hopes to grow in dental professionalism needs to learn to look beyond his or her own development and reflect carefully on the impact of his or her actions on the future of dentistry. In addition, if there are any in dentistry who look at the description of professionalism and conclude that it is permanently beyond their reach or who have somehow entered the profession without a concern for its commitment to ethics and professionalism, they too should take these challenges seriously if they want there to be a dental profession where they can continue to practice in the future.

A CASE FOR CONSIDERATION: FEAR OF DROWNING

Jonathan Levinson is an eight-year-old patient who recently came to the practice of Dr. Nathan Silverman. From his first visit to a dentist at age four until two months ago, Jonathan's dentist has been a young pedodontist, Dr. Edwin Samuels. Jonathan's parents find Dr. Samuels considerate and caring, and a neighbor had recommended him, so they assumed that Jonathan would relate to him easily, just as they had when interviewing him. But Jonathan claims from the first visit that Dr. Samuels is "mean" and "doesn't like me." Every checkup is resisted, and it takes great persistence by Jonathan's parents to get him to go. Routine diagnostic work and prophylaxis in the office are traumatic, and restorative work requires one or both of Jonathan's parents to be at chairside restraining him. Eventually, Dr. Samuels speaks to Jonathan's parents after a particularly difficult visit and recommends that they call Dr. Silverman.

"Dr. Silverman is one of my heroes," Dr. Samuels explains to Jonathan's parents. "He was a young pedodontist when I was a kid and my parents just happened to take me to him. I didn't give dentists trouble when I was young, but as I grew up I became aware that many kids needed a dentist with a special gift for reaching them, and Dr. Silverman has it. He is one of the reasons I am a pedodontist. I think about him often and I hope that someday I will be able to help kids the way he does. So I'm sure he will know how to help Jonathan."

Jonathan's mother mentions to Dr. Silverman's receptionist that Dr. Samuels has recommended that they contact Dr. Silverman and that Dr. Samuels has found Jonathan "difficult," even though he is a very nice child. This prompts Dr. Silverman to call Dr. Samuels to talk about Jonathan.

"Both of Jonathan's parents have high dental anxiety," says Dr. Samuels. "I think they passed it on to Jonathan unconsciously before he ever set foot in my office. He was distrustful from the start. I talked to him a lot, as I do with all my patients, explaining things and trying everything I could to get him to relax in the chair, but I'm afraid he had it in for me from day one.

"He would clamp his mouth shut, turn his head away, even push me away with his arms, just for routine probing and examinations of his dentition. Heaven help us when it came to cleaning! He wouldn't actually push Joyce away, maybe because she is a woman, but he would shout and yell out whenever he could feel her instruments touching tissue of any sort. Thank goodness I didn't have to do much restorative work, even though his hygiene was not very good. He must have very strong enamel. But when restorations were needed, he would resist and resist until finally I would give up and bring in his mother or father—once, actually, both of them—to try to calm him down and a couple of times to actually hold him down so I could get the work done. After a few rounds of that—plus he's eight years old now, and you'd expect more understanding and self-control—I decided I'd better refer him to you. He needs someone with a lot more experience than I have at this point."

"Well, we certainly need to find other ways to help him," says Dr. Silverman. "Thanks for sending his records over. I'm going to see him tomorrow afternoon."

"Well, I wish you luck with Jonathan," says Dr. Samuels. "Starting over with a new dentist is probably a good idea in any case, and he's a pretty smart kid. But you're the best pedodontist I know, so I hope it goes well."

"Thanks for the compliment, Ed," says Dr. Silverman. "I'll do my best."

At his first visit, Dr. Silverman meets Jonathan in the waiting room, shakes his hand and his father's, and invites Jonathan into his office. "These are more comfortable chairs for talking," he says, "and I'd like to get an idea of what you think of dentists before we talk about anything else."

Jonathan's opinion of dentists is not very high. Dr. Silverman asks him what he thinks of regular dental self-care and whether he has ever had a toothache and what that was like.

Jonathan admits that he has had a couple of toothaches and doesn't like them and that Dr. Samuels's work had ended the pain. He says that he knows brushing his teeth is something he should do, but he says he doesn't like having anything in his mouth except food, so he only brushes his teeth when his mother or father are actually watching him, and that still makes him gag.

"Does it hurt your mouth to have a toothbrush in it?" asks Dr. Silverman. "I only ask because a lot of people, even people with very small mouths, don't usually find it a problem. Do you have any idea why it bothers you?"

"When I was four," says Jonathan, "I fell off a pier where I was playing with my friends at a lake, and I almost drowned. Whenever anything blocks up my mouth, I think about that and it scares me and it makes me gag. I was really scared. I was under the water a long time, and I couldn't breathe."

"That sounds terrible," says Dr. Silverman. "You must have been very frightened. How were you saved? Did someone dive in and pull you out, your parents or someone?"

"My parents never knew about it. I haven't told anyone about it before you because when I got out—I finally climbed up the logs that made up the pier—I was screaming that I almost drowned and my friends were laughing at me. They said that the water was only up to my waist, but I was so bent over that I just thought I was drowning, and all I had to do was stand up. They thought it was funny. So I never told anyone about it. I was really scared, but I thought anyone else would just laugh at me like they did."

"Well, I appreciate your telling me about it, Jonathan," says Dr. Silverman. "I certainly can understand how frightened you were, no matter how deep the water was. Not being able to breathe is one of the most terrifying things that can happen to a human being. I am very sorry that your friends laughed at you; they certainly wouldn't have laughed if the same thing had happened to them. It was mean of them to laugh at it."

"That's how I felt," says Jonathan. "But I couldn't tell anyone. If they had been there, maybe they would have understood, but I figured anyone else would just laugh at me."

"Would you be willing to try out some special, small-sized toothbrushes that I've got? We could try them out here, where you can experiment without anyone knowing, and if we can find a brush that's comfortable for you, you can just take it home and use it and no one will ever know that you were really concerned about suffocating. Would that be a good idea?"

Jonathan agrees and follows Dr. Silverman into one of the operatories, where Dr. Silverman pulls out a box of toothbrushes of different sizes and styles. Jonathan experiments with a couple of them and finds one he is comfortable with. Dr. Silverman asks him if he would mind hopping into the chair so he could take a quick look to see how hard he would need to brush, since Jonathan hadn't been doing it very regularly lately. "I won't put any instruments in your mouth, I promise. You just open wide and I'll take a look around," Dr. Silverman says. Jonathan gets into the chair and opens his mouth.

"Well, everything I can see looks pretty good, Jonathan. Why don't you take a look?" He gives Jonathan a mirror so he can look into his own wide-open mouth.

"Now I want to show you something, back here in my office," Dr. Silverman says. They return to the more comfortable chairs. "What you saw in the mirror is just what I saw, looking in. It's pretty much what you can see if I hold this model of a set of teeth right in front of you, except this doesn't have any cheeks in the way. But let me ask you something, how would you go about looking at the back side of the teeth."

Jonathan reaches out to turn the model around, and Dr. Silverman says with a laugh, "You're now looking through the back of this patient's head. I haven't had a patient yet that would let me do that. What do you think?"

"I don't know," says Jonathan.

"Do you think it would be good if a dentist could see the back sides of the teeth?"

"Sure," says Jonathan. "What if they have something wrong with them?"

"Right! Now let me show you something else," says Dr. Silverman, picking up a pediatric mouth mirror. "This mirror is actually smaller than that toothbrush you chose, but it is plenty big enough to let you see most of the back of the teeth. Here, try it."

Jonathan inspects the back of the model's teeth using the mirror. "Let me ask you something, Jonathan," says Dr. Silverman. "The next time you come in, could I use a mirror like this to look at the back sides of your teeth, to make sure there's nothing wrong with them?"

"You can look right now if you want," says Jonathan.

"Are you sure?"

"Yeah. But do I have to sit in that weird chair in the other room? It smells funny in there."

"If you wouldn't mind," says Dr. Silverman. "I know it's a strange chair and the room smells funny. The smell is because of what we have to clean it with, and the chair has a special light we can use to see into your mouth. Regular room lights don't light up the inside of your mouth enough."

They return to the operatory and Dr. Silverman inspects Jonathan's teeth with the mirror, reporting in detail on what he sees, which is a mouth in need of cleaning but otherwise nothing that needs immediate attention.

"I have some more instruments here in this cabinet," says Dr. Silverman, "all of them smaller than that toothbrush. If it turns out—after you try it out at home—that the toothbrush is okay to use, then I'd like to ask you to come back and I can show you how some of these other instruments are useful for checking out your teeth, too."

Jonathan nods.

"So you'd be willing to come back and see how I can use them? This one we use to give teeth a special cleaning. You probably saw one like it before. If you are comfortable with it when you come back, cleaning your teeth would be a very good idea, and we can talk about preventing new cavities. But I promise you that I will not put any instrument or anything else in your mouth that makes you uncomfortable or that you don't understand what it's for and what job we're going to do with it. Would that be something you'd be willing to come back for in a couple of weeks so we can give it a try?"

Jonathan nods but then looks at the toothbrush in his hand and studies it for a moment. Then he says, "That's okay, but can we talk in your regular office first, in the comfortable chairs?" he asks.

"Sure," says Dr. Silverman.

Two months pass. Jonathan completes four visits to the dentist. He receives a complete prophylaxis, sealants, and a small restoration on one of his deciduous molars. His oral hygiene is now very good, and he chats comfortably with Dr. Silverman at each visit about his many interests—school, sports, and stamp collecting—and also about his desire to learn to swim some day.

SELF-FORMATION IN PROFESSIONALISM: THE FIRST STEPS

Professionalism is the internalized and habitual ways of thinking and acting that characterize the life and practice of the most admirable members of the profession. This is not something that a dental student can accomplish in the four years of dental school. It is, in fact, something that even the most committed dental student will only accomplish years into the future. Besides, a lot of a dental student's time and attention is—and should be—focused on learning the information and developing the technical skills needed to graduate and be authorized to practice without supervision. But this does not mean that a dental student does not need to do anything about growing in professionalism. There are some "first steps" in the process of growing in professionalism that every dental student needs to take in order to be ready for the "next steps" that characterize the work of professionalism for the now-graduated dentist in the first years of practice. There are five of these "first steps": (1) a preliminary step that ideally happens before the student begins dental school; (2) a factual learning step; (3) a habit-forming step; (4) a reflective, "exploratory" step; and (5) a self-assessment step that, ideally, has begun to become a habit by the end of dental school.

The preliminary step is for the person who is going to strive for professionalism in dentistry or any other profession to establish a *personal ethical commitment* to *keep the commitments he or she makes*. Becoming a professional means making a commitment to the larger community—and also to the other members of the profession—to conform one's conduct to the ethical standards of the profession. A person who comes to dental school because he or she wants to have a career with a lot of independence, likes hard work, can get along with people or even enjoys helping them, and wants to make a good living—or just some combination of these reasons—but who is not committed to keeping the commitments he or she makes cannot be a dentist. They may pass through dental school successfully, graduate, get licensed, and start practicing. But this person would not be a professional and therefore would not be a dentist, for a professional is someone who makes a commitment to the larger society to live and practice in a certain way, and dentists are professionals who are committed to living and practicing in accord with dentistry's ethical norms and its commitment to professionalism.

Obviously, any dental student who arrives at dental school without already having fulfilled this preliminary step needs to do some serious thinking about whether he or she really wants to be a professional and a member of the dental profession. If so, learning what it means to make a personal ethical commitment and what keeping the commitments one makes requires of a person needs to be the student's first and most important goal (and if learning these things requires others' help, the student needs to seek that help out right away).

It is beyond the scope of this book to survey the ethical standards appropriate to the role of being a student and a member of a group of students studying and learning together. But it is important to point out that there are such standards and that failure to live and learn according to them is likely to be an indicator of how genuinely a student is committed to keeping the commitments he or she makes. For related reasons, since this commitment is a prerequisite to the student's truly becoming a professional, a school that responds merely punitively to a student's shortfalls in this respect, rather than framing the response in accord with that student developing such a commitment, is probably missing an opportunity to guide the student more constructively.

Once this "preliminary step" is in place, the student is ready to begin the factual learning step—that is, to learn the *ethical minimums* of the dental profession. This is a *factual* learning step because students will not be able to form habits of conforming to the ethical minimums (i.e., the next step in the process) unless they know what the ethical minimums are. They also will not have the intellectual background they need to understand the more complex ethical questions that practice situations will present them with or to develop more complex ethical habits to respond properly to these situations without knowing what the minimal ethical expectations of the profession are.

There is a myth that is held by many people—including many professionals and, unfortunately, by some of the people involved in professional ethics education—namely, that ethics is supposed to be simple and ethical habits are supposed to be simple to develop. This is plain nonsense, as anyone who has thought carefully about ethical issues that arise in dental practice knows from experience. The only things that are simple about dentistry's ethics are *some* of the statements of *some* of dentistry's *ethical minimums*, examples of which can be found in the American Dental Association's *Principles of Ethics and Code of Professional Conduct* (hereafter ADA Code) and in other dental organizations' codes and in the chapters of this book. But many of the ethical minimums in the codes or in this book cannot be stated simply. In this book, for example, consider the Interactive Relationship, the ranking of dentistry's Central Practice Values, and the Relative Priority of the Patient's Well-Being. These are ethical minimums, but they are far too complex to state simply. Similarly, in section 4.C, "Justifiable Criticism," in the ADA Code, how is "justifiable" to be understood? *Justifiable* is hardly a simple concept. Neither is what counts as "false or misleading" in the description of norm 5-E on professional announcements easily understood, and so on.

The reality is that developing an adequate factual understanding of dentistry's ethical minimums—that is, just learning what they require and what the words stating them mean in relation to the ethically simplest situations in dental practice, requires genuine effort, discussion of actual cases in detail, and, ideally, identifying and weighing the reasons *why* these norms are the ones that the dental profession and the larger community in dialogue have adopted for dentists to live and practice by.

The third component of these "first steps" in self-formation in professionalism is that, once they are caring for patients, the students must not only act in accord with the ethical minimums but must also begin to deliberately form *ethical habits* so their practice is dependably shaped by them. That is, it is not enough that dental students only understand what the ethical minimums are and how they apply in simple instances of dental practice; it is necessary that they begin to form habits of acting accordingly.

Dental education is deliberately designed so dental students *habituate* the basic technical knowledge and skills that are needed for safe and effective care of patients. This is because only if these things have become habitual can the dentist be depended on to respond properly in real time to the technical needs of the specific patient and oral cavity in front of him or her. As chapter 1 and other parts of this book have stressed, the same is true regarding the formation of ethical habits of living and practice according to dentistry's ethical minimums. Only if these become habitual aspects of the student's practice can that student be depended on to respond properly in real time to the ethical requirements of caring for and relating properly to the specific patient and situation in front of him or her. It takes time and practice, as well as the kind of self-assessment that comprises the fifth component of these first steps to self-formation as a professional, to develop such habits, so the goal here is to *begin* to deliberately form *ethical habits* because it would be a mistake to think that this process will be fully completed by the time the students graduate.

The fourth component of self-formation in professionalism for dental students involves deliberately "exploring" among the dentists (or other persons) known to the student to identify admirable exemplars of professionalism and then begin the "reflection" on what aspects of these persons and/or their practice of dentistry makes them admirable. The goal is for the student to begin to build up an imaginative "picture," as well as actual memories, of the characteristics that the student might, over time, imitate and, if appropriate, make habitual in order to grow in professionalism themselves. (This kind of reflection, if directed at exemplars of ethically inappropriate conduct but with sympathy rather than anger, can also enhance the student's understanding of what professionalism requires. But positive examples are more constructive for growth than negative ones.)

Those who teach and administer in dental schools or interact with dental students in other capacities should be sensitive to this component of the future dentist's growth. While presuming that one is invariably an admirable role model is probably a sign that one isn't, it is always worth keeping in mind that the students are not only watching but *should be* watching and remembering. This should motivate faculty, administrators, and other staff to deliberately pay attention to their own conduct and ask whether it conforms to the same ethical standards and aspirational goals they hope the students will adopt.

For the same reason, it is important for faculty, staff, and especially administrators to remember that how the institution and its policies deal with students should also model what they hope the students are learning about ethics and professionalism.

The fifth component of the "first steps" of dental students' formation in professionalism is a self-assessment step that, ideally, has become a habit by the end of dental school. This is the most forward looking of the five components because all further growth in professionalism throughout the dentist's career depends on it. What the activity of self-assessment consists of is for the student to regularly—and to have the best results, daily—stop to ask how effectively he or she is achieving the other four components of professional growth at this stage of his or her life as a dental professional. The student who is conscientious about growing in professionalism will regularly assess how well he or she is learning the ethical minimums in order to employ them in practice, how successful he or she has been (since the last assessment) in making conformity to the ethical minimums a matter of habit, and what he or she is learning by searching for exemplars of professionalism and reflecting on what has been learned from them.

In addition, because habituating this activity of self-assessment is itself a goal of the first steps of growth in professionalism, the student needs to regularly *assess* his or her efforts at self-assessment and the self-criticisms and self-commendations to which they lead. Such self-assessment of efforts at self-assessment, especially if reinforced by successful growth and appropriate experiences of productive self-correction and positive continuations, can make it possible for truly constructive (versus guilt-producing) self-assessment to itself to become habitual for the student by the end of dental school. For if the press of daily activities causes this periodic self-assessment to temporarily disappear from the student's life, it and its benefits will be missed and will need to be reinstituted.

Those who teach professional ethics and professionalism in the dental schools would do well to note the importance of helping young dentists learn the skills of self-assessment, self-criticism and self-commendation. Many young adults have had little opportunity to learn these skills outside of punitive contexts or, at least, a focus on guilt for one's faults. Providing supportive training in these skills is likely to prove very useful to the learners when they are practicing independently and, in many cases, in settings in which communicating with others about such matters is difficult.

The most direct challenge to growing in these five ways during dental school is the pressure to master the technical information and skills needed to graduate and become authorized to practice without supervision. Today's dental school education is extremely expensive, and most dental students feel the burden of huge indebtedness well before they graduate and are expected to begin paying the debts off. In addition, their hope for—and the difficulties of finding—a good position in which to begin practicing after graduation only adds to these concerns, which are certainly related to and often experienced as pressures to be successful in the dental marketplace. Stories by practicing dentists who teach in the dental school about the challenges of succeeding in the dental marketplace even after obtaining a position can further reinforce the feeling that growing in dental professionalism will have to be put in second place, at least until the young dentist is fairly well established, if that can ever happen.

So the dental student's efforts to form himself or herself in professionalism may appear to be doomed by pressures from outside the dental school that the student will face soon enough and the student's current sense of indebtedness. It takes considerable courage and commitment on the part of a dental student to take advantage of the four years of dental school to try to build up enough knowledge and habitual practice of ethical conduct and habits of self-assessment and self-formation before these pressures make themselves fully felt. It is also important for the faculty and administrators and the practicing dentists who interact with dental students during these years to recognize that doing this does take courage and to commend it. They need to focus on supporting students' growth in professionalism rather than increasing the impact of their fears with stories about the pressures that await them.

The suggestion sometimes heard (and echoed in Dr. Prentice's comments to Jack Williamson in the case in chapter 2) that growing in professionalism in dental school is not practical or realistic—severely misrepresents the reality of becoming a professional. Rather, dental students should be encouraged to do as much growing in professionalism as possible while in dental school so that when they are out in actual practice they will be more likely to have the resources they need to stay true to their professional commitments to the larger community—and to other dentists and the dental profession as a whole—to dependably live and practice according to dentistry's ethical standards.

THE FIRST YEARS OF PRACTICE

During the first years of practice, the young dentist will find that the technical knowledge and skills needed to care safely, effectively, and ethically for patients will solidify into highly dependable habits, so maximizing dentistry's Central Practice Values will get easier. This will also make more and more energy and attention available to them to deal effectively with circumstances that are unusual or particularly complex in ordinary dentistry. They will encounter patients of many different types and personalities. They will grow familiar with adapting their communication skills to work with a wide range of patient types effectively, achieving the fullness of the Interactive Relationship with some and getting as close to that goal as possible with many. If all goes well for them, they will also be able to pay off some of their debts while supporting themselves and those they are responsible for in fairly dependable ways. And over time, each of these achievements will become more and more secure.

But what about their growth in professionalism? They will in fact be facing the fiscal pressures mentioned above. For some of them, the optimistic scenario of the previous paragraph wherein they are able to pay down their debts and earn a living may not pan out so dependably. In addition, the elements of the commercial marketplace described in chapters 10 and 13 may have become part of their daily lives. So at a minimum, the dentist in the first years of practice must certainly begin asking the question posed throughout chapter 13 and many other times in this book: Is the message I am sending to the larger community one that puts the emphasis on dentistry as a profession or one that makes people wonder if dentistry is becoming just another player in the commercial marketplace?

Regularly asking this question and applying the skills of self-assessment described above is the first component of what growth in professionalism requires of the dentist during the first years of practice. It is the version of the "What kind of dentist am I?" and "What kind of dentist do I want to be?" questions that gets at the details of daily practice most concretely. Moreover, asking this question and responding accordingly may be made more complex if the dentist is practicing as someone else's employee in those first years. This is because deciding what to do about any mirroring of the commercial marketplace in the practice may be done exclusively or almost exclusively by the owner(s). Asking this question effectively may require learning how to prompt someone else to ask it. Initiating a proper response may require skillful communication with an employer about what might need changing, either in what is in fact being done or in how it is being communicated to the public so that the message being sent about dentistry is more appropriate.

The processes of self-formation in professionalism that begins in dental school also needs to be continued and built on. The component of learning dentistry's ethics should be continued by deepening one's understanding not only of the ethical minimums but also of the ethics of more complex clinical situations—especially, of course, if the dentist is encountering these in practice. This may be through continuous education programs or making use of the print and online resources that are available for ethics self-education; it may be through a study group, especially if one can be found or formed to focus on cases embedded with complex ethical issues. But however it is done, a dentist who is now encountering more complex clinical situations should not assume that the dental student's level of ethical knowledge will be sufficient to meet his or her needs in practice. (Of course, if the dentist realizes that what should have been learned about the ethical minimums in dental school is in fact missing, then that would be the place to start.)

It goes without saying that besides learning the standards of dental ethics at a more sophisticated level, the dentist should also be reinforcing the habits of practicing ethically that are initially learned in the clinic so that practicing in conformity with dentistry's ethical commitments becomes more and more "second nature" for the dentist. Thus, as the dentist grows in habitual ethical practice, he or she will also become more and more sensitive to subtler ethical questions, a sensitivity that, ideally, should motivate additional efforts at learning.

The practicing dentist is very likely to recognize early on that he or she needs someone to talk with about the ethically challenging matters that arise. Many dentists who have spouses or life partners turn to them for someone to dialogue with about such situations. For many, these conversations become an important component of the process of self-assessment described earlier, especially when they can be conducted in a genuinely supportive environment. Dentists who do not have the benefit of dialogue "at home" in this way should consider identifying dental colleagues or sympathetic friends with whom such conversations can be safely (and with appropriate commitments to confidentiality) undertaken. But this does not mean that personal efforts are no longer needed for regular, even daily, self-assessment, self-commendation with a view to making a habit of what is working well, and self-criticism and imaginative work toward self-correction.

The activity of seeking positive role models described as exploratory and reflective in the section on dental students is one that the dentist in early years of practice should continue. With any luck it will be easier for the dentist in practice than for a student to find role models because the dentist in practice, through local or regional professional organizations, informal study groups, community programs, and so forth, will ordinarily have more opportunities to meet and reflect on the characteristics of more experienced dentists. In addition, the dentist who gradually builds up experience over several years is likely—even if encountering no admirable exemplars—to begin to construct in his or her imagination a "picture" of an admirable member of the profession that, through self-assessment and efforts at personal growth in professionalism, the dentist can aspire to imitate.

Why stress the ways in which self-formation in professionalism can happen most effectively as the years of practice build up? One reason is that there will be plenty of other challenges during these years, especially for dentists who have young children, aging parents, or other weighty responsibilities outside their dental practice. The other reason relates to two themes that have been stressed often in these pages but have special bearing on the topic of continual self-formation in professionalism: patient trust and the message dentists send to the larger society. Very few people who think about it carefully would expect that a recently graduated dentist would already be fully formed in professionalism. So what would their likely reaction be if a dentist said to each new patient, "Now that I am in practice, I don't have to worry any more about growing in my skills and my conduct as a professional. I mastered all that in school and I've fine-tuned it now in practice. I'm a fully formed professional and consider myself the equal of the most experienced and admired members of the profession!"

No dentist would say this, of course. Thoughtful, ethical dentists would know that they still have growing to do. But the other reason for not saying it is the view that such a dentist's patients would form about him or her and the message that such a statement would send to the larger society about dentistry. It's possible that the dentist's patients might not doubt his or her basic competence or ability to avoid violating dentistry's most basic ethical standards (Trust That and Trust What). But there is little chance that they would trust such a person to be already fully committed to the priority of his or her patients' well-being (Trust the Person). In a similar way, such a statement would challenge dentistry's claim that, as a profession, it differs sharply from the marketplace because it can be trusted (Trust the Person) to give priority to the well-being of all those it serves. Actualizing that kind of professional commitment—and therefore earning that kind of trust as an individual dentist and as a profession—depends on continual growth in professionalism: each year, each month, each day.

THE MATURE, WELL-EXPERIENCED DENTIST

If the mature, well-experienced dentist has continued his or her learning about ethics and regularly dialogued with colleagues about complex ethical questions that arise in practice, the natural next step would be for this dentist to begin to teach about ethical practice, either at a dental school, by hosting a study group, through a continuing education program, or in some other way. A number of dental journals have occasional articles or regular features on dental ethics where such a person's insights might be most welcome. On the other hand, if the ethics learning of the previous stages of professional growth has not been completed, this dentist should start there.

Further reinforcement of even well-established ethical practice habits needs to continue through continued self-assessment. And if the growth processes appropriate to earlier stages of self-formation have not been accomplished, then they need the dentist's attention now. But if this dentist's ethical practice habits are indeed well established—and his or her technical skills similarly—and trusted colleagues confirm the dentist's self-assessments in these respects, then he or she might make an excellent chairside mentor at a dental school. This is especially true because so much carefully reflected on experience would likely mean that such a person could guide students wisely through otherwise unnoticed ethical complexities in the cases they are addressing. But it is worth mentioning that a person who is an excellent technical dentist and highly effective in ethical discernment and conduct at chairside is not necessarily a good teacher. Getting advice about teaching from experienced educators, perhaps with some work in a quasi apprentice role with evaluation by admirable teachers of ethics, would be advisable.

By this point in a dentist's career, the elements of the commercial marketplace described in chapters 10 and 13 that have become connected to his or her practice could easily be simply taken for granted. But that does not mean that the message they are sending to the larger community is one that strongly reinforces dentistry's commitments as a profession rather than suggesting that dentists are increasingly like participants in the competitive commercial marketplace. In addition, as senior members of the profession—who are very often the dentists who have come to be the most active in organized dentistry and in other social roles that are influential in the larger community—these well-experienced dentists are more likely than dentists earlier in their careers to have significant influence both on the profession and on the views of the larger community. Therefore, first of all, they need to be asking the question about what kind of message—a message emphasizing professionalism or a message emphasizing the ways of thinking, valuing, and acting characteristic of the commercial marketplace—their own practices and ways of conducting themselves are sending. Second, they should be using their influence in the profession and in the larger community to counter messages that weaken dentistry's acceptance as a profession by the larger community and to support dentistry's efforts to communicate its commitment to professionalism, not only in word but also in action.

In addition, by this point in a dentist's career, the dentist has probably identified the handful of dentists whom he or she considers exemplars and has probably been gradually trying to imitate their best characteristics already. If this process is already being done carefully and reflectively, the best thing to do is to keep it up. But a dentist at this point in his or her career may also have begun to look for exemplars who have achieved retirement and the status of senior citizens in admirable ways and to reflect on what these dentists' experiences might mean for them. This seems like something to seriously consider since many professionals continue to view themselves as members of their profession even after they have ended their full-time practice of its work.

THINKING ABOUT THE CASE

From the perspective of a dental student, much that has been said about the well-experienced dentist will probably seem to be far in the future, and even the activities of self-formation that are appropriate for the early career dentist may seem remote and impractical. These descriptions have been included here, however, in part to underline the fact that the growth in professionalism that a dentist needs to do in order to dependably live and practice ethically cannot be completed in dental school (much less accomplished before entering dental school). It is a lifelong process. But it is a lifelong process that requires laying down the foundations as soon as one starts learning about dentistry. And, as indicated in the section on first steps, the foundations that need to be laid down during dental school involve much more than learning a few rules.

In the case offered earlier in the chapter, Dr. Samuels makes it clear that he considers Dr. Silverman an exemplar, his hero, and a truly admirable member of the dental profession. Readers of the case may agree with him or not, and the Dr. Silvermans of the world probably don't think they deserve admiration, because they know they still have important growing to do. But one point of the case is that identifying dentists who are special examples of how to practice ethically and build the best kind of relationships with patients and then reflecting on what makes them special and using self-assessment skills to reinforce these characteristics in our own lives is the best way to keep growing in professionalism. And if what we learn from doing this is then applied to making sure the message dentistry is sending to the public is that dentistry is a profession, first of all, committed to giving priority to the well-being of the patients it services and living up to its commitments to the larger community, then dentistry's future as a profession is secure.

CONCLUSION

The purpose of this book has not been to offer the last word on anything but rather to provide a detailed, concrete impetus to more thoughtful and more extensive conversation about the dental profession's ethical commitments and professionalism. Our aim above all has been to stimulate reflection and conversation about the contents and the grounds of the obligations and aspirations of individual dentists, of dental organizations, and of the dental profession as a whole. Such reflection and conversation is needed in every profession and it is always important. But the context of dentists' work has gone through significant changes in recent decades, and these changes have made reflection and conversation about dentistry's ethics and professionalism even more important.

If this book prompts more thoughtful conversations between individual dentists about professional-ethical matters in dentistry, then that would be a fine outcome. If it prompts conversations within and between groups of dentists and dental organizations, especially if the conversation crosses geographic lines and specialty divisions, then that would be wonderful. If it prompts conversation from every corner of the dental community, from the most powerful in organized dentistry and the most respected in academic dentistry and dental research to the most experienced in chairside practice, then that would be outstanding. But this would still not be all that dentistry needs.

Our hope is that this discussion of professional-ethical issues in dentistry will also stimulate conversations about dental ethics between dentists and their patients, between dental organizations and groups within the lay community, and between the dental profession and the larger community. Then all parties to the dialogue about dentistry as a profession and about dental ethics and professionalism will be actively involved. Then, too, there will be a broad enough base of relevant experience that the answers that are the fruit of that dialogue—about how men and women who are committed to caring for others' oral health ought and ought not to act—will likely be the best possible.

APPENDIX

※※※※※※※※※※※※※※※※※※※※※※※※※※※※※※※※※

Resources for Dental Professional Ethics and Professionalism Education

Online Resources

1. **American College of Dentists (www.acd.org):** Most of the online ethics resources of the American College of Dentists (ACD) are directly available at www.dentalethics.org. These include fifty-two ethical dilemmas originally authored by the late Thomas Hasegawa in the *Texas Dental Journal* and a series of ethical dilemma videos, both of which will be found in the Resources section of the website, as well as a number on online dental ethics courses and many other useful items. In addition, each issue of ACD's quarterly journal, the *Journal of the American College of Dentists* (*JACD*), includes an Issues in Dental Ethics section that is edited by members of the American Society for Dental Ethics. To view these, go to www.acd.org and click on General, then Publications, then JACD, then Previous Issues, and scroll to the desired year and issue number.

2. **American Dental Association (www.ada.org):** A number of ethics resources are available on the American Dental Association (ADA) website at www.ada.org /en/about-the-ada/principles-of-ethics-code-of-professional-conduct/ada-ethics -resources. These include the Ethical Moment articles from the *Journal of the American Dental Association* that examine a wide variety of dental ethics issues as well as information about the ADA's ethics hotline, statements from the ADA's Council on Ethics, Bylaws, and Judicial Affairs, and information about online resources for continuing ethics education.

3. **Student Professionalism and Ethics Association in Dentistry (SPEA;** www .speadental.org): The SPEA website's Resources section includes thirty-three case studies in dental ethics, a blog, and a "start-up" kit for establishing an SPEA chapter at a dental school that does not yet have one.

Online Bibliographic Resources for Dental Ethics Literature

1. **NLM (National Library of Medicine):** A typical search would be for "dental ethics" at www.nlm.nih.gov/libserv.html.

2. **PubMed:** Typical search strategies would include "ethics, dental AND professional-patient relations"; "ethics, dental AND conflict of interest"; "ethics, dental AND personal autonomy" at www.ncbi.nlm.nih.gov/pubmed. It is also possible to set up a "save search" strategy to notify a user when materials are added to the PubMed database on a topic that is of interest.

3. **BELIT (Bioethics Literature Database at the German Reference Centre for Ethics in the Life Sciences [DRZE]):** This is a very large database that draws on international bibliographic resources, including from France (1970–2009) and the United States (1974–2011). There is a bioethics thesaurus at: www.drze/bioethics-thesaurus. For help in searching, go to www.drze.de/belit-1/search-2/help.

4. **Kennedy Institute of Ethics: Bioethics Research Library:** This is a useful and easily accessible resource for materials on dental ethics up until 2011. Search "dental" or "dentist" at this site: https://bioethics.georgetown.edu.

Other Online Resources for Professionalism Education

1. ***DocCom.org: An Interactive Learning Resource for Healthcare Communication:*** This is a website resource sponsored by the American Academy on Communication in Healthcare. It offers forty-two multimedia modules that demonstrate fundamental and advanced communication/interactional skills. The professionals in the modules are physicians and medical students, but the skills taught in most of the modules are fully transferable to dental care. Four free demonstration modules show how *DocCom*'s self-teaching process works at www.doccom.org/Resources/Demo-Modules.

2. ***ProfessionalFormation.org (PFO):*** This is an online resource for teaching, learning, and assessing professionalism in health care education. In collaboration with the Academy for Professionalism in Health Care and the American Academy on Communication in Healthcare, Drexel University College of Medicine created PFO. Supported by a 2014 Arthur Vining Davis Foundations grant, PFO currently includes thirteen interactive modules complemented with a sophisticated learning management system. Its goal is to become a comprehensive resource for education, assessment, remediation, and research in health care professionalism. Here, too, the professionals in the modules are physicians and medical students, but the skills taught in most of the modules are fully transferable to dental care. It can be accessed at www.professionalformation.org.

Professional Organizations

1. **Academy for Professionalism in Health Care (APHC; www.academy -professionalism.org):** This is an interdisciplinary organization of health professionals and professional school faculty whose national meetings and website focus on understanding the elements of professionalism in the health professions and on how to learn and teach them more effectively.

2. **American College of Dentists (www.acd.org):** Dental ethics and ethics education are a major focus of the American College of Dentists (ACD). In addition to its online resources, each issue of ACD's quarterly journal, the *Journal of the American College of Dentists* (*JACD*), includes an article about dental ethics in the Issues in Dental Ethics section, which is edited by members of the American Society for Dental Ethics. *JACD* also regularly includes other important articles and research on dental ethics, as well as articles on these topics by the journal's editor, David Chambers. The ACD also sponsors an ethics workshop at its annual meetings and provides support and assistance through the ACD Foundation for other ethics projects.

3. **American Dental Association (www.ada.org):** In addition to its online resources and the *Journal of the American Dental Association*'s Ethics Moment articles, searching the archives of the *Journal of the American Dental Association* for "ethics" or "ethics consultation" will yield an even broader range of articles on ethics-related topics. The ADA also sponsors workshops and other ethics-related events from time to time.

4. **American Society for Bioethics and Humanities (ASBH; www.asbh.org):** This is the principal interdisciplinary North American organization for the study and teaching of ethical issues in all aspects of health care, biomedical research, and the interface of the humanities and health care, which is the focus of its annual meetings and website. ASBH's special interest group (Affinity Group) for dental ethics has met annually at ASBH's national meetings since 1987.

5. **American Society for Dental Ethics (ASDE; www.societyfordentalethics.org):** This is the principal national organization for teachers and scholars in dental ethics. It works closely with the American College of Dentists, of which it is a Section, and also sponsors its own workshops on topics in dental ethics and ethics teaching.

6. **Association for Practical and Professional Ethics (APPE; http://appe-ethics .org):** This is the principal international interdisciplinary organization for teachers and scholars of professional ethics across all the professions. Its meetings and other activities focus on interprofessional collaboration in understanding, learning, and teaching professional ethics.

7. **International Dental Ethics and Law Society (IDEALS; www.ideals.ac):** IDEALS is an international organization with members in Europe, the United States, Canada, and many other countries. It was founded to foster an international

dialogue on the values guiding the practice of oral health care. It sponsors international conferences on dental ethics and law every two or three years.

8. **Student Professionalism and Ethics Association in Dentistry (SPEA; www .speadental.org):** Formally founded in 2011 after four years of planning, the Student Professionalism and Ethics Association in Dentistry is a national, student-driven association that was established to promote and support students' lifelong commitment to ethical behavior in order to benefit the patients they serve and to further the dental profession. SPEA sponsors annual meetings, and its chapters in many US dental schools also sponsor their own regular meetings and ethics-related activities.

Bibliography

"ADA Practical Guide to Associateships Book." American Dental Association, Chicago, IL, 2017.

ADA Principles of Ethics and Code of Professional Conduct. American Dental Association, Chicago, IL, 2016. www.ada.org/en/about-the-ada/principles-of-ethics-code-of-professional-conduct.

"Advancing Oral Health in America." Report brief. National Academy of Science, Washington, DC, April 2011. http://nationalacademies.org/HMD/Reports/2011/Advancing-Oral-Health-in-America.aspx.

American College of Dentists. "Special Feature: Codes of Ethics." *Journal of the American College of Dentists* 82, no. 4 (2015): 17–59.

———. "Special Feature: Varieties of Chairside Perspectives on Practice." *Journal of the American College of Dentists* 82, no. 2 (2015): 6–24.

———. "Special Feature: Varieties of Dental Services Organizations—Management Perspective on Practice." *Journal of the American College of Dentists* 82, no. 1 (2015): 5–29.

"American College of Dentists Core Values & Aspirational Code of Ethics." American College of Dentists, Gaithersburg, MD, 2017. www.acd.org/aspirationalcode.htm.

American Dental Education Association. "Professional Promises—Hopes and Gaps in Access to Oral Health Care." Edited by Frank Catalanotto, Donald Patthoff, and Carolyn Gray. Special issue, *Journal of Dental Education* 70, no. 11 (2006): 1117–1247.

Appelbaum, Paul S., and T. Grisso. *Assessing Competence to Consent to Treatment: A Guide for Physicians and Other Health Professionals.* New York: Oxford University Press, 1998.

"ASDA Student Code of Ethics." American Student Dental Association, Chicago, IL, 2002. Revised in 2008, 2009, and 2010. www.asdanet.org/utility-navigation/about-asda/leaders-and-governance/current-statements-of-position-or-policy/dental-education-administration/statement-on-policy/E-8.

"ASDA White Paper on Ethics and Professionalism in Dental Education." American Student Dental Association, Chicago, IL, 2009, 2012.

"ASDO Code of Ethics." Association of Dental Support Organizations, Arlington, VA, 2014. http://theadso.org/value/code-of-ethics/.

Baab, D. A., and Muriel J. Bebeau. "The Effect of Instruction on Ethical Sensitivity." *Journal of Dental Education* 54 (1990): 44.

Baker, Jim. "We Have Your Back." *Journal of the American College of Dentists* 82, no. 1 (2015): 26–29.

Barnard, David. "Vulnerability and Trustworthiness: Polestars of Professionalism in Healthcare." *Cambridge Quarterly of Healthcare Ethics* 25 (2016): 288–300.

Bayles, Michael D. *Professional Ethics.* 2nd ed. Belmont, CA: Wadsworth, 1989.

Bebeau, Muriel J. "Enhancing Professionalism Using Ethics Education as Part of a Dental Licensure Board's Disciplinary Action: Part 1. An Evidence-Based Process." *Journal of the American College of Dentists* 76, no. 2 (2009): 38–50.

———. "Enhancing Professionalism Using Ethics Education as Part of a Dental Licensure Board's Disciplinary Action: Part 2. Evidence of the Process." *Journal of the American College of Dentists* 76, no. 3 (2009): 32–45.

———. "Influencing the Moral Dimensions of Dental Practice." In *Moral Development in the Professions: Psychology and Applied Ethics*, edited by James Restand Darcia Narváez, 121–46. Hillsdale, NJ: Erlbaum Associates, 1994.

Bebeau, Muriel J., D. O. Born, and David T. Ozar. "The Development of a Professional Role Orientation Inventory." *Journal of the American College of Dentists* 60, no. 2 (1993): 27–33.

Bebeau, Muriel J., and Jeffrey P. Kahn. "Ethical Issues in Community Dental Health." In *Community Dental Health*, 4th ed., edited by Anthony W. Jong, 287–306. St. Louis, MO: Mosby, 1998.

Bebeau, Muriel J., and Verna E. Monson. "Professional Identity Formation and Transformation across the Life Span." In *Learning Trajectories, Innovation and Identity for Professional Development*, edited by Anne Mc Kee and Michael Eraut, 135–63. Dordrecht, Neth.: Springer, 2012.

Bebeau, Muriel J., and Stephen J. Thoma. "The Impact of a Dental Ethics Curriculum on Moral Reasoning and Student Attitudes." *Journal of Dental Education* 58 (1994): 684–92.

Beemsterboer, Phyllis L. "Educating the Developing Dental Student in Ethics and Professionalism." *Journal of the American College of Dentists* 83, no. 1 (2016): 9–12.

———. *Ethics and Law in Dental Hygiene.* 3rd ed. St. Louis, MO: Elsevier, 2017.

Berg, Jessica W., Paul S. Appelbaum, and Charles Lidz. *Informed Consent: Legal Theory and Clinical Practice.* New York: Oxford University Press, 2001.

Boden, David F. "What Guidance Is There for Ethical Records Transfer and Fee Charges?" *Journal of the American Dental Association* 139 (2008): 197–98.

Boerschinger, Thomas H. "Dentists' Advertising: Patient Welfare or Caveat Emptor." *Dental Practice Administration* 9 (1989): 5–9.

Boyd, Marcia A., Kathleen Roth, Stephen A. Ralls, and David W. Chambers. "Beginning the Discussion of Commercialism in Dentistry." *Journal of the California Dental Association* 36, no. 1 (2008): 57–65.

Bramson, J. B., D. E. Noskin, and J. D. Ruesch. "Demographics and Practice Characteristics of Dentists Participating and Not Participating in Managed Care Programs." *Journal of the American Dental Association* 128 (1997): 1708–14.

———. "Dentists' Views about Managed Care: Summary of a National Survey." *Journal of the American Dental Association* 129 (1998): 107–10.

Brown, Ronald S., and Michael Mashni. "Emerging Dental Specialties and Ethics." *Journal of the American College of Dentists* 82, no. 3 (2015): 31–38.

Buchanan, Allan E., and Dan W. Brock. *Deciding for Others: The Ethics of Surrogate Decision Making*. New York: Cambridge University Press, 1989.

Chambers, David W. *Building the Moral Community: Radical Naturalism and Emergence*. New York: Lexington, 2016.

———. "Do Patients and Dentists See Ethics the Same Way?" *Journal of the American College of Dentists* 82, no. 2 (2015): 31–47.

———. "The Ethics of Experimenting in Dental Practice." *Journal of the American College of Dentists* 81, no. 3 (2014): 31–40.

———. "Interim ACD Gies Ethics Project Report: Is Professionalism a Contact Sport or a Spectator Sport?" *Journal of the American College of Dentists* 83, no. 4 (2016): 27–42.

———. "Moral Communities." *Journal of Dental Education* 70, no. 11 (2006): 1226–34.

———. "Moral Courage." *Journal of the American College of Dentists* 71, no. 1 (2004): 2–3.

———. "The Professions." *Journal of the American College of Dentists* 71, no. 4 (2005): 57–64.

———. "The Separation of Treatment from Management." *Journal of the American College of Dentists* 82, no. 1 (2015): 2–4.

Chan, Steven D. "Being Professional in the Social Media World." *Journal of the American College of Dentists* 79, no. 4 (2012): 48–55.

Chiodo, Gary T., and Susan W. Tolle. "Can a Rational Patient Make an Irrational Choice? The Dental Amalgam Controversy." *General Dentistry* 40 (1992): 184–87.

———. "Diminished Autonomy: Can a Demented Patient Consent to Dental Treatment?" *General Dentistry* 56 (2004): 372–73.

"Code of Ethics." Alexandria, VA: International Association for Dental Research, 2009. www.iadr.org/IADR/About-Us/Who-We-Are/Code-of-Ethics.

Davis, Michael. "Conflicts of Interest." In *Encyclopedia of Applied Ethics*, vol. 1, edited by R. Chadwick, 585–95. London: Academia Press, 1998.

d'Oronzio, J. C. "Practicing Accountability in Professional Ethics." *Journal of Clinical Ethics* 13, no. 4 (2002): 257–64.

Drane, James F. "The Many Faces of Competency." *Hastings Center Report* 15 (1985): 17–21.

Dufurrena, Quinn. "Dental Support Organizations." *Journal of the American College of Dentists* 82, no. 1 (2015): 21–25.

Duhigg, Charles. *The Power of Habit*. New York: Random House, 2012.

Dummett, Clifton O., and Lois Doyle Dummett. *The Hillenbrand Era: Organized Dentistry's Glanzperiode*. Bethesda, MD: American College of Dentists, 1986.

"Ethics Handbook for Dentists." American College of Dentists, Gaithersburg, MD, 2016. www.acd.org/ethicshandbook.htm.

Faden, Ruth, Thomas Beauchamp, and Nancy M. P. King. *A History and Theory of Informed Consent*. New York: Oxford University Press, 1986.

Feinberg, Joel. "Social Justice." Chap. 7 in *Social Philosophy*. Englewood Cliffs, NJ: Prentice-Hall, 1973.

Freidson, Eliot. *Professionalism: The Third Logic*. Chicago: University of Chicago Press, 2001.

Garetto, Lawrence P., and Wendy E. Senour. "Using an Ethics across the Curriculum Strategy in Dental Education." *Journal of the American College of Dentists* 73, no. 4 (2006): 33–37.

Gesko, David S. "Managing for Quality Rather Than Profit." *Journal of the American College of Dentists* 82, no. 1 (2015): 12–16.

Gilbert, John A. "Ethics and Esthetics." *Journal of the American Dental Association* 117 (1988): 490.

Gilbert, John A., and Mary Ellen Waithe. "Esthetic Dentistry: A Case and Commentary." In *Dental Ethics*, edited by Bruce D. Weinstein, 195–206. Philadelphia: Lea and Febiger, 1993.

Gorlin, Rena A. "Health: Allied Health, Chiropractic, Dentistry, Medicine, Mental Health, Nursing, Pharmacy, Social Work." In *Codes of Professional Responsibility: Ethics Standards in Business, Health, and Law*. 4th ed. Washington, DC: Bureau of National Affairs, 1999.

Graham, Bruce S. "Is Dentistry a Business or a Profession?" *Journal of the American College of Dentists* 71, no. 4 (2005): 8–10.

Graskemper, Joseph P. "Ethical Advertising in Dentistry." *Journal of the American College of Dentists* 76, no. 1 (2009): 44–49.

———. *Professional Responsibility in Dentistry: A Practical Guide to Law and Ethics*. Chichester, UK: Wiley-Blackwell, 2011.

Hammer, Dan. "New Leaders in Dentistry: Dental Students." *Journal of the American College of Dentists* 77, no. 3 (2010): 10–13.

Hasegawa, Thomas K. Jr. "Ethical Issues of Performing Invasive/Irreversible Dental Treatment for Purposes of Licensure." *Journal of the American College of Dentists* 69, no. 2 (2002): 43–46.

Hasegawa, Thomas K. Jr., and Jos V. M. Welie. "The Search for a Common Ethic: The Ethics Alliance of Oral Health Organizations." *Journal of the American College of Dentists* 67, no. 2 (2000): 21–22.

Hernandez, Lyla, et al. *Oral Health Literacy—Workshop Summary*. Washington, DC: National Academy of Science, 2011. http://nationalacademies.org/HMD/Reports/2013/Oral-Health -Literacy.aspx.

Hirsch, A. C., and Bernard Gert. "Ethics in Dental Practice." *Journal of the American Dental Association* 113 (1986): 599–603.

Hobhouse, L. T. *The Elements of Social Justice*. London: George Allen and Unwin, 1922. See esp. chap. 9.

Institute of Medicine. *To Err Is Human: Building a Safer Health System*. Edited by Linda T. Kohn, Janet Corrigan, and Molla S. Donaldson. Washington, DC: National Academy of Science, 2000. https://doi.org/10.17226/9728.

Jenson, Larry. "Restoration and Enhancement: Is Cosmetic Dentistry Ethical?" *Journal of the American College of Dentists* 72, no. 4 (2005): 48–53.

Jerold, Laurance, and Hengameh Karkhanehchi. "Advertising, Commercialism, and Professionalism: A History of the Ethics of Advertising in Dentistry." *Journal of the American College of Dentists* 67 (2000): 32–44.

Jong, Anthony W. "Dental Care for the Cognitively Impaired: An Ethical Dilemma." *Gerodontics* 4 (1988): 172–73.

Kahn, Jeffrey P., and Thomas K. Hasegawa. "The Dentist-Patient Relationship." In *Dental Ethics*, edited by Bruce D. Weinstein, 53–64. Philadelphia: Lea and Febiger, 1993.

Katz, Jay. *The Silent World of Doctor and Patient*. New York: Free Press, 1984.

Koelbl, James J. "HIV-Positive Health Care Professionals: Should They Still Provide Patient Care?" *Journal of Law and Ethics in Dentistry* 4 (1991): 63–72.

Koka, Sreenivas. "Conflict of Interest: The Achilles Heel of Evidence Based Dentistry." *International Journal of Prosthodontics* 21 (2008): 364–68.

Kramer, Matthew. "Dentists in Private Practice Settings Provide Free or Reduced-Fee Care." *Journal of the American College of Dentists* 79, no. 4 (2012): 72–79.

Kuskey, G. F. "Health Care, Human Rights, and Government Intervention." *California Dental Association Journal* 1 (1973): 10–13.

Loader, Clifford F., and Shigeo Ryan Kiski, eds. *Legacy, the Dental Profession: The Philosophies and Thoughts of Selected Dental Leaders Worldwide.* Bakersfield, CA: Loader/Kiski, 1990.

Logan, Mary K. "The HIV-Infected Dental Professional: A Challenge to Law, Ethics, and the Dental Profession." *Journal of Dental Practice Administration* 6 (1989): 162–68.

Marshall, Patricia. "Reducing Emotional Distress Associated with Childhood Illness." *Comprehensive Therapy* 15 (1989): 3–7.

McCullough, Laurence B. "Ethical Issues in Dentistry." In *Clinical Dentistry*, vol. 1, rev. ed., edited by J. W. Clark, 1–14. Philadelphia: Harper and Row, 1983.

Meru, Michael. "Following Your Moral Compass: Ethics in Dental School." *Journal of the American College of Dentists* 77, no. 1 (2010): 4–9.

Morreim, Haavi. "Am I My Brother's Warden? Responding to the Unethical or Incompetent Colleague." *Hastings Center Report* 23 (1993): 19–27.

Nash, David A. "Can Dentistry Have Two Contracts with the Public?" *Journal of the American College of Dentists* 82, no. 3 (2015): 4–11.

———. "Ethics in Dentistry: Review and Critique of Principles of Ethics and Code of Professional Conduct." *Journal of the American Dental Association* 109 (1984): 597–603.

———. "A Larger Sense of Purpose: Dentistry and Society." *Journal of the American College of Dentists* 74, no. 2 (2007): 27–33.

———. "Professional Ethics and Esthetic Dentistry." *Journal of the American Dental Association* 117 (1988): 7E–9E.

Nisselson, Harvey S. "What Ethical Considerations Are Involved in Offering Introductory Discounts to Attract New Patients?" *Journal of the American Dental Association* 139 (2008): 769–71.

Odom, John G., and Donald F. Bowers. "Informed Consent and Refusal." In *Dental Ethics*, edited by Bruce D. Weinstein, 65–80. Philadelphia: Lea and Febiger, 1993.

Owsiany, David J. "The Intersection of Dental Ethics and Law." *Journal of the American College of Dentists* 75, no. 4 (2008): 47–54.

Ozar, Anne C. "The Plausibility of Client Trust of Professionals." *Business and Professional Ethics Journal* 33 (2014): 83–98.

———. "Trust as a Moral Emotion." In *Emotional Experiences: Ethical and Social Significance*, edited by John Drummond and Sonja Rinofner-Kreidel, 137–153. Lanham, MD: Rowman and Littlefield, 2018.

Ozar, David T. "Basic Oral Health Needs: A Public Priority?" *Journal of Dental Education* 70 (2006): 1159–65.

———. "Conflicts of Interest." *Journal of the American College of Dentists* 71, no. 3 (2004): 30–35.

———. "Dentistry." In *Encyclopedia of Bioethics*, 4th ed., edited by Stephen Post, 831–37. New York: Thomson/Gale, 2014.

———. "Ethical Issues in Dental Care for the Compromised Patient." *Special Care in Dentistry* 16 (1990): 206–9.

———. "Ethical Issues in Pediatric Dentistry." *Pediatric Dentistry* 13 (1991): 374.

———. "Ethics, Access, and Care." *Journal of Dental Education* 70 (2006): 1139–45.

———. "Ethics in Dentistry: The Ethical Importance of Preferred Patterns of Professional Practice in Dentistry." In *Dental Horizons*, edited by Rajiv Saini and Santosh Saini, 313–26. New Delhi: Paras Medical Publisher, 2011.

———. "Professionalism: Challenges for Dentistry in the Future." Supplement, *Journal of Forensic Odonto-Stomatology* 30, no. S1 (2012): 72–84. www.iofos.eu/Journals/JFOS%20sup1 _Nov12/IDEALS%208-118.pdf.

———. "Professions and Professional Ethics." In *Encyclopedia of Bioethics*, 4th ed., edited by Stephen Post, 2526–37. New York: Thomson/Gale, 2014.

———. "What Should Count as Basic Health Care." *Theoretical Medicine* 4 (1983): 129–41.

Ozar, David T., and David A. Baab. "Whistle-Blowing in Dentistry." *Journal of the American Dental Association* 125 (1994): 199–205.

Ozar, David T., Jessica Berg, Patricia H. Werhane, and Linda Emanuel. *Organizational Ethics in Health Care: Toward a Model for Ethical Decision-Making by Provider Organizations*. Chicago: American Medical Association, 2000.

Ozar, David T., and Donald E. Patthoff. "Exploring Preventive Ethics in Dentistry: Viewing Colleagues in a Competitive World." *AGD Impact (A Journal of the Academy of General Dentistry)* 43, no. 8 (2015): 21–23.

———. "Looking Inward: Determining What Professionalism and Self-Formation Mean to Us." *AGD Impact (A Journal of the Academy of General Dentistry)* 44, no. 3 (2016): 20–24.

———. "Moral Distress: When Others' Decisions Trouble Us." *AGD Impact (A Journal of the Academy of General Dentistry)* 44, no. 8 (2013): 22–24.

———. "Proactively Preventing Bad Outcomes." *AGD Impact (A Journal of the Academy of General Dentistry)* 44, no. 12 (2013): 26–29.

———. "Professionalism in the Office: Part One: What It Means to Your Practice." *AGD Impact (A Journal of the Academy of General Dentistry)* 40, no. 9 (2012): 26–28.

———. "Professionalism in the Office: Part Two: Understanding Staff Roles and Working Together." *AGD Impact (A Journal of the Academy of General Dentistry)* 41, no. 4 (2013): 25–28.

Ozar, David T., and James Sabin. "Access to Dental and Mental Health Services." In *Medicine and Social Justice: Essays on the Distribution of Health Care*, 2nd ed., edited by Rosamond Rhodes, Margaret P. Battin, and Anita Silvers, 401–11. New York: Oxford University Press, 2012.

Parker, Lisa S., and Jeffrey Holloway. "Professional Responsibilities toward Incompetent or Chemically Dependent Colleagues." In *Dental Ethics*, edited by Bruce D. Weinstein, 101–16. Philadelphia: Lea and Febiger, 1993.

Parker, Lisa S., and Valerie B. Satkoske. "Conflicts of Interest: Are Informed Consent an Appropriate Model and Disclosure an Appropriate Remedy?" *Journal of the American College of Dentists* 74, no. 2 (2007): 19–26.

Patthoff, Donald E. "Balancing Business with Professionalism." *Journal of the American Dental Association* 134 (2003): 1434–38.

———. "Defining the Ethical Organization in Oral Health Care." *Journal of the American College of Dentists* 65, no. 3 (1998): 24–26.

———. "Ethics and Mediation: Part One." *Dentistry: Journal of the American Student Dental Association* 13, no. 4 (1993): 8–15, 17, 25.

———. "Ethics and Mediation: Part Two: The Role of Power." *Dentistry: Journal of the American Student Dental Association* 14, no. 1 (1994): 24–31.

———. "How Did We Get Here? Where Are We Going? Hopes and Gaps in Access to Oral Health Care." *Journal of Dental Education* 70 (November 2006): 1125–32.

———. "The Need for Dental Ethicists and the Promise of Universal Patient Acceptance: Response to Richard Masella's 'Renewing Professionalism in Dental Education.'" *Journal of Dental Education* 71 (2007): 222–26.

Patthoff, Donald E., and Bruce V. Corsino. "Acceptance, Universal Patient Acceptance, and Access to Care: An Update." *Linacre Quarterly* 76, no. 1 (2009): 47–67.

———. "The Ethical and Practical Aspects of Acceptance and Universal Patient Acceptance." *Journal of Dental Education* 70 (2006): 1198–1201.

———. "Universal Patient Acceptance: Ethics Pipe Dream or Key to Improved Access in Dentistry?" *Journal of the American College of Dentists* 68, no. 4 (2001): 39–43.

Patthoff, Donald E., and John G. Odom. "The Continuing Education of Professional Ethics in Dentistry." *Journal of the American College of Dentists* 59, no. 2 (1992): 32–36.

Pellegrino, Edmund D. "The Commodification of Medical and Health Care: The Moral Consequences of a Paradigm Shift from a Professional to a Market Ethic." *Journal of Medicine and Philosophy* 24 (1999): 243–66.

Pellegrino, Edmund, and David Thomasma. *For the Patient's Good: The Restoration of Beneficence in Health Care.* New York: Oxford University Press, 1988.

Peltier, Bruce N. "Discursive Ethics, Conflicts of Interest, and the Elephant in the Reception Area." *Journal of the American College of Dentists* 67, no. 2 (2000): 17–18.

———. "Painless Parker's Legacy: Ethics, Commerce, and Advertising in the Professions." *Journal of the History of Dentistry* 55, no. 3 (2007): 150–59, see especially the discussion, 171–85.

———. "White Coat Principles." *Journal of the American College of Dentists* 71, no. 4 (2005): 53–56.

Peltier, Bruce N., and James S. Dower Jr. "The Ethics of Adopting a New Drug: Articaine as an Example." *Journal of the American College of Dentists* 73, no. 3 (2006): 11–19.

Peltier, Bruce N., Alvin Rosenblum, Muriel J. Bebeau, and Anne Koerber. "A Case of Collegial Communication and a Patient Who Does Not Pay." *Journal of the American College of Dentists* 78, no. 1 (2011): 33–34.

Perrin, E. C., and P. S. Gerrity. "There's a Demon in Your Belly: Children's Understanding of Illness." *Pediatrics* 67, no. 6 (1981): 841–49.

Pickering, Stephen R. "Group Practices and Partnerships: A Traditional Model That Fits Many Situations." *Journal of the American College of Dentists* 82, no. 1 (2015): 5–7.

Pollack, Burton R., and R. D. Marinelli. "Ethical, Moral, and Legal Dilemmas in Dentistry: The Process of Informed Decision Making." *Journal of Law and Ethics in Dentistry* 1 (1988): 27–36.

Reddy, Akhil. "Looking for the Right Balance between Dentist as Manager and Dentist as Care Provider." *Journal of the American College of Dentists* 82, no. 1 (2015): 8–11.

Rest, James, and Darcia Narvaez, eds. *Moral Development in the Professions: Psychology and Applied Ethics.* Hillsdale, NJ: Lawrence Erlbaum Associates, 1994.

Rest, James, Darcia Narvaez, Muriel J. Bebeau, and Stephen J. Thoma. *Postconventional Moral Thinking: A Neo-Kohlbergian Approach.* Mahwah, NJ: Lawrence Erlbaum Associates, 1999.

Rosenblum, Alvin B., and Steve Wolf. "Dental Ethics and Emotional Intelligence." *Journal of the American College of Dentists* 81, no. 2 (2014): 26–35.

Roucka, Tony M., Pamela Zarkowski, Evelyn Donate-Bartfield, and Donald E. Patthoff. "Ethical Obligations and the Dental Office Team." *Journal of the American College of Dentists* 80, no. 4 (2013): 49–58.

Rule, James T. "How Dentistry Should Approach Its Problems: A Vote for Professionalism." *Journal of the American College of Dentists* 77, no. 4 (2010): 59–67.

Rule, James T., and Muriel J. Bebeau, *Dentists Who Care: Inspiring Stories of Professional Commitment.* Chicago: Quintessence, 2005.

Rule, James T., and Robert M. Veatch. *Ethical Questions in Dentistry*. 2nd ed. Chicago: Quintessence, 2004.

Rule, James T., and Jos V. M. Welie. "The Dilemma of Access to Care: Symptom of a Systemic Condition." In *Dental Clinics of North America* 53, no. 3 (2009): 421–33.

———. "Justice, Moral Competencies, and the Role of Dental Schools." In *Justice in Oral Health Care*, edited by Jos V. M. Welie, 233–60. Milwaukee, WI: Marquette University Press, 2006.

Scheirton, Linda S. "Professional or Commercial Enterprise? An Ethical Analysis of Dental Advertising." *Texas Dental Journal* 190 (1992): 19–27.

Scholl, R. H. "The Privilege of Practice." *Journal of the American Dental Association* 98 (1979): 159–60.

Schwartz, Barry. "A Call for Ethics Committees in Dental Organizations and in Dental Education." *Journal of the American College of Dentists* 71, no. 2 (2004): 35–39.

———. "Errors in Dentistry: A Call for Apology." *Journal of the American College of Dentists* 72, no. 2 (2006): 26–32.

———. "The Evolving Relationship between Specialists and General Dentists: Practical and Ethical Challenges." *Journal of the American College of Dentists* 74, no. 1 (2007): 22–26.

Schwartz, Barry, Larry E. Jenson, Toni M. Roucka, and Donald E. Patthoff. "Writing Off the Copayment." *Journal of the American College of Dentists* 78, no. 2 (2011): 26–33.

Segal, Herman, and Richard Warner. "Informed Consent in Dentistry." *Journal of the American Dental Association* 99 (1979): 957–58.

Shampaine, Guy S. "State Dental Boards and Public Protection Fulfilling the Contract." *Journal of the American College of Dentists* 82, no. 3 (2015): 25–30.

Sharp, Helen M., Raymond A. Kuthy, and Keith E. Heller. "Ethical Dilemmas Reported by Fourth Year Dental Students." *Journal of Dental Education* 69 (2005): 1116–22.

Shue, Henry. *Basic Rights*. 2nd ed. Princeton, NJ: Princeton University Press, 1996.

Shuman, S. K. "Ethics and the Patient with Dementia." *Journal of the American Dental Association* 119 (1989): 747–48.

Sokol, David J., "Endodontic Intervention—Is It Paternalism?" *Journal of the American Dental Association* 117 (1988): 5.

———. "Informed Consent in Dentistry." *Journal of Dental Practice Administration* 6 (1989): 157–61.

———. "Informed Consent in Dentistry: The Impact of 'Who Pays the Bills.'" *Journal of Law and Ethics in Dentistry* 2 (1989): 64–68.

———. "Some Aspects of the Emerging Dental Malpractice Crisis." *Journal of Law and Ethics in Dentistry* 1 (1988): 22–26.

Sokol, David J., and Carol K. Sokol. "A Review of Non-intrusive Therapies Used to Deal with Anxiety and Pain in the Dental Office." *Journal of the American Dental Association* 110 (1985): 217–22.

Thucydides. *History of the Peloponnesian War*. Translated by Richard Crawley. Book 2, Chap. 7. http://classics.mit.edu/Thucydides/pelopwar.2.second.html.

Tiller, Chrissy. "Dentistry and Ethics by the Road Less Traveled." *Journal of the American College of Dentists* 78, no. 3 (2011): 11–13.

"Toward a Common Goal: The Role of Dental Support Organizations in an Evolving Profession." White paper and code of ethics, Association of Dental Support Organizations, Arlington, VA, 2014. http://theadso.org/download/toward-common-goal-role-dsos-evolving-profession/?wpdmdl=5183.

Turner, Sharon P. "A Dental Dean's Perspective on Ethical Remediation of Practitioners." *Journal of the American College of Dentists* 76 (2009): 37–41.

United States Department of Health and Human Services. "Oral Health in America: A Report of the Surgeon General." Report of the U.S. Department of Health and Human Services, National Institute of Dental and Craniofacial Research, and National Institutes of Health, Rockville, MD, 2000. www.nidcr.nih.gov/DataStatistics/SurgeonGeneral/sgr/welcome.htm.

United States Federal Trade Commission. "Final Order on Ethical Restrictions against Advertising by Dentistry." *Journal of the American Dental Association* 99 (1979): 927–93.

US Centers for Disease Control and Prevention. "Universal Precautions for Preventing Transmission of Bloodborne Infections: 2007 Guideline for Isolation Precautions: Preventing Transmission of Infectious Agents in Healthcare Settings." The National Institute for Occupational Safety and Health (NIOSH), Atlanta, GA, September 2016. www.cdc.gov/niosh/topics/bbp/universal.html.

Weber, Leonard J. *Business Ethics in Healthcare: Beyond Compliance.* Bloomington: Indiana University Press, 2001.

Weinstein, Bruce D., ed. *Dental Ethics.* Philadelphia: Lea and Febiger, 1993.

Welie, Jos V. M. "The Dentist as Healer and Friend." In *The Health Care Professional as Friend and Healer: Building on the Work of Edmund D. Pellegrino*, edited by David C. Thomasma and Judith Lee Kissell, 35–48. Washington, DC: Georgetown University Press, 2000.

———. "Is Dentistry a Profession? Part 1: Professionalism Defined." *Journal of the Canadian Dental Association* 70 (2004): 529–32.

———. "Is Dentistry a Profession? Part 2: The Hallmarks of Professionalism." *Journal of the Canadian Dental Association* 70 (2004): 599–602.

———. "Is Dentistry a Profession? Part 3: Future Challenges." *Journal of the Canadian Dental Association* 70 (2004): 675–78.

———, ed. *Justice in Oral Health Care: Ethical and Educational Perspectives.* Milwaukee WI: Marquette University Press, 2006.

Werhane, Patricia H. "Business Ethics, Stakeholder Theory, and the Ethics of Health Care Organizations." *Cambridge Quarterly of Healthcare Ethics* 9 (2000): 169–81.

White, Becky Cox. *Competence to Consent.* Washington, DC: Georgetown University Press, 1994.

Wikler, Dan. "Paternalism and the Mildly Retarded." In *Paternalism*, edited by Rolf Sartorius, 83–84. Minneapolis: University of Minnesota Press, 1983.

Winslow, Gerald. "Integrity and Compromise in Dental Ethics." *Journal of the American College of Dentists* 70, no. 2 (2003): 25–30.

Index

About the Authors

David T. Ozar, PhD, FACD (hon), FACLM (hon), taught professional and social ethics in the Philosophy Department of Loyola University Chicago from 1972 until his retirement in 2015. He was also director of Loyola's Center for Ethics and Social Justice, 1993-2006. He was founding president of the American Society for Dental Ethics and he is an honorary Fellow of the American College of Dentists. He has lectured and published widely on the ethics of the dental profession.

David J. Sokol, DDS, JD, FAGD, deceased, was a general dentist in private practice for many years in Highland Mills, New York, where he also practiced dental and medical health and malpractice law.

Donald E. Patthoff, DDS, FACD, MAGD, has been a dentist in government and non-profit settings and in private practice in Martinsburg, West Virginia, since 1971. He is a frequent author and lecturer and a former president of the American Society for Dental Ethics and has served in leadership roles in other ethics organizations and in organized dentistry at local, state, national, and international levels.